WHAT PEOPLE ARE SAYING ABOUT DR. CUTLER AND WINNING THE WAR AGAINST IMMUNE DISORDERS & ALLERGIES

"Chronic Fatigue, Fibromyalgia, environmental illness and other immune disorders can be reversed permanently using NAET. The enzyme therapy enhances NAET since all patients with allergy and immune disorders suffer from enzyme deficiency. It is a unique combination to lead you quickly to the castle of health! *Winning the War Against Immune Disorders & Allergies* says it all and teaches you to find the Road to your Castle of Health." *Devi S. Nambudripad, D.C., L.Ac., R.N., O.M.D., Ph.D., NAET Originator and author of* Say Goodbye to Illness.

"A unique and easy-to-read book that may help many people with yeast problems and other chronic health disorders." *William G. Crook, M.D., Author of* The Yeast Connection Handbook.

"Dr. Ellen Cutler's innovative technique for natural health care has helped thousands of people reverse food and environmental sensitivities and achieve optimum health . . . something that we all deserve. In simple layman's terms, she instructs you have to improve your health and conquer these illnesses for a lifetime." *John Gray, Author of* Men Are From Mars, Women Are From Venus.

"A clear and comprehensive alternative approach to treating some of our most common chronic ailments. Dr. Cutler provides the reader with a multitude of self-healing tools, while documenting some of the dramatic success stories from her own practice. Congratulations!" *Robert S. Ivker, D.O., President, American Holistic Medical Association, and author of the best-selling* Sinus Survival: The Holistic Medical Treatment for Allergies, Asthma, Bronchitis, Colds, and Sinusitis.

"Dr. Cutler's impressive body of knowledge and extensive research is a great contribution to the field of Immunology and Allergy. This is the kind of 'cutting edge' innovative thinking medicine needs." *Elizabeth Chen Christenson, M.D., Fellow-College of American Pathology, Medical Acupuncture, and Director, Comprehensive Health Innovations Medical Center, Inc.*

Winning the War Against Immune Disorders & Allergies

To my children, whom I adore, Aaron and Gabrielle

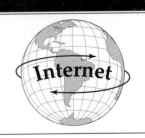

Winning the War Against Immune Disorders & Allergies

BY ELLEN W. CUTLER, D.C.

Delmar Publishers

I⊤P™ An International Thomson Publishing Company

Albany • Bonn • Boston • Cincinnati • Detroit • London •
Madrid • Melbourne • Mexico City • New York • Pacific Grove
Paris • San Francisco • Singapore • Tokyo • Toronto • Washington

NOTICE TO THE READER

Consulting Editor: Claire Pogue   Author Photograph: Courtesy of Linda J. Russell

Epigraphs for all chapters, copyright ® 1998 by Marie Henry, excerpted from poems by Marie Henry, from The Grounding of a Long-Distance Swimmer, reprinted courtesy of the poet.

Copyright© 1998
by Ellen W. Cutler, D.C.
a division of International Thomson Publishing Inc.
The ITP logo is a trademark under license.

Printed in the United States of America

For more information, contact:

Delmar Publishers
3 Columbia Circle, Box 15015
Albany, New York 12212-5015

International Thomson Publishing Europe
Berkshire House
168-173 High Holborn
London WC1V 7AA
United Kingdom

Nelson ITP, Australia
102 Dodds Street
South Melbourne
Victoria, 3205 Australia

Nelson Canada
1120 Birchmont Road
Scarborough, Ontario
M1K 5G4, Canada

International Thomson Publishing France
Tour Maine-Montparnasse
33 Avenue du Maine
75755 Paris Cedex 15, France

International Thomson Editores
Seneca 53
Colonia Polanco
11560 Mexico D. F. Mexico

International Thomson Publishing GmbH
Königswinterer Strasse 418
53227 Bonn
Germany

International Thomson Publishing Asia
60 Albert Street
#15-10 Albert Complex
Singapore 189969

International Thomson Publishing Japan
Hirakawa-cho Kyowa Building, 3F
2-2-1 Hirakawa-cho, Chiyoda-ku,
Tokyo 102, Japan

ITE Spain/Paraninfo
Calle Magallanes, 25
28015-Madrid, Espana

Library of Congress Cataloging-in-Publication Data
Cutler, Ellen W.
       Winning the war against immune disorders & allergies : a drug-free
    cure for allergy sufferers / by Ellen W. Cutler.
          p.   cm.
       Includes index.
       ISBN 0-7668-0059-8
       1. Allergy—Alternative treatment.   2. Chronic diseases-
    -Alternative treatment.   3. Applied kinesiology.   4. Acupuncture.
    5. Acupressure.   I. Title.
    RC585.C88   1998
    616.97'06—DC21
                                                                98-23746
                                                                CIP

TABLE OF CONTENTS

ACKNOWLEDGMENTS

This book would never have been written if it wasn't for the many patients I have seen in my clinic over the past 20 years. They helped me write this book and they have been the inspiration and motivation for my service and research over the many years. They come to me for knowledge and assistance, and in the end, they open my heart to the instinct and revelation of true healing. They are my gift in life, and I treasure the work I do in this field.

I express my sincere gratitude to:

Stephan Bodian, who skillfully and patiently edited the manuscript, who expressed my words perfectly, and whose attention to detail, precision, and expression created a body of work that reflects my intuition and incentive.

Greg Vis, whose vision, support, and patience helped in this book's publication.

The staff of Tamalpais Pain Clinic, Doris, Becky, Sara, and Susan, who are there for me and keep my clinic balanced and human so that I am able to work in a healing environment. I truly respect them. And my dear associate Barbara Wolf, who I love, respect, and value so very much. And my wonderful husband, Steven, who is part of the clinic and part of me, and who provides all the love and support anyone could ever desire. If it wasn't for his patience, his sustenance, and his help at all times and in so many ways, this book could never have been written. I love and appreciate him very much.

Ariana Garfinkel, who helped research, edit, and prepare this manuscript, and who has become a permanent fixture in the "Winning the War" series. I thank her especially. She is an intelligent and creative person with a great future ahead of her.

Janis Callon, who edited and researched the text on CFIDS.

All the NAET practitioners, especially my sister-in-law, Dr. Deborah Cutler, who have written to me over the past two years with their support, backing, and appreciation, first for *Winning the War Against Asthma and Allergies,* and now for this book, *Winning the War Against Immune Disorders and Allergies.* Thank you all for your confidence.

Devi Nambudripad, D.C., L.Ac., the founder of NAET. She is my mentor, my friend, and truly an extraordinary and brilliant woman. Dr. Nambudripad has created a healing tool incomparable to any other. Allergies are at the core of chronic illness. This has been proven to me over and over, and Dr. Nambudripad has given the world a wonderful breakthrough treatment to eliminate allergies and therefore heal those with chronic illnesses. Not a day goes by that I don't praise the work of Dr. Devi Nambudripad and thank her for what she has taught me and what I am able to do in service to all those who are in need.

Howard Loomis, D.C., who not only saved my life but gave me the tools to save many others. He is brilliant, dedicated, and a true pioneer in the field of nutrition. His research in enzyme therapy and his enzyme formulas have enabled me to help save life, increase longevity, and restore the immune system.

Finally, Claire Lussler-Pogue, my friend, my sister, and my inspiration. She is a true example of the wonders of alternative therapy, and because of her, the "Winning the War" series became possible. I will always be indebted to her for her constant heartfelt devotion to this work, and her consistent faith in my efforts as a healer and an author. Thank you, Claire, for always being there.

Marie Henry, who wrote the epigraphs that appear at the beginning of each chapter, is a writer and musician living in San Rafael, California. Her poetry and short fiction have appeared in numerous literary journals and anthologies, including *Yellow Silk, Exquisite Corpse, Alcatraz, Apalachee Quarterly,* and *Full Court: A Literary Anthology of Basketball.*

FOREWORD

"Yes, Virginia, there is a Santa Claus!" That is what you, the reader, will be proclaiming after reading Dr. Ellen Cutler's second book, *Winning the War Against Immune Disorders and Allergies.*

Like Dr. Cutler, I was also introduced to NAET through a colleague and had difficulty believing that such a simple technique could have such success. I delayed taking Dr. Devi Nambudripad's seminars for over two years until I read Dr. Sandra Denton's personal story in the foreword of Dr. Devi's book, *Say Goodbye to Illness.* Although I did not know Sandra personally at the time, we had many colleagues in common, so I knew her story was true, and I made up my mind, right then and there, to put an end to my skeptical curiosity and check it out for myself. Even after meeting Dr. Devi and taking her Basic Seminar, where I heard her own incredible story firsthand, I was still skeptical. On the plane coming home that Sunday night in October 1994, I decided to attend the Advanced Seminar the following month, treat myself first, and then if it worked on me, treat a few of my most difficult allergy cases to give this strange, new approach the true "acid test" (see "Allergy Elimination IS Possible!" in the AHMA Journal, *Holistic Medicine*, at the AHMA web site, http://www.HolistMed@aol.com).

Curing my own long-standing, exercise-induced , left sacroiliac pain with one treatment (amino acids) defi-

nitely got my attention in a hurry, especially when I had
been so certain that the origin of my discomfort was
structural, not allergic. How is that possible? I argued
with myself. I was never taught in medical school, even
osteopathic medical school, that hip pain could originate
from an allergy. "So much for book-learning," my amazing 93-year-old grandmother said to me shortly thereafter,
when I shared my "miraculous" healing experience with
her in excited anticipation of perhaps finally being able
to treat her age-old arthritic aches and pains effectively.
"What matters most, honey, is that the pain is gone and
hasn't come back . . . isn't that so?" Yes, Grandma, the al-
leviation of suffering in any form really is what matters
most, when all is said and done, or at least what should
matter most.

In the innocent plain-spoken words of my own dear
grandmother, I was abruptly reminded of the following
ancient words of wisdom of Hippocrates (historically, the
"Father of Medicine"), whose oath all physicians take
upon graduation from medical school: ". . . the physician
has but one task: to cure; and if (s)he succeeds, it matters
not a whit by what means (s)he has succeeded . . ."
(circa 400 B.C.).

In a day and age when conventional physicians are
leaving their careers in droves, discouraged by the lack
of long-term effectiveness of their craft in all but the most
emergent of cases, and 51 percent of the health care dollar is being spent out-of-pocket on alternative therapies
that may prove to be still only a safer treatment of symptoms versus truly eliminating the cause of chronic pain
and chronic illness, hope is finally emerging on the
health care scene for physicians and patients alike in the
form of Dr. Ellen Cutler's "Winning the War" series.
Those who have read her first book in the series,
Winning the War Against Asthma and Allergies, will be
even more inspired by her second book, as she and her
patients recount the myriad of success stories contained

in these pages, primarily using NAET and enzyme therapies to treat major immune disorders such as CFIDS,
fibromyalgia, Crohn's disease, colitis, Hashimoto's thyroiditis, Candida, herpes, lupus, Gulf War Syndrome, MS,
Sjorgrens, and HIV. Dr. Cutler's information is sound, her
documentation is thorough, and most important, she has
lived up to her sacred oath and passed with flying colors
Hippocrates' own rigorous mandate to the healing arts:
"first, do not harm." No greater challenge is necessary or
required of any physician. Bravo, Dr. Cutler!

May all who have "eyes to see and ears to hear"
read this book. I cannot endorse it (or these therapies)
highly enough. It is both a privilege and an honor to play
a small part in helping Dr. Cutler spread the word regard-
ing her success in achieving every physician's ultimate
task, goal, and dream: to cure the ills of those whom we
serve. Dr. Cutler and her patients *are* winning the war
against asthma, allergies, and immune disorders.

Remember, we all have the possibility of changing
our lives by opening our minds and hearts to new ways
of thinking and being. Today *can* be the first day of the
rest of your life as it has been for so many practitioners
and patients who have embraced these therapies. If you
could conceive of the possibility of a cure for immune
disorders, allergies, or other medical maladies, wouldn't
you at least want to know about it? Turn the page.
Astonishing results await you.

—Ann McCombs, D.O.
Bellevue, WA
April 1998

PREFACE

When most people think of allergies, they think of itchy, watery eyes, sneezing, and congested sinuses. What many do not know is that you might have allergies and never experience those typical allergic symptoms. In fact, allergies can be behind a whole range of seemingly unrelated health conditions. You might be suffering from debilitating fatigue or pain in nearly every muscle in your body, and not realize that allergies are the cause.

Ellen Cutler, D.C., like other alternative medicine physicians, looks for the root causes of a health condition in order to provide treatment that goes beyond symptomatic relief to a more lasting solution. From her many years of clinical experience, she has discovered that allergies are the culprits in a multitude of health problems. In this book, she focuses on those having to do with immunity.

Chronic immune disorders are one of the specialties of alternative medicine. Whereas conventional medicine throws up its proverbial hands, not knowing what to do for systemic illnesses such as chronic fatigue syndrome, fibromyalgia, and candidiasis, among others, the alternative medicine model of treatment is exactly what these conditions require: find the imbalances and deficiencies in the body, correct them, strengthen the body to support its innate healing capacity, and the health problem will be resolved.

Enzyme therapy and the Nambudripad Allergy Elimination Technique (NAET), the methods Dr. Cutler uses to accomplish this, embody the alternative medicine principle of natural, noninvasive, safe, and effective treatment. In this book, you will learn how these therapies can help you recover your health.

I'm here to tell you that you don't have to live with illness, even when you've been told that's your only choice.

God bless.

—Burton Goldberg

AUTHORS' INTRODUCTION

We have all had the experience of feeling fatigued and unable to get out of bed in the morning and function. It is not a pleasant feeling. Now imagine feeling this way every day, as well as experiencing flu-like symptoms, severe muscle and joint pain, depression and mental confusion, spaciness, sore throat, and swollen lymph nodes. It can be torture.

Whenever I feel this way for a day or two, I reflect on the fact that more and more people feel this way 365 days a year. To make matters worse, most physicians still don't recognize that there is a problem worth investigating. Despite the lack of acknowledgment from the mainstream medical community, chronic fatigue, fibromyalgia, and other immune disorders have become the most common illnesses of our time, and their symptoms overlap. Among private insurers, Chronic Fatigue Immune Disorder Syndrome (CFIDS) is the fastest rising cause of disability for men and women. We must understand the impact of these illnesses and not just brush them off as "yuppie diseases" or as merely psychosomatic.

Many of the people who contract immune disorders were energetic, highly motivated individuals who woke up one day to find that their bodies had "crashed." I listen to this scenario in my office every day from high-powered executives, teachers, investment bankers, and accountants whose health unraveled overnight and who are now barely able to walk, let alone think and function as they once did. Their lives have been devastated, and the economic and social impact is overwhelming for them and for their families and friends.

As a practitioner of NAET and enzyme therapy, I have the good fortune of helping people win the war against immune disorders such as chronic fatigue, fibromyalgia, colitis, thyroiditis, candidiasis, and herpes.

"As a person with CFIDS for seven years," wrote one of my patients, "I've had to fight a daily battle with severe fatigue, lethargy, feeling out-of-balance and fluish. I would stay in bed most of the time, feeling debilitated. My former life, which was filled with jogging, hiking, lunches with friends, dinner parties, activities with the children, and intimate times with my husband, has dwindled to almost nothing. I was often depressed and wondered if I would ever feel normal again. No doctor was able to diagnose my illness; instead, they just classified me as clinically depressed and recommended psychiatric help and medications.

Three years ago a psychologist I want to see recommended NAET treatment. With NAET and enzyme therapy I've been able to win not only the battles, but the war itself. I am able to function again, go out to lunch with friends, enjoy time with my husband and children, exercise, and most importantly, smile and feel good about myself."

The road to complete recovery is short and easy for some patients, long and arduous for others, but it is a journey that is well worth every challenge.

My work with allergies and nutrition started almost 20 years ago, and over the years my compassion for people who suffer from chronic illness and are unable to live full and energetic lives motivated me to search for answers to these dibilitating disorders. This continuous, undeviating effort to help people strengthen their immune systems and create resilient, balanced bodies led me to write this book, in which I share my knowledge and research.

In my clinical experience with all types of chronically ill individuals, three contributing factors have repeatedly presented themselves: poor digestion, dietary stress, and allergies. Although this book focuses on the relationship between allergies and immune disorders, it can also benefit those who suffer from allergies or other chronic health problems.

Individuals with immune disorders live with symptoms every day of their lives. Most of them experience extreme fatigue and find themselves struggling to perform even basic life functions. People develop immune disorders in response to poor digestion and absorption, and basic allergies to foods, molds, chemicals, and other environmental factors including infectants such as viruses and bacteria, fluoride in water, hydrocarbons in car exhaust, and natural substances such as textiles, pollens, feathers, yeast and fungi, mercury amalgams in teeth, and emotions. These reactions accumulate over time and create a heavy load on the body which can overburden the immune system and cause an eventual collapse. All immune disorders have their roots in allergies.

This book is divided into five main sections: Part I, Allergies; Part II, Immune Disorders; Part III, Nambudripad Allergy Elimination Technique (NAET) Therapy; Part IV, Adjunctive Therapy; and Part V, Resource Guide. The case histories scattered throughout the book document the results of NAET treatment and enzyme therapy and are based on patients I have treated. They demonstrate why the information presented in this book is a must-read for all individuals with immune disorders, their families and friends, and all allergy sufferers.

Chapters 1–3 explain the types, origins, and causes of allergies, and summarize the various allergy testing and treatment approaches, including NAET. They also feature a detailed, self-help emergency treatment and muscle response allergy test that could save your life.

Chapters 4–13 educate the reader about the immune system and the diagnoses of immune disorders, and provide a review of immune disorders in general (a complete explanation of chronic fatigue immune disorder syndrome [CFIDS], fibromyalgia, thyroiditis, Crohn's disease and ulcerative colitis, candidiasis, and herpes), and list the numerous allergens that can cause each disorder. These allergens include food, hormones, glands, vitamins, fungi, viruses, bacteria, cold and heat, molds, pollen, dust, chemicals, vaccines, metabolic imbalances, genetic factors, aspirin, and the drugs and antibiotics individuals ingest. Once the allergens are pinpointed by a

NAET practitioner, the allergies can be eliminated, along with the problems they cause.

Chapter 14 is a complete guide to creating an allergy-free environment for allergy sufferers. Once people have completed NAET treatment, many of these suggestions no longer need be followed. But until the allergies are eliminated, this chapter can be extremely helpful.

Chapters 15–17 describe in detail the revolutionary allergy elimination technique that has transformed the lives of thousands of people. My patients often ask me why NAET is not the mainstream approach to treating allergies and immune disorders. These three chapters delineate the most common treatment protocols for immune disorders in general and for each individual disorder.

Chapter 18 discusses stamina and the effects of NAET treatment on exercise, energy levels, sleep habits, and mental health. Individuals with immune disorders suffer from poor digestion, including constipation, bloating, irritable bowel, loss of appetite, hypoglycemia, and overall toxicity. Many are sugar and starch intolerant and are deficient in life-supporting enzymes that are needed for every chemical reaction in the body. These enzymes are critical in the process of building and rebuilding the body from proteins, fats, and carbohydrates; no vitamin or mineral can function without their support. Of the more than 5,000 enzymes that have been discovered, four are food enzymes found in raw food and 22 are digestive enzymes secreted by the pancreas. The rest are metabolic enzymes that involve all the different systems of the body that help to maintain a healthy immune system.

I first learned about enzymes from Dr. Howard Loomis, who along with Dr. Edward Howell, is one of the foremost pioneers of enzyme therapy. Their research initiated an exciting new phase in the study of nutrition and its implications for chronic health problems. According to Loomis, all individuals with immune disorders suffer enzyme deficiency as a result of poor digestion, which eventually compromises immune system function. Chapter 19 is a complete overview of enzyme therapy, including how it is used, why it is important for individuals with immune disorders, and why proper digestion and utilization of foods is paramount for health and vitality.

Chapter 20 is a Resource Guide that includes all necessary ingredients for proper NAET treatments, food guides for
the allergens, diets for the different enzyme deficiencies and
food intolerances, and a complete recipe guide for the enzyme
formulas recommended in the book. This chapter also features
a glossary of terms and other important resources for both
health practitioners and sufferers of immune disorders.
Glossary terms are printed in bold type the first time they appear in the book. This book has an on-line companion on our
internet site (http://www.allergy2000.com) which features new
research findings, an "Ask the Experts" column, an updated list
of trained NAET professionals, and more.

The information presented in this book can help you
identify and eliminate the true cause of your illness and it can
enable you to see yourself not as an average allergy sufferer
but as an individual with your own unique biochemical
makeup, allergies, and needs. For example, most people with
CFIDS have been told that it is a chronic problem they will
have to contend with for the rest of their lives. This book
shows that CFIDS can be cured, not miraculously and instanta-
neously, but inevitably and permanently, once the allergies
and metabolic imbalances that cause it have been eliminated.

Every person with CFIDS, fibromyalgia, and other immune disorders should be able to lead a normal, drug-free life.
If you are a person with an immune disorder who wants to
overcome your condition and prevent your children and loved
ones from developing immune disorders, read this book and
discover how you can secure optimal health and win the war
against disease. If you are a health practitioner dealing with
the immune disorders and allergies of your patients, this book
will introduce you to a new approach that may revolutionize
your practice.

As we approach the Twenty-first Century, the growing incidence of immune disorders reflects an increase of chemical
pollutants in our environment and food, a decline in adequate
nutrition caused in large measure by poor absorption of vitamins, minerals, and other nutrients, and an exponential rise in
the use of pharmaceutical drugs that weaken and suppress the
immune system. At the same time, the dawn of the new century heralds a new awakening to drug-free alternative ap-

proaches to chronic health problems. People are disillusioned
with the medical establishment and are demanding remedies
that enliven their bodies and minds and encourage rather than
suppress their own healing forces. We all need a chance to reclaim control and responsibility for our health.

This book offers new understanding of the symptoms
and causes of chronic fatigue syndrome, fibromyalgia, candidiasis, Crohn's disease and colitis, thyroiditis and herpes. It offers hope to those afflicted with these disorders, and it
empowers everyone by providing an alternative approach for
overcoming them, now and forever. There are many other disorders, such as HIV-AIDS and rheumatoid arthritis that could
have been included in this book and some of my colleagues
encouraged me to do so. However, after careful thought, I decided that they deserve to be treated in separate volumes of
the "Winning the War" series. Although my research in these
areas is not complete, I can report that I and other NAET and
enzyme therapy practitioners have treated patients with these
disorders with extraordinary success. The simplicity and clarity
of this approach complements and promotes the pure healing
force that is within each one of us.

I | ALLERGIES: TYPES, CAUSES, SYMPTOMS, TESTING, AND TREATMENTS

1 | DEFINING ALLERGIES

Hansel and Gretel didn't get roasted,
they died from inhaling oven cleaner fumes.
Death among Brillo Pads, ammonia and mothballs.
Mop & Glo your way to morbidity—
wipes out dirt and brain cells
in one fell swoooosh.
Excuse me a moment
I have to take a nap.
—from "Case Study of Cognitive Dysfunction
in 3.5 Million CFIDS Patients"

Jocelyn

Jocelyn, age 45, came to see me with chronic fatigue syndrome. Her symptoms were constant tiredness, intermittent nausea, severe postnasal drip and/or stuffiness, and frequent coughing. After experiencing a bitter divorce, she noticed that her symptoms became more severe and she needed to rest more often. In addition to noting a low-grade infection, she reported that she was premenopausal and had been experiencing moderate hot flashes, constipation, insomnia, and irregular menstruation. Acupuncture and Chinese herbs had proved somewhat helpful for limited periods of time. Her main reason for coming to see me was to treat the chronic fatigue and to strengthen her immune system so she could fight off infections.

After a lengthy history and consultation, I performed an abdominal diagnostic exam and urinalysis which revealed poor sugar metabolism and absorption, Vitamin C deficiency, and difficulty digesting fats. Her 24-hour urinalysis showed dietary stress with fat meaning poor digestion and absorption of fats. Her assimilation of sugars was poor, and she exhibited low calcium. When I see signs of calcium deficiency, I usually suspect that a calcium allergy is preventing the person from absorbing the calcium properly. She was also mildly deficient in Vitamin C. In addition, her urine tended to be acidic which often indicates a deficiency in bicarbonate and therefore an inability to absorb sugars, which she showed. Her kidney function and electrolytes appeared normal. I immediately prescribed an enzyme that helps to digest fats and and to successfully assimilate sugars (see Biliary Enzyme).

Allergy testing revealed that she was allergic to calcium, Vitamin C, B vitamins, sugars, iron, minerals, and salt and I began to treat her for these basic allergens. We did a combination of minerals with thymus gland. This is important for the immune system in that the thymus produces specific anitbodies to fight infection. I also treated her for severe allergies to coffee, chocolate, and caffeine. After treating her for the basics, I prescribed an adrenal enzyme, a calcium enzyme (para), and Vitamin C enzyme (opt). (See the Resource Guide for a listing of enzymes.) At this point, her energy had improved noticeably and she had more stamina and clarity at work.

After coffee, chocolate, and caffeine, I treated for the Epstein-Barr virus, alone and in combination with lactic acid. This combination is common in people who exercise and feel concomittant muscle or joint pain. I also treated for Epstein-Barr in combination with grains and sinus. Anytime Jocelyn exercised and ate grains or foods with lactic acid such as milk or some fruits, she would immediately awaken the link with Epstein-Barr and experience severe fatigue. With any chronic health problem, my approach, after strengthening the immune system and treating for the basics and some foods, is to treat for the infectant causing the major symptoms, whether it is a fungus, a bacteria, or a virus such as Epstein-Barr or herpes.

After treating for Epstein-Barr, I treated her for the adrenal gland, the adrenal cortex, and the adrenal medulla. I then treated her for food additives, including MSG, hydrolyzed vegetable protein, BHA, and BHT as well as for nerve tissue which is often helpful to people who experience irritation, debility, long-standing nerve problems, MS, lupus, fibromyalgia, insomnia, and PMS. I then treated her for sinus which was probably the most dramatic treatment, because her chronic congestion and runny nose disappeared overnight. Afterwards, in combination with sinus, I treated sinus mucous and nasal mucous to complete the treatment.

Next we treated for gluten which cleared wheat, barley, rye, and oats and allowed her to eat those foods again. After clearing the bacteria, including *strep pneumoniae, hemophilus influenzae, aerobacter aerogenes,* and *Barnaloides,* we treated her for dairy, cheese, yogurt, the rest of the grains, vegetables, beverages including red and white wines, herbs and spices, food coloring, and animal and vegetable fats. Then I began to treat some of the environmentals, especially tree mix and tree pollen, which turned out to be one of Jocelyn's most difficult and rewarding allergy treatments for chronic fatigue. It took more than ten sessions to clear the trees, including combinations with different emotions, organs, and foods. I learned that she loved trees and experienced severe emotional symptoms and Candida outbreaks when she didn't clear. These Candida symptoms were severe thrush or coating on her tongue, a metallic taste in her mouth, and skin eruptions. We treated all the trees at once and then treated individual trees separately. Once the trees cleared, she was a different person. She hasn't had a reaction to trees for two years now, even during pollen season.

We then treated for *Candida albicans.* As I mentioned earlier, I require patients to wear a mask and gloves, avoid skin-to-skin contact, get new underwear, shoes, socks, maybe even new clothes, and otherwise be careful as one can easily expose oneself to the fungus and lose the treatment. After we treated for Candida, she lost the metallic taste, the coating in her tongue changed, and her fatigue all but disappeared.

We went on to treat for hormones in order to reduce some of the premenopausal symptoms. All the hormones, including cortisone, DHEA, estradiol, estriol, insulin, progesterone, testosterone, and T_2, T_3, and T_4 cleared easily and she began to use a natural hormone progesterone cream. We then treated for the phenolics including indol, norepinephrine, coumarin, glutamine, acetaldehyde, alanine, butyric acid, and menadione to clear any foods that might be left. Next we treated for the thyroid gland itself which usually gives one an energy boost. We treated for the viruses, including rhinovirus and echovirus, pesticides and herbicides, the remaining fruits, berries, vinegar, other organs such as the parotid gland, immune mediators such as IgG, IgM, and RF factor. Finally we treated for dust, radiation, and some of the organs. Jocelyn is no longer plagued with chronic fatigue and is radiantly healthy.

BROAD DEFINITION OF ALLERGIES

In this book I explore the relationship between allergies and immune disorders and I would like to begin by defining the term allergy. An **allergy** is an abnormal, adverse physical reaction of the body to certain substances known as **allergens** (or **antigens**). These substances can be toxic (exhaust fumes or other petrochemicals) or nontoxic (pollens or food) and allergy sufferers will react to quantities that are harmless to most people.

When exposed to allergens, allergic individuals develop an excess of an **antibody** called **immunoglobulin E (IgE)**. The IgE antibodies react with allergens to release **histamines** and other chemicals from cell tissues that produce various allergic symptoms. In other words, the **immune system** mistakenly identifies harmless substances as dangerous invaders and activates antibodies to defend the body. The development of an allergy begins with sensitization to the substance on first contact, usually without symptoms. A second exposure to the substance, however, allows the previously created antibodies to become active and produce symptoms.

Although a person can develop allergies to practically any substance, the most common allergens include pollen, dust, **dust mites**, animal dander (skin, saliva, hair, or fur), feathers, cosmetics, mold, insect venom, certain chemicals, drugs, medicines (especially penicillin), and foods. The most troublesome foods are usually peanuts, other tree nuts, shellfish, milk, eggs, wheat, and soy. Allergens may cause a reaction following inhalation, injection, ingestion, or contact with the skin. Allergic reactions can involve any part of the body, but most frequently affect the nose, chest, skin, and eyes. The rarest and most dangerous type of allergy is called **anaphylactic shock**. It can affect many organs at once and is evidenced by rapid decreases in blood pressure, rash or hives, breathing difficulties, abdominal pain, swollen tongue or throat, diarrhea, fainting, asphyxiation and, too often, death.

It is estimated that between 35 and 50 million people in the United States suffer from allergies. Allergies can emerge suddenly at any age without prior warning. Many studies have shown conclusively that parents with allergies tend to have children with allergies. Some research suggests that the tendency to develop an allergy of some kind is inherited, although not the tendency to a particular allergy. However, I have repeatedly seen in my practice that a child's allergic tendencies are often related to those of his or her parents, and I often have treated parents and their children for the same allergies. Some people tend toward allergic reactions (these individuals are known as atopic). Once a person develops one allergy, others commonly follow.

Part of the difficulty in determining the number of allergy sufferers lies in how broadly or narrowly one defines the term. Medical doctors and scientists often support a narrow definition, asserting that the only true allergies result from the activation of IgE antibodies. Millions of people, however, experience allergic symptoms without the antibody reaction. These people are said to have an intolerance or a **hypersensitivity** to particular substances. Although the causes may differ, the diagnosis and treatment of allergy and intolerance often overlap. As a result, allergy research and information benefits more people than those with traditional allergies alone.

In my clinical work I have found that the measurements and treatments for allergies and intolerances are exactly the same and I use the terms interchangeably. For example, many asthmatics are *intolerant* to sugars and *allergic* to animal dander. **Muscle response testing** with these two substances yields identical results, and I treat them in the same way.

Allergies can cause a predisposition to colds and the flu by compromising the immune system and lowering resistance. Once the body becomes host to viruses and bacteria, it is difficult to distinguish a cold from an allergic reaction, especially since the two often occur simultaneously. Allergies don't generally cause fever, however, and colds, unlike allergies that refuse to go away, do not linger for more than a week or two.

In this book, I take the wider view of an allergy as any negative or abnormal response in the immune system. For example, I believe there is no such thing as a simple cold. A cold is the response of a challenged immune system, whether it is to a food, a pollen, or a virus. Because a virus is also an allergen, I treat a cold like an allergy, and experience excellent results.

TYPES OF ALLERGIES

Allergies can be classified according to the causative substance or the resulting symptoms. There are also active (acute) allergies and hidden (chronic) allergies.

The first category includes the following subtypes:

- ingestants, also referred to as food allergy
- inhalants such as dust
- contactants such as latex or chemicals
- injectants such as drugs
- infectants such as viruses or bacteria
- physical agents such as cold or heat
- organs
- autoimmune allergies such as those to hormones that can include thyroid, estrogen, testosterone, cholesterol, and adrenaline
- insect allergies

Allergies defined by symptoms include:

- hay fever
- **asthma**
- skin conditions (**eczema**, hives, rashes)
- headaches and migraines
- stomach upset
- chronic fatigue
- depression
- chronic pain
- conjunctivitis
- anaphylactic shock
- the most widespread allergy-related diseases.
- autoimmune disorders

Active or acute allergies can be of the "immediate type" in which symptoms appear within seconds of contact after every exposure (for example, hives, itching, vomiting, coughing, wheezing) and usually subside within an hour. Or they can be of the "delayed type" in which the reaction occurs hours or days after contact because the allergen is not the food itself, but instead a chemical by-product of digestion.

Hidden or chronic allergies can cause severe developmental and functional problems, deficiencies, or chemical imbalances. For example, an allergy to B vitamins can cause B vitamin deficiencies and result in chronic health problems such as **chronic fatigue syndrome**, **attention deficit disorder (ADD)**, depression, digestive problems, asthma, and headaches. An allergy to calcium (Ca.) can cause joint or arthritic problems. The diagnosis and treatment of chronic allergies is the focus of this book.

Food Allergy

A food allergy is the immune system's response to a certain food during which IgE-mediated chemicals trigger an allergic reaction. After ingesting foods to which he or she is allergic, a person may experience vomiting, stomach pain, swelling and bloating, diarrhea, constipation, eczema or hives, an asthmatic attack, breathing difficulties, joint pain, chronic fatigue, migraines and, on occasion, anaphylaxis. In extreme cases, an individual can have an allergic reaction to minute amounts of the allergen such as skin contact with the food, or kissing someone who has eaten the food. For example, an infant allergic to milk can have a reaction to a diaper rash cream that contains an ingredient derived from milk. The eight foods that cause ninety percent of all allergic reactions are milk, eggs, wheat, peanuts, soy, tree nuts, fish, and shellfish. Peanuts, nuts, fish, and shellfish commonly cause the most severe and dangerous reactions.

Conventional medicine has no cure for food allergies, except strict avoidance of the allergens. The **Nam-**

budripad Allergy Elimination Technique (NAET) approach described in this book is an efficient, effective, and permanent method of allergy desensitization. People can determine which foods they are allergic to through an elimination diet, skin or blood testing, and muscle response testing (refer to the section on muscle testing in Chapter 2).

Children and adults with food allergies experience a wide variety of symptoms including abdominal pain, headaches, chronic fatigue, fibromyalgia, eczema, muscle pain, runny noses, asthma, chronic coughing, attention problems, and behavioral problems. Many feel these allergies disappear as a child matures to adulthood, but in reality they do not. Often, some of the acute symptoms lessen over time, but the allergy becomes chronic or hidden, and has the potential of causing developmental or functional problems and persistent maladies.

Twenty-five percent of adults believe they have food allergies but conventional medicine claims that only one or two percent are actual allergy sufferers. Those who do not have allergies, according to the limited definition of mainstream medicine, have what is usually called a food intolerance, which can be equally uncomfortable. The difference is that a genuine food allergy is caused by antibodies that can be identified by blood testing, whereas food intolerance is a broader term encompassing many illnesses caused by food. Food intolerance does not register on conventional allergy tests although it can be measured using muscle response testing.

Some causes of food intolerance are chemicals such as caffeine and food colorings (tartrazine) that do not produce adverse effects in the majority of the population, but do trigger allergic symptoms in some people. A deficiency of enzymes (the chemicals that help digestion) can cause problems as well. If a person lacks one or more enzymes, or is deficient in one or more of these enzymes, he or she can experience digestive problems such as diarrhea and stomach pain after consuming the food the missing enzyme digests. For example, people who have difficulty drinking milk are deficient in the enzyme that digests lactose, the sugar in milk. In my clinical practice, I have found that people who are "lactose intolerant" are essentially allergic to lactose. When we treat patients for lactose intolerance, they are fully able to tolerate milk with no side effects. In fact, a complete clinical study on milk allergy showed that the NAET method is ninety-nine percent effective.

Finally, studies indicate that taking antibiotics can increase the chances of food intolerance in some people. The antibiotics apparently kill some types of bacteria in the large intestine and allow others to flourish, causing an abnormal reaction during digestion that produces various unpleasant chemical by-products and associated symptoms. Antibiotics can also cause an abnormal amount of yeast, or Candida, in the intestines that leads to an imbalance of other healthy intestinal flora or microorganisms. I have had successful results in treating Candida and other abnormal **pathogens** with NAET. These will be discussed later in this book.

Drug Allergy

A severe, even life-threatening reaction to certain drugs and chemical additives, particularly penicillin, occurs in a small percentage of people. Other problematic drugs include aspirin, vaccines, insulin, and illegal drugs. Most often, the allergic reaction appears as a skin condition such as itching, hives, rashes, swelling, or peeling skin. Other symptoms can include incontinence, headache, dizziness, high blood pressure, moodiness, depression, agitation, edema, insomnia, hyperactivity, heart palpitations, bloating, constipation, diarrhea, blurred vision, hot flashes and, of course, drug dependence and addiction. For example, 5,000 men and women who participated in Operation Desert Storm experienced severe side effects, probably allergic reactions, to a drug they were instructed to take every day called pyristigimide bromide. This medication was supposed to protect them from harmful exposure to nerve gas. These men and women developed numerous health problems from tearing eyes and runny noses to chronic fatigue, twitches, cramps, blurred vision, incontinence, diarrhea, and other serious maladies. Even now, five years later, they continue to experience these symptoms and show signs of suppressed immune systems and long-term muscle damage. This drug was developed in 1955 for myasthenia gravis and was approved only for investigative use.

Insect Allergy

In general, the normal toxic reaction and discomfort that follow an insect sting is not considered an allergy. However, many people have severe allergic reactions to bee and wasp stings that can sometimes be fatal. These IgE-mediated reactions induce rashes, runny noses and eyes, swelling of the throat, asthma attacks, and anaphylactic shock.

Occupational Allergy

This term refers to allergies that develop in people as a result of working with industrial dusts, vapors, gases, fumes, nickel, chromium, rubber, dyes, formaldehyde, glues, in heat, and the like. Symptoms can manifest themselves within weeks, or take years of repeated exposure before they appear. The least protected parts of the body (hands, arms, face) are affected most frequently. Protective masks, gloves, and clothing can help prevent a reaction and even save a life. For example, bakers who handle different foods can prevent reactions by wearing gloves and masks if necessary.

Latex Allergy

Often categorized as an occupational allergy because it is frequently found among health-care workers, latex allergy is surfacing in increasing numbers among the general population as well. The offending material can be found in balloons, gloves used for washing dishes or handling food, dental and medical gloves, condoms, clothing and shoes, carpets, rain slickers, pacifiers, baby-bottle nipples, and air pollution. Symptoms include swelling, welts, itchiness and hives after contact, sneezing and nasal congestion, watery and itchy eyes, chronic fatigue, and occasionally anaphylactic shock. Generally, the people with the highest risk of developing latex allergy are those with high levels of exposure to latex, a history of allergies, multiple surgeries as children, or food allergies. Studies have shown also that people with allergies to certain fruits and vegetables—particularly bananas, kiwis, raw potatoes, tomatoes, celery, carrots, stone fruits, figs, avocados, papayas, passion fruit, hazelnuts and water chestnuts—are more likely to develop latex allergy. NAET has been very successful in treating latex allergy.

Skin Conditions

The most common skin condition, eczema, is a rash or irritation that can be either wet or dry, occasionally chapped, and most often accompanied by severe itching. Although the cause isn't always clear, the condition often appears in children of families with a history of allergic disease. Milk and woolen clothes are possible contributors to the condition. Eczema usually begins in the first year of life as a facial rash and is often a precursor of asthma. Later in life it can appear on the insides of the elbows, the backs of the knees, the neck, ankles, wrists, and the backs of the hands.

Contact eczema has similar symptoms to common eczema, but can be traced to direct contact with a variety of substances including nickel found in coins, stainless steel, chromium found in cement and leather, rubber found in gloves and boots, and preservatives found in creams, ointments, and cosmetics.

Hives, or urticaria, is evidenced by a warming of the skin with redness and itching, or white raised wheals. It can appear very suddenly and may last for hours or a whole day.

NAET is quite effective in treating eczema and other skin conditions in all age groups. I usually find that eczema in children is caused by an allergy to wheat, corn and B vitamins. In adults, the allergens can range from foods, clothing, animals, chemicals, and creams to fungus, yeast, and bacteria. Acne also responds, sometimes dramatically, to treatment of those basic allergies, milk and yeast, and then the bacteria in the system.

Conjunctivitis

The main symptoms of conjunctivitis include redness of the eyes and itchiness. It most often affects adults. Treating environmental allergies early with NAET can help prevent this condition.

Anaphylaxis

The most severe and life-threatening allergic reaction, anaphylactic shock, is usually a sudden response of the immune system to foods, insect stings, or medication. Symptoms can include any combination of the following: swelling, difficulty breathing, hives, vomiting, diarrhea, cramps, and a drop in blood pressure. An anaphylactic reaction can occur in as little as five to 15 minutes and medical attention is needed immediately. When waiting for medical assistance, stimulation of the respiratory acupuncture points can provide some relief of the symptoms and improve breathing (refer to the emergency treatment procedures in Chapter 9).

Hay Fever (Allergic Rhinitis)

Hay fever is a condition that afflicts millions of Americans. Symptoms range from runny or stuffy nose, sneezing, swelling of mucous membranes, and itchiness of the throat, palate, and eyes to loss of smell and taste. Primary causes are airborne inhalants such as grass, weeds, tree pollens, and mold spores. Hay fever can be seasonal or intermittent. NAET has been extremely successful in handling these type of allergies. In our clinic I have seen symptoms reverse immediately after NAET treatment for ragweed or other pollens, and these results have been replicated by other practitioners.

Asthma

During an asthma attack, an individual's bronchial tubes swell periodically and the muscles surrounding the tubules go into spasm. This obstructs the flow of air to the lungs, leading to wheezing, coughing, and difficult, labored breathing. Asthma may begin at any age and has the potential to recur and become chronic. It is an allergic disease that is always triggered by allergens. These allergens include not only foods, pollens, and environmental factors such as perfume, animal dander, and chemicals but also bacteria, climactic conditions, and emotions. When these allergies are active from birth, asthma can be diagnosed early in life, even in infancy. When the allergies are hidden and chronic, they can cause other chronic functional and developmental problems such as fatigue, coughing, or headaches. Tissues break down slowly with chronic allergies, with minimal secretion of immune mediators that cause minor muscle contraction, swelling, and increased mucus secretion. When other stressful factors are added to the system—menopause, emotional stress, medication, or gastritis—the allergic load is increased and late-onset asthma can occur (see *Winning the War Against Asthma and Allergies*).

ORIGINS AND CAUSES OF ALLERGIES

An allergic reaction can be IgE mediated or non-IgE mediated. An IgE-mediated allergy is the traditional type recognized by most medical doctors in which immunoglobulin E antibodies are produced in response to environmental allergens and foods. Typical symptoms are hay fever and some forms of eczema. A non-IgE-mediated allergy, not always recognized as an allergy by conventional physicians, is a negative change in the immune system that can cause a variety of symptoms. Allergens that are non-IgE mediated may affect the sympathetic and parasympathetic nervous systems. For example, an individual with colitis, an irritation of the colon caused by food or bacterial allergies, may stimulate the parasympathetic nervous system to secrete acetylcholine. Acetylcholine increases peristalsis which causes undo spasm and cramping and triggers an attack of colitis.

Allergens such as bacteria, viruses, or certain foods seem to create antigen-antibody complexes by combining with **T cells** and **B cells**, the adaptive defenses of the body produced in bone marrow. These antigen-antibody complexes lodge themselves in certain tissues of the body (for example, in the muscles, joints, and glands). When trying to destroy these complexes, the immune system brings about an **autoimmune reaction** that inflames and destroys healthy tissue. This inflammation triggers an autoimmune reaction and creates a chronic condition until the allergens and complexes are removed.

The most common cause of allergies is genetic. The probability of a child developing an allergy is increased if one or both parents suffer from any type of allergic condition, and is the strongest factor for predicting future allergies. If one parent suffers from allergies, the child will develop allergies seventy-five percent of the time. If both parents have allergies, the child will develop allergies one hundred percent of the time.

The second most common cause of allergies is poor digestion. If a food is not properly digested, it will eventually trigger an allergic reaction.

Chemotherapeutic drugs, excessive antibiotics, steroids, or exposure to toxic chemicals or radiation are also important factors in the development of allergies or depressed immune reaction. For example, when antibiotics and steroids are used concurrently over a long period of time, the antibiotics destroy the good microflora of the intestines, and strengthen and increase the longevity of bad microflora or yeast. This leads to **candidiasis**. A suppressed immune system is unable to destroy these yeast cells that can eventually scar the intestinal villi. This allows toxins, undigested food, and yeast to enter the bloodstream through the intestine and leads to a systemic yeast problem, which, in turn, stimulates the creation of **circulating immune complexes (CICs)** and autoimmune reactions.

When an expectant mother is exposed to various toxins such as chemicals or radiation, or suffers an illness such as a flu or an infection, allergies will often occur in the child. Altered cells do not carry over the genetic codes and do not undergo normal development. As a result, organs and tissues may develop nonfunctional sensory nerve receptors that are unable to conduct messages to and from the spinal cord and brain. In some people these nerve receptors become hyposensitive toward certain items; in other people they become hypersensitive. When hyposensitive fibers predominate, few allergic reactions are seen but poor growth, chronic fatigue, and poor functioning of body and mind are evident also. Active, acute allergies result from hypersensitivity, whereas hidden or chronic allergies result from hyposensitivity.

Finally, chronic or severe malnutrition can also cause allergies. If the body is deficient in protein, vitamins, and minerals, enzymatic and metabolic processes cannot occur. This results in undigested food and an increase in the production of toxic metabolites that can eventually lead to allergies. These vitamins and minerals are also needed for effective immune function to protect the body when fighting off infections.

ALLERGIC LOAD PHENOMENON

In my estimation, over ninety percent of the population has allergies or intolerances, most of which are genetic in origin. However, in the majority of people, these allergies are hidden or inactive. It is the allergic load phenomenon that activates these allergies in certain people. If, over a period of time, one confronts other, more active, or acute allergens, and one is physically, mentally, or emotionally stressed—lacks sufficient sleep or eats poorly—these chronic hidden allergies become pronounced and the body falls prey to other problems. Resistance breaks down, the immune system cannot keep these allergies in check, and chronic emotional, functional, or developmental problems arise. Then, for the first time, one can experience chronic fatigue, arthritis, swelling, chronic pain, headaches, and asthma.

For example, last week a woman came into my office complaining of chronic fatigue. About two months ago, when she started a very stressful, high-pressured job, she had a bad case of the flu. Around the same time, her mother died of cancer and she was beginning to develop premenopausal symptoms. After a complete examination I began some allergy testing. I found she was very allergic to hormones, flu viruses, certain environmental and chemical substances, many foods including sugar, dairy products, grains, and many other foods. She was particularly intolerant of sugars and carbohydrates and was unable to absorb these foods.

It soon became apparent that she was experiencing the allergic load phenomenon. She was living on pasta and breads, and had never fully recovered from the flu virus to which she was also allergic. The death of her mother added to her stress, and her premenopausal state caused hormonal fluctuations. With her immune system compromised, certain hidden allergies manifested themselves, her system became overly sensitive, and she developed chronic fatigue. It didn't happen overnight, however; in fact, most of the allergies were there from the beginning.

ILLNESSES AND CHRONIC DISEASES RELATED TO ALLERGIES

We don't usually imagine that allergic reactions can play a role in seemingly unrelated medical conditions. Many experts, however, are drawing connections between a history of allergies and numerous other chronic conditions from alcoholism to obesity. Allergies also are considered partially responsible for some types of behavioral or emotional problems. We have had excellent results in cases of obesity, as well as those of depression and exhaustion, of seeing the problem as rooted in allergies and using NAET to clear the allergies.

Alcoholism

The concept of alcoholism is that alcoholics might be allergic to the ingredients in alcoholic beverages. This causes deficiencies of those ingredients and leads to strong cravings for such beverages. The substances people are usually allergic to are B vitamins, sugar, grapes, brewer's yeast, malt, or corn and become addicted to an alcoholic beverage that contains any or all of the allergens.

I have treated alcoholics successfully with NAET. Eileen, an alcoholic in her early thirties, was referred to me by her parents, both of whom had excellent results with the method (her father with hay fever and her mother with menopausal symptoms). Their daughter had been an alcoholic for ten years. During this time she suffered some near-fatal car accidents and financial disasters because of her drinking, and she had tried a number of treatment facilities and therapists with no success. People usually crave the foods to which they are allergic, and Eilleen hoped that I might be able to help her with her intense craving for alcohol which then would enable her to make better use of traditional treatments.

I performed a full examination that included a complete enzyme evaluation and allergy testing protocol. Like most alcoholics, she was especially allergic to all the B vitamins, all sugars, and alcohol. I prescribed an enzyme for sugar digestion and began to treat her for the basic allergies, including the B vitamins and sugars. Then I treated her for alcohol. Six hours after the treatment, she called to tell me she was drunk. I immediately felt disappointed. But then she added that she was drunk not because of the alcohol or sugar, but simply as a result of the process of clearing the allergy. The difference was that this time she was completely cognizant of everything that was happening which was never the case when she was actually drunk. I imagine that she was detoxifying the alcohol. She also noted how good she felt.

The next day, when I retested her, she was no longer allergic to alcohol. She then attended a three-week alcohol treatment program, and I didn't hear from her again until three years later when she called to tell me how grateful she was. She said she hadn't had a single drink since the allergy clearing which was a breakthrough for her.

Obesity

Similar to alcoholics, people who struggle with excessive weight may be allergic to their favorite foods and unable to resist indulging their intense cravings. Additionally, some people have noticed that hunger can be a symptom of an allergic reaction. For example, when sufferers of a wheat allergy eat a wheat-heavy meal, they may feel strong cravings to eat again within a short period of time, even though they no longer need the nutrition. NAET reverses cravings by clearing the basic allergies. People's addictions and cravings are diminished. Then the various individual diets based on specific food intolerances (located in the Resource Guide) can be followed easily and weight loss is natural, easier, and effective. I've seen frustrated, overweight persons lose 9–10 pounds within 10 days after the basic allergies were treated with NAET.

Arthritis

Arthritis has been attributed partially to an allergic reaction in the joints to common foods. When some arthritic patients avoid certain foods or environmental allergens, their symptoms diminish. Acid foods seem to be especially troublesome, as are the nightshades which include tomatoes, white potatoes, eggplant, peppers, and tobacco (refer to Part 6). I have also found arthritic patients to be allergic to bacteria and parasites that can trigger the autoimmune reaction.

I have had many successes with arthritis sufferers. A woman with severe arthritis in her sacroiliac and hips came to me seeking help with her extreme chronic pain and migraine headaches. Unfortunately she was a housekeeper and cook. This caused her to be on her feet most of the day and to be very active. When I performed a full examination and allergy testing I found her to be highly allergic to all the basic allergens, acid-forming foods, the nightshade family, and fifteen different bacteria. She was unable to digest proteins and fats, yet she was eating large amounts of protein because she was trying to lose weight. The uric acid content in her urine sediment was quite high, generally an indicator of high protein consumption. I recommended an **enzyme** to help her digest fats and proteins, and I prescribed a diet lower in protein and fats and higher in complex carbohydrates. I treated her with NAET for all the basic allergies, acid foods, and all the bacteria.

After all the bacteria were cleared, her hip and sacroiliac pain almost completely subsided and her flexibility improved by seventy-five percent. In addition to being able to take care of her household responsibilities, she now walks three miles a day and has lost thirty pounds. She also smiles a lot when I see her.

Migraines and Headaches

Allergies are a common culprit in recurring headaches. Research has found again and again that some migraine sufferers can eliminate their symptoms by avoiding certain triggering foods, particularly milk, eggs, wheat, aged cheese, MSG, chocolate, oranges, tea, coffee, beef, corn, cane sugar, yeast, and alcoholic beverages.

A sensitivity to extreme weather, smoke, exercise, pollen, chemical fumes, and stress can also cause chronic headaches. The woman with arthritis experienced headaches daily and migraines weekly. No remedy worked for her headaches. While treating for the arthritis, I also treated her with NAET for female hormones, estrogen, progesterone, thyroid hormones T_3 and T_4, and adrenaline. I had to treat her for progesterone three times before it completely cleared. I even had her treat herself at home for this allergen because it was so severe. After completing the hormone clearing, her headaches disappeared and never returned.

Psychological and Behavioral Conditions

Perhaps some of the least recognized but most interesting effects of allergies are psychological conditions. Evidence is mounting that in some people certain allergens can actually result in, or aggravate, emotional and behavioral problems including depression, hyperactivity, learning difficulties, anxiety, irritability, and schizophrenia. NAET practitioners have had excellent results with atten-

tion deficit disorder (ADD), hyperactivity, and other behavioral problems in children and adults. Children with
attention deficit disorder are treated for the following:

- the basic allergies

- possibly mercury and fluoride

- thyroid and thyroid hormones

- yeast or Candida

- foods such as wheat, dairy, sugar, artificial sweeteners, food additives, food coloring, and chocolate

- environmental allergies such as radiation, dust,
  chemicals, mold, and pollution

- emotional traumas

I also supplement these children with enzymes and minerals and make strong dietary recommendations based
on an individual evaluation. Treating children with NAET
is fulfilling and rewarding because the changes in their
physical and emotional health are immediate and profound.

2 | ALLERGY TESTING

And as for those put-down, flip-talking,
denying sons-of-bitches who claim
if you don't look sick,
you ain't,
so stop malingering and
get off your duff . . .
Tell them I'm putting on my Joe Louis trunks
and lacing up my gloves.

—from "Declaration of Intention"

Sharon

Sharon, 43, was referred to me by an addiction rehabilitation facility for help with her allergies, obesity, and fatigue. Since having a hysterectomy several years before because of fibroids and endrometriosis, her general health and energy level had declined. She had developed fungal infections and skin eruptions, she had become depressed, and she had gained 30 pounds.

Since the hysterectomy, Sharon had been on Premarin®, which had caused high blood pressure and a number of other symptoms such as bloating and weight gain. She was hoping I could help her with her energy level and depression, her Candida infection, her skin problems, and her weight. Since the hysterectomy, she had also been experiencing hot flashes six or seven times a day.

On her first visit, I performed an abdominal diagnostic enzyme evaluation to determine what nutritional and enzyme supplementation she might need. On the fasting part of the exam, I found a positive epigastric reflex, usually a sign of gastritis, which may be the a result of an allergy to a synthetic hormone. I also found that she had trouble absorbing sugars, which she craved. She was low in calcium, a significant indicator for all women, especially those who have had a hysterectomy. And I found positive kidney and liver reflexes, suggesting possible water retention and toxicity, common side effects of Premarin®.

On the nonfasting part of the exam, I again found a positive epigastric reflex and a problem digesting sugars. I prescribed an enzyme to calm the gastritis (stm) and recommended the diet for sugar intolerance found in this book.

Allergy testing revealed that Sharon was allergic to all the basic allergens except most of the minerals. The only mineral to which she was allergic was chromium, and this was severe. I treated her for eggs and chicken, calcium, and vitamin C, which we needed to treat in combination with hormones, estrogen, progesterone, and testosterone. Then we treated her for all the B vitamins and all the sugars. After we treated her for iron in combination with acid, she no longer experienced an acid stomach and gastritis when eating iron-rich foods. This allowed me to switch her to an enzyme more appropriate for sugar-intolerant people (pan). I also added enzymes for Vitamin C (opt) and calcium (para), and an adrenal enzyme supplement (adr). After a woman goes through menopause or a hysterectomy, the adrenal glands are important in the production of estrogen and progesterone. These supplements reduced the frequency of her hot flashes by almost 50 percent.

The trace mineral chromium helps the body metabolize sugar by optimizing the utilization of insulin. Most people eat a diet low in chromium. Foods that are high in chromium include tomatoes, pineapple, white potatoes, and grains. Chromium helps people who are sugar intolerant to avoid the predisposition to diabetes. If you are allergic to this mineral, you are not absorbing it from food and can become deficient. Once people are cleared of the allergy and given a chromium supplement, they need less insulin to process sugar. It can also lower blood cholesterol levels and reduce the craving for sugar. After being treated for for B vitamins, sugars, and chromium, Sharon stopped craving sugars and was able to go on the sugar-intolerant diet I had given her. Soon her weight began to drop naturally and her depression began to lift.

Next, we treated Sharon for yeasts, molds, and other fungi, including *Aspergillis fumigatus, Aspergillis niger, Candida albicans, Candida pseudo tropicalis, Candida rugosa, Schimmelpilz 1 and 2*, and *aflatoxin*. In doing the treatment, she wore gloves and lived in a mold-free environment for 25 hours. Not long after she had cleared, her skin problem disappeared and her fatigue significantly diminished. Then I prescribed an antifungal enzyme (AllerZyme C™), which worked so well for her that she stayed on it permanently.

Then we began treating her for hormones because she still had a hormonal imbalance, and was still experiencing hot flashes. This was no small task in a woman who had had a hysterectomy at age 40. First I treated her for Premarin and talked at great length with her about it. I find that most women are extremely allergic to this medication. Symptoms include weight gain, headaches, and depression, which Sharon had been experiencing since her hysterectomy. Because I am not a medical doctor, I do not feel I have the right to take anyone off a prescription medication. However, I will recommend that they talk to their physician. I gave Sharon some information about Premarin® and urged her to read it.

First introduced in the United States in 1949, Premarin was the first available oral estrogen, and is still the most commonly prescribed drug of its kind in this country. A mixture of about 20 different equine estrogens drawn from a pregnant mare's urine, Premarin has estrogen-like effects on the human female even though it is not natural to the human body. Dr. Christiane Northrup points out that Premarin® can be of concern because its metabolic breakdown products, called "dodder compounds," can be stronger than the estrogens themselves. "When you use a hormone that is native to the female body, such as estradiol, the body will metabolize it into weaker and weaker 'dodder' compounds," writes Northrup. "But with Premarin® they get stronger and have the potential to cause more side effects." I have found that Premarin can cause headaches, irritability, breast swelling, weight gain, severe depression, bleeding, and cramping. Often the drug can be linked to a yeast or fungus allergy, which may develop over a period of years and may cause severe bloating.

Another patient on Premarin® had numerous tests and an ultrasound to help determine the cause of her bloating. When I treated her for Candida and hormone, it completely disappeared. Her gynecologist was astounded.

After treating Sharon for Candida and fungus, I began to treat her for her own hormones, including estrogen, progesterone, and testosterone. Women like Sharon who are allergic to these hormones tend to have hormonal imbalances and irregular menstrual cycles, with symptoms ranging from premature menopause and irregular periods to infertility and severe PMS. After reading the materials I gave her and discussing the matter with her physician, Sharon discontinued the Premarin and began taking a natural hormonal replacement. I also prescribed some natural progesterone oil which she used 10 to 14 days out of the month to help balance her estrogen and progesterone levels. Her hot flashes completely disappeared with the combination of the clearing of the hormones and the natural progesterone.

Treating her for Vitamin E and hormones in combination with heat and sugar restored her energy even more, but she was still concerned about her depression and mood swings. I decided to do a basal temperature test which revealed an average temperature of 96.2. This is quite low and suggests an allergy to thyroid. Further testing revealed she was allergic to T_3

and T$_4$. After prescribing a thyroid enzyme (AllerZyme thy™), I treated her for thyroid, mercury, Vitamin F, fatty acids vegetable fat, animal fat, and the amino acids tryptophan and tyrosine.

After these treatments, Sharon began noticing a significant change in her depression, and she was able to get off Prozac, which she had been taking since shortly after her hysterectomy. Now that her hormones were more balanced, she felt the desire to exercise, and she gradually lost 26 pounds. She comes in occasionally to check her enzymes but she has basically been doing well ever since. Sharon's case shows the importance of chromium, hormones, yeast, and thyroid for people with chronic fatigue. I have also found that women with fibroids and endometriosis, which are generally caused by a hormone imbalance, respond well to treatment for yeast, hormones, and thyroid as well as for sugar.

In addition to self-assessment questionnaires that help determine whether or not a person has the symptoms commonly associated with allergies, there are a number of frequently used allergy tests administered by qualified health professionals. These include skin reaction tests, blood tests, pulse test, muscle response test, and electronic test.

SELF-ASSESSMENT QUESTIONNAIRES

The following self-assessment questionnaire helps determine the presence of symptoms that commonly raise suspicion of allergies. A significant number of "yes" answers to the following questions would indicate further testing and/or consultation with a doctor.

1. Do any blood relatives suffer from allergy syndromes (hay fever, asthma, skin rashes, severe reactions to drugs or insect stings), food allergies, addictive disorders (alcohol or drug abuse, compulsive eating), diabetes or low blood sugar, arthritis, headaches, or digestive disorders? Were any blood relatives hyperactive, learning-disabled, or bed wetters as children?

2. Did your mother experience severe stress during her pregnancy with you? Was your birth difficult or complicated?

3. As an infant, did you have any problem tolerating bottle formula or breast milk? Did you have problems with weight gain, colic, or vomiting?

4. As an infant, did you suffer from frequent digestive, respiratory, or skin problems?

5. Were you "difficult" in infancy and/or childhood, often crying or irritable, overactive or underactive? Did you have problems sleeping, trouble learning, or paying attention at school?

6. As a child, were you often sick, plagued by ear infections, sore throats, swollen glands, colds, bronchitis, croup, stomach aches, constipation, diarrhea, or headaches?

7. As an adult, are you always tired even though you get enough sleep (six to eight hours)?

8. Do you frequently have puffy eyes? Wrinkles or dark circles under your eyes? Itchy, red, watery, burning, painful or light-sensitive eyes? Blurred vision? Baggy, swollen eyelids?

9. Do you often have a stuffy, watery, runny nose? Sneeze several times in a row? Rub nose upwards or wiggle nose? One cold after another, without feeling sick? Nosebleeds? Excessive mucus?

10. Do you have asthma or wheezing? Do you cough or wheeze with laughter, exercise, cold air, cold drinks, at night, or when it's damp outside?

11. Do you have skin rashes such as eczema or atopic dermatitis? Itchy rashes or hives, especially

in arm or leg creases? Cracked toenails or fingernails? Acne? Dandruff? Loss of hair?

12. Do you have recurrent earaches? Fluid behind
your eardrums? On and off hearing trouble? Ears
popping or ringing? Flushed, red earlobes? Dizziness? Itchy ears? Drainage from ear?

13. Do you suffer from digestive problems? Swelling or
soreness of face and lips? Itchy roof of mouth?
Canker sores? Bleeding gums? Bad breath? Nausea
and stomach aches? Excess gas, diarrhea, or constipation? Belching? Itchy rectal area? Ulcers? Colitis?

14. Do you have difficulty gaining or losing weight?
Binge eating?

15. Do you have repeated bladder infections, difficulty urinating, or water retention?

16. Is your pulse or heartbeat irregular after eating?

17. Have you ever had seizures?

18. Do you have sinus problems, earaches, or sore
throats? Headaches, dizziness, convulsion? Insomnia? Leg or muscle aches, back pain, swollen or
stiff joints, arthritis? A constant low-grade fever,
feeling flushed or chilled, excessive sweating,
fainting spells?

19. Do you have dark circles under your eyes, a pale
complexion, a bloated or puffy face?

20. Are you a picky eater? A binger?

21. Do you feel like you are high one moment, low
the next, with depression appearing for no reason?

22. Do you have trouble concentrating, sometimes
feeling confused and spacy? Are you hyperactive,
overly nervous, frequently anxious, quick to
anger?

23. Does a change in your surroundings or the seasons change how you feel?

SCRATCH TEST OR SKIN REACTION TEST

Some tests for allergies involve provoking an allergic reaction on the skin by exposure to a minute amount of an allergen. Most commonly, this is accomplished by applying drops of an allergenic extract to the skin surface that has been pricked or scratched. Other possibilities include:

- introducing a small quantity of allergenic extract with a needle between the layers of skin (intradermal test)
- placing a piece of gauze soaked in a suspected allergen over the skin for a prolonged period of time (patch test)
- putting a drop of allergenic extract in the eye (conjunctival test, rarely used today)

If the test is positive, the site of the injection or exposure swells and the surrounding area becomes inflamed. This is generally not useful to determine food intolerance but is a simple method of detecting sensitivity to inhalant allergens. A reaction can occur after 15 minutes and up to 24 to 48 hours later.

RADIOALLERGOSORBENT TEST (RAST)

The radioallergosorbent test (RAST) is an initial laboratory test administered to a patient's blood sample to measure the amount of IgE antibodies in blood. The number of antibodies increase with the severity of the allergy. The blood sample is tested for specific IgE antibodies against likely allergens in the patient's environment.

PULSE TEST

Pulse testing for allergies measures the heart rate before and after exposure to a suspected allergen and is an effective method for determining allergic reactions to foods. Pulses can be felt at various points. The radial artery at the wrist is the most common and probably the simplest to locate. Three fingers are placed lightly over the artery on the inside of the wrist, slightly above the thumb. Other areas to read the pulse are located at the temporal region of the skull, the popliteal region in back of the knee, the pedal pulses behind the malleolus of the ankle, the carotid artery in the neck, and the femoral pulse in the groin area. A normal pulse should be even and forceful, at a regular rhythm, with no delays, interruptions, or other irregularities.

The pulse generally deviates from normal in allergic patients. It usually becomes faster and more forceful, but can also become slower and weaker. This test can be helpful in detecting a food allergy. Unfortunately, if one eats several foods at a time, which, of course, we all do, it is hard to determine exactly which food is causing the allergic reaction. Many of my patients come into my office already knowing they have food allergies because they used this method of diagnosing themselves.

MUSCLE RESPONSE TEST

Also known as applied **kinesiology**, this test was developed in 1964 by Dr. George Goodheart, a chiropractor, to diagnose or read certain blockages in the body. Muscle response testing is also a method of using the relative strength of the muscles to uncover allergies, nutritional imbalances, and structural misalignments in the body.

This method identifies blockages in the electromagnetic energy fields when one is exposed to, or in contact with, an allergen. Muscle testing bypasses the conscious and subconscious minds. When a suspected allergen is held in the hand, a strong muscle will weaken if an allergy to the substance is present.

The person to be tested generally lies down or sits up and extends an arm at a ninety-degree angle, thumb down, in front of him. The facilitator pushes against the arm to establish the strength of the testing muscle (indicator muscle) while the subject resists. When the person holds a food or other substance to which he or she is allergic, the indicator muscle will immediately and markedly weaken. People can learn to perform this technique on others, and can teach others to test them. Muscle testing procedures can detect both hidden and active or acute allergies and can indicate which substances should be avoided.

SURROGATE MUSCLE TEST

This technique is used to determine allergies in infants, young children, and elderly, weak, or physically incapac-

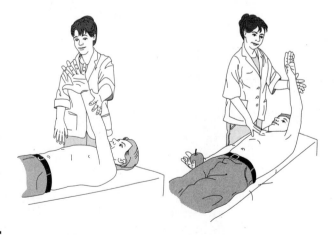

Figure 2–1   Muscle testing for identifying allergies.

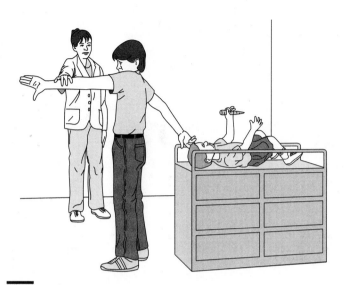

Figure 2–2 Surrogate muscle test for identifying allergies in infants, toddlers, or weak individuals.

itated adults. It utilizes energy conductivity to diagnose allergies in a person who otherwise could not be muscle tested. The surrogate touches the skin of the person being tested and the facilitator muscle tests the surrogate. When the one being tested holds a particular item, the surrogate's response indicates whether that person does or does not have an allergy to the item.

O-RING TEST

People can be taught to test themselves using a method similar to muscle testing. The tester makes a circle by opposing his little finger and thumb on one hand. Then, with the other index finger, he or she tries to separate the two opposing fingers. They should be strong and inseparable. If they are not strong, there can be structural misalignment or carpal tunnel syndrome that renders the technique ineffective. If they are strong, the potential allergen is held in

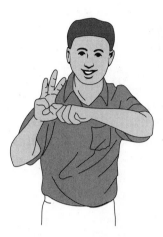

Figure 2–3   O-Ring test for self-testing allergies

the hand being tested, with the fingertips touching the allergen. If the circle is strong, the person is not allergic to the substance. If the fingers weaken and the circle separates, they are allergic to the substance. This technique takes practice to learn, but it can be a survival tool for severely allergic individuals who can use it to test their foods before eating.

ELECTRONIC TEST

Electronic devices have been used for more than a century in the treatment and diagnosis of patients. Two German scientists, Voll and Werner, designed and built an instrument to chart and verify the relationship of acupuncture points to their corresponding organs and systems. This instrument can directly infer the functional status of these structures. Specific acupuncture points are charged with approximately one volt of direct current, resulting in measurements of resistance along particular meridians. A meter is used to show readings of irritation to the electromagnetic pathways or organ systems (for example, blockages in the flow of electromagnetic energy). Electronic devices work by reading the galvanic skin response, a measure of this flow. Because this process is still considered investigational, these meters have been approved for investigational use only by the Food and Drug Administration (FDA) in the United States.

Electronic devices such as the one developed by Voll and Werner are used for food and environmental allergy testing. Correlations with other test procedures have shown that the electro-acupuncture device (EAV) test is accurate in detecting sensitivities to foods, chemicals, pesticides, herbicides, environmental irritants, dental irritants, fungi, bacteria, and viruses as well as dysfunctions of organs and systems. The method causes little or no discomfort because there are no needles or puncturing of the skin. A low-level electric stimulus (not perceptible by the subject being tested) is passed through the body while the patient holds a brass handle in one hand and a metal probe is placed against acupressure points on the hands and feet. A reading is taken for each point and stored in the computer for future analysis.

3 | TYPES OF ALLERGY TREATMENTS

What did I swallow in that mad ocean years ago?
Or was my sin in emerging and returning to the land?
—from "Suspended Animation"

Cynthia

Cynthia, age 44, came to see me complaining of chronic fatigue, allergies, headaches, occasional colds, frequent sinus infections, and postnasal drip. After a complete case history, I performed a full enzyme and diagnostic exam and found moderate pancreas and small intestine dysfunction, with abdominal bloating, pain, and gas one or two hours after eating. There were also symptoms of severe hypothyroid, including low appetite, low sex drive, constipation, hemorrhoids, dry skin, and depression as well as signs of adrenal hypofunction including water retention, rapid mood swings, oversensitivity to sugar, and irritability under stress. Besides the nasal and sinus congestion, allergy symptoms included sneezing, itchy eyes, and feeling worse after eating certain foods. In addition, Cynthia suffered from some severe menstrual and premenstrual symptoms (PMS), including weight gain, depression, irritability, sore and swollen breasts, a craving for sweets, painful cramps, and lower back pain.

The diagnostic exam and a 24-hour urinalysis revealed that Cynthia had difficulty digesting and absorbing sugars and fats, and a positive thyroid reflex indicated the possibility of low thyroid. In fact, she had been diagnosed seven years before with Hashimoto's thyroiditis and had been taking synthroid, a synthetic thyroid hormone, ever since. To assess her thyroid problems more thoroughly, I recommended that she do a basal axillary temperature test to record her axillary temperature. I also found some liver toxicity which shows up in the upper right quadrant, as well as a calcium deficiency and low adrenals, as revealed in the urinalysis and in three specific places on the abdominal palpation exam. The urinalysis pointed to poor digestion and assimilation of sugars and a severe Vitamin C deficiency.

Based on these findings, I recommended an enzyme (pan) to help digest and absorb sugars, a liver detoxification enzyme (lvr), a kidney enzyme (kdy) especially good for allergies and lymphatic congestion, characterized by swelling and water retention, an adrenal enzyme (adr) that helps absorb sugars and increases energy, and an enzyme used to reduce her PMS problems (fem) and AllerZyme CFS for chronic fatigue. These enzymes are listed in the Resource Guide. As we cleared and desensitized her to certain allergies, I adjusted her regimen of enzymes and supplements.

The two most important symptoms I wanted to address with Cynthia were the chronic fatigue and the frequent sinus infections. She had been taking antibiotics every other month for the sinus infections, but this simply exacerbated the postnasal drip and caused more headaches and fatigue. First, I treated her for the basic allergens, including calcium, which was especially important because she was deficient in this mineral. Next, we treated all the B vitamins plus some individual B vitamins like PABA, B_{17}, and folic acid. Then I treated her for the sugars and the salt mix which concluded her basic allergy treatments.

After the basic allergies, I treated her for corn and grain mix, spices, vegetable fat, amino acids, and Vitamin E. We went on to treat for all the different hormones which completely cleared up her premenstrual symptoms as well as some hot flashes and hormonal imbalances. Because she experienced frequent headaches, we treated her for wheat, vinegar, shellfish, chocolate, caffeine, coffee, and cold which are common causes of headaches. In doing the allergy treatment for clearing the hormones, I commonly combine hormones with heat and sugar which will permanently relieve women of menopausal symptoms. Sometimes a particular allergen can be linked with another allergen in the body. Until you clear both of them together, the primary allergen will not be completely eliminated. These are called the combination treatments. For example, caffeine and chocolate have to be treated with hormones, so the hormone allergy is not complete until that dynamic combination is done. Once this initial series of treatments had been completed, we proceeded to treat for allergens specifically related to the chronic fatigue, sinus infections, and Hashimoto's thryoiditus.

For chronic fatigue, we first treated Cynthia for the different viruses, including herpes I, shingles (herpes zoster), Epstein-Barr, CMV, coxackie B, infectious mononucleosis, polio, adenovirus, and varicella. When I treat for the viruses, I make sure the person being cleared gets no closer than four to six feet from other people. Sometimes they need to wear a mask because even contact with a telephone mouthpiece can cause exposure to a virus such as Epstein-Barr.

For example, one woman I treated for the Epstein-Barr virus had a massage afterwards and started to feel more fatigued. Apparently the masseuse or the previous client had the virus. In any case, the patient lost the treatment and became severely ill. If you expose yourself to the allergen during the 25-hour period, you will lose the treatment and may become ill. The Epstein-Barr virus is often found linked to tissues or organs and in combination with other foods or infectants.

Cynthia needed two to three weeks to clear Epstein-Barr from her system. The virus had to be treated with a number of different combinations including alcohol, sugar, the brain, and several emotions. Ultimately it was not until I had her take the virus vial home and treat herself three times a day for two weeks that the virus completely cleared. Almost immediately she noticed a dramatic improvement in her chronic fatigue: greater clarity, fewer headaches, less achiness, improved concentration, and more energy. Of all the allergens we treated, Epstein-Barr was probably the most important.

Before being treated for the herpes virus, Cynthia frequently developed sores around her nose and mouth. Since her treatment, she has not had a single outbreak. Between these treatments we also treated her for other foods including alcohol, cheese, tomatoes, peppers, red wine, and food additives, as well as for mercury, a common ingredient in dental amalgams.

Next we addressed the chronic sinus infections. In such cases, I generally focus first on clearing all the bacteria and fungi, and then treat for environmental factors. Once Cynthia had been treated for all the bacteria together, we found some that did not clear and needed to be treated again, either separately or in combination, including *strep faecalis, hemophilus vaginal, Klebsiella pneumoniae, scarlatinum, Tuberculocidinum Klebs, proteus*, and *Staphlococcus aureus*. While clearing these bacteria it is important to use only distilled water, to refrain from bathing, from touching or eating raw food, to avoid contact with anyone who might be infected with bacteria, and to use plastic gloves when going to the toilet. Many of the bacterial infections that plague people with chronic sinusitus are those that have been repeatedly suppressed with antibiotics. These drugs usually do not eliminate the bacteria; instead, they suppress the symptoms and create allergic reactions or links with other allergens in the body. Once you clear these bacteria, the person can resist new infections and never contract sinus infections as long as their immune system is kept strong through the use of enzymes and a balanced diet (see listing for AllerZyme B in the Resource Guide).

Other important factors in chronic sinus infections are Candida and other fungal infections. We spent a great deal of time treating Cynthia for fungi. Once the allergy is completely cleared and we know there are no more combinations, I recommend an antifungal diet and enzymes (see recipe section in the Resource Guide for specific enzymes). The anitfungal diet is a 10-day diet to clean and detoxify the body. The necessary diet and enzymes are also important to detoxify and clean the liver and to restore healthy intestinal flora and homeostasis.

Since clearing the bacteria and fungus three years ago, Cynthia has not had a single sinus infection. Conventional medications such as antibiotics do not correctly deal with the problem. Instead, they suppress it and exacerbate the hidden allergy. NAET recognizes the allergy and eliminates it from the body and the enzymes restore homeostasis, help digestion, and strengthen the immune system to prevent developing other allergies.

Next we addressed Cynthia's Hashimoto's thyroiditis. Even though she had been on synthroid for years, she still experienced strong hypothyroid symptoms including dry skin, dry brittle hair, severe fatigue, low energy (although her energy improved considerably after we treated for the Epstein-Barr virus), a tendency to gain weight easily, constipation, cold hands and feet, depression (which had plagued her for years), low sex drive, and difficulty concentrating although that seemed to change after the Epstein-Barr treatment. Her basal temperature, taken during her menstrual cycle so it would not be influenced by ovulation, averaged 96.4, which was quite low. Without taking her off any medications, I began to treat her for specific allergens commonly involved with thyroiditis. The first was her own prescription synthroid and the various thyroid hormones: thyroglobulin, T_2, T_3, and T_4. Many people are also allergic to the thyroid gland itself, and their energy may change dramatically after they have been treated. An allergy to the thyroid suggests a glandular imbalance or dysfunction and treatment will generally strengthen the gland and restore normal functioning.

I then treated for mercury and amalgam in combination with animal fat and vegetable fat. I treated for Hashimotos thyroiditis itself. Treating for the disease is a treatment for the sensitivity to the electromagnetic energy of the particular problem.

It helps to reduce the emotions related to the disease and helps reduce the severity of symptoms. Thyroiditis is an inflammation caused by an allergy to your own thyroid hormones, and clearing the allergy to the hormones will frequently eliminate the Hashimoto's. We also treated for iodine, a key allergy in thyroid problems. Then we treated for fluoride and made sure that all the viruses and fungi were still clear. At this point, most of her thyroid symptoms had diminished or disappeared. Although she continues taking synthroid, her dosage has been substantially diminished.

While treating for sinus congestion and sinusitis, I also treated for parasites (and recommended AllerZyme P), which can cause stress to the immune system, as well as for environmental allergies such as newspaper ink, mold, grasses, trees, weeds, shrubs, and certain plants she had growing in her house. Most of the sinusitis had been cleared by treating the infectants, but some of the mucus and drainage problems did not clear completely until we treated the environmental airborne allergies. Now Cynthia does not experience chronic fatigue and is no longer susceptible to infections. Her depression also has lifted. The psychologist who referred her to me was so impressed that she has since sent me many patients who suffer from depression and anxiety.

Because Cynthia had a history of incest and molestation that complicated some of the food allergies, I had to treat her with a specific chiropractic manipulation and this proved to be helpful in reducing the low back pain she had experienced for years. When I examined her back, I found that her coccyx was out of alignment, a common symptom of childhood molestation or trauma. When children are molested, pressure is put on that area that can eventually misalign the coccyx, and in conjunction with a fall or accident, may result in chronic low back pain and severe emotional and physical blockages. Until the misalignment is adjusted and relieved, the person will not have complete freedom in the area and may experience ongoing pain. I have also found that clearing the basic allergies is not successful until this treatment is done. The treatment, an internal coccyx adjustment, can help clear some of the trauma as well as pave the road to complete allergy elimination. For Cynthia the adjustment and subsequent emotional clearing was crucial to her progress.

Although I have treated similar cases, this one was especially significant because Cynthia was constantly taking antibiotics and was extremely fatigued and depressed when she first came to see me. Her recovery was dramatic. Now she considers herself healthy and normal for the first time in many years. She has plenty of energy, exercises regularly, and can read without getting confused or distracted. We still need to do some maintenance adjustments and treat some allergies here and there, but the bulk of her treatment occurred as I've described in this case history.

The simplest and most effective approach to treating allergies is to avoid the allergenic substance entirely. When avoidance is difficult or even impossible, as with environmental allergens, a number of other treatments are available.

MEDICATION

Medication is probably the most commonly used treatment for allergies. There are **antihistamines** to relieve itching, hay fever, and irritation from airborne allergens; **bronchodilators** or inhalers for asthma symptoms; decongestants; steroids; **corticosteroids**; and cromolyn, taken orally before eating to prevent gastrointestinal (GI) symptoms. Used primarily to suppress symptoms, these medications can have many side effects including drowsiness, anxiety, frequent and painful urination, nausea, dry mouth, vomiting, loss of appetite, abdominal discomfort and cramps, constipation or diarrhea, headaches, loss of sexual libido, depression, and fatigue.

ALLERGY SHOTS

Allergy shots, or immunotherapy, are another commonly used treatment approach. Allergy shots desensitize the person to the allergen by injecting a small amount of an extract of the substance under the skin's surface. The dose is gradually increased until a maintenance dose is obtained. After three years or the allergy has been eliminated, the injections are generally stopped.

Allergy shots are often effective in treating allergies to pollen, dust, and animal dander, but they have not proven useful for allergies to food. Additionally, food shots may cause side effects including sore arms, hives, throat spasms and, on occasion, even death. By controlling reactions to airborne allergens, however, shots can reduce the load effect and thereby reduce the allergic response to foods.

For many years, doctors have tried using allergy shots, primarily for pollens, to treat people who suffer asthma attacks. Studies have shown that while these people were receiving the shots they suffered fewer asthmatic symptoms, but the effects diminished over time and disappeared entirely after two years. In addition, the shots were extremely expensive.

ROTATION AND ELIMINATION DIETS

Elimination and **rotation diets**—also called exclusion or simplification diets—are widely used by physicians and individuals to diagnose and eliminate allergic reactions. These regimens remove all potential allergens from the diet and then reintroduce them one at a time at different intervals while observing their effects. Although they can be helpful in detecting hidden allergies, rotation diets are difficult to sustain and generally fail.

HOMEOPATHY

Homeopathic treatment appears to have a positive effect in treating allergic individuals and disorders related to immune function. Homeopathy is based on the concept that a substance, prepared from plants, animal sources, vitamins, minerals, and even toxic substances actually heals the exact symptoms it produces. For example, bee venom can cause swelling and inflammation, but as a homeopathic remedy in diluted form, helps to reduce swelling and inflammation in joints. So substances that normally cause symptoms of immune deficiency, with homeopathic preparation and treatment, actually treat infection, stimulate immune function, repair and generate healing, detoxify and decongest areas of swelling and inflammation, and increase energy.

ENZYME POTENTIATED DESENSITIZATION (EPD)

Enzyme potentiated desensitization (EPD) is a method of immunotherapy developed by Dr. Leonard McEwen of London in the mid 1960s. It involves desensitization using a series of injections containing a combination of mixed allergens and the enzyme beta-glucoronidase administered every two to three months at first and then less frequently over time. Because many allergens are treated at once, only nine or ten injections are required and the results are reportedly longer lasting than are conventional allergy shots. Beta-glucuronidase in combination with other allergens causes T-suppressor cells to multiply and differentiate and allows them to recognize the allergen originally injected. These T-cells then supposedly suppress any adverse reaction when the individual is then exposed to the allergens.

BEE POLLEN

An antiallergic product that has gained some popularity in recent years is bee pollen. The pollen is actually a mixture of bee digestive enzymes, nectar, and reproductive dust from the flowers visited by the bees. Because bee pollen contains some of the airborne grass and ragweed pollens to which people are most allergic, it can act the same as allergy shots to desensitize an individual with a small quantity of the substance to which he or she is allergic. But allergy shots deliver pollen in an undiluted form, whereas oral dosages are broken down by enzymes during the digestive process. The patient might have to take up to 10,000 times as much pollen orally as he or she would through injection to achieve the same results. The other disadvantage of taking bee pollen is that one never knows exactly what it contains because it varies from week to week and from beehive to beehive. Also, bee pollen in large dosages can cause unpleasant side effects or be contaminated with environmental pollutants.

CHIROPRACTIC CARE

Chiropractic care has been known to help strengthen the immune system by strengthening the nervous system. A healthy immune system means resistance to disease, allergies, and chronic illness, and one that is free of spinal musculoskeletal misalignments. "Chiropractic is able to hypothesize that skeletal disrelations, particularly in the complex spinal structures, can lead to the loss of nervous system integrity and, hence, to the loss of health elsewhere in the body" (*Essential Principles of Chiropractic* by Virgil V. Strang). Many studies have observed the effect of a healthy nervous system on immune system health. In one study, for example, people under chiropractic care for five years or more were found to have a two hundred percent greater immune system competence than people who had not received chiropractic care.

ACUPUNCTURE

Extensive research has shown that acupuncture helps people with a variety of conditions including pain, anxiety, immune disorders, arthritis, eczema, migraines, and allergies by promoting natural healing and improving bodily functions. Developed and practiced in China over the past 2,000 years, acupuncture treats the whole person rather than a particular disease, attempts to address the root cause of the problem rather than symptoms alone, and works to restore balance between the physical, emotional, and spiritual aspects of being. Instead of treating standard points for specific allergies, the acupuncturist treats each allergic individual differently depending on the diagnostic picture that emerges after examining the pulses, the tongue, and other indicators.

Acupuncture has proven successful in reducing the sensitivity of allergic individuals. In *The Journal of Traditional Chinese Medicine* 1993 (Dec. 13, [4]: 243–8), acupuncture and desensitization were compared in the treatment of 143 cases of type I allergies. The results proved that acupuncture therapy provided remarkable success against type I allergic reactions. The curative effect was higher in the acupuncture group with allergic asthma, allergic rhinitis, and chronic urticaria.

NAMBUDRIPAD ALLERGY ELIMINATION TECHNIQUE (NAET)

NAET was developed by Dr. Devi Nambudripad, a registered nurse, chiropractor, and acupuncturist who has done extensive research in the areas of allergies. NAET is a revolutionary new technique that utilizes chiropractic, acupuncture, and kinesiology to permanently desensitize a person to an allergen. Much of this book on allergies and immune disorders, as well as the upcoming books in this series, will focus on NAET. This approach is based on a thorough understanding of the body as bioenergy, and a recognition that the body consists not only of matter but also of electromagnetic pathways and currents. This concept, along with a detailed description of NAET, is presented in Chapter 9.

When an allergen is encountered by an allergic individual, it can cause certain blockages in the electromagnetic pathways or U currents. These blockages are connected to certain organs, cells, or systems and cause what we call allergic symptoms. For example, certain allergenic foods can cause blockages in the digestive system through energy pathways, and these blockages in turn create digestive symptoms such as bloating, flatulence, and pain. NAET clears these blockages by reprogramming the nervous system and neutralizing the body's immune mediators, thereby permanently desensitizing a person to the allergen. Any allergen can be treated in this way.

EMERGENCY TREATMENT

In the event of anaphylactic shock or other allergic emergencies, it is crucial that the patient receive first aid treatment within the first 10 to 15 minutes. People who are prone to severe allergic reactions should carry an allergy kit with antihistamines and a syringe containing the drug epinephrine (a bronchodilator that opens the airways and restores blood pressure to normal) for immediate emergency self-treatment. Applying a tourniquet above an insect sting will slow the circulation and absorption of blood, and placing ice on the sting area reduces swelling. The patient should lie on his or her side with the head turned to one side to avoid choking if vomiting occurs. If the person stops breathing, mouth-to-mouth resuscitation should be performed by someone who knows how to do it. As soon as possible, the person should be taken to a hospital emergency room or doctor's office.

In an emergency, the NAET treatment can help save the life of a patient who is waiting for medical assistance. It can be self-administered. By using the acupressure points of NAET, the symptoms can be reduced or eliminated almost immediately. Stimulation of the acupressure points while the subject holds the suspected allergen starts to reverse the allergic reaction and allows the immune system to recover. For example, if you eat a cookie that causes abdominal pain or wheezing and coughing, hold the cookie in your hand and treat yourself by using the acupressure points, preferably every ten minutes until symptoms subside or medical assistance is available. Refer to the Self-Treatment section of Chapter 5 for complete instructions on how to perform the NAET self-treatment.

II | IMMUNE SYSTEM: IMMUNE DISORDERS

4 | IMMUNE DISORDERS

The doctors tell me
my antibodies have gone berserk—
little soldiers with big guns.
Their job is to attack.
They always do
what they are told.
But these troops are confused—
they don't know who the enemy is.
                    —from "The Language of War or
                        T-Cell Immunology, 1A"

Richard

Richard, 45 and HIV positive, was referred to me by a good friend of his whose food allergies had responded well to enzymes and NAET. He wanted to increase the strength of his immune system and reduce the sluggishness and chronic eczema he had been experiencing since being diagnosed with HIV.

I have had excellent results treating HIV-positive people. One of the most important things I do is to help establish a healthy digestive system by regulating or decreasing the amount of circulating immune complexes (CICs) in the body. This reduces stress on the system and thereby reduces the amount of autoimmune activity. I then use NAET to eliminate food and environmental allergies and any other allergies that might compromise the immune system so that the body is fully available to fight the HIV virus.

With Richard, I started by doing an abdominal diagnostic exam and a urinalysis evaluation. The abdominal exam revealed that he had mild to moderate liver/gallbladder toxicity and a problem with decreased respiration characterized by an inability to exhale fully. He also had a positive thyroid reflex that sometimes indicates hypothyroid (which runs in his family), as well as the possibility of a yeast, mold, fungus, or Candida infection which he suspected to be the cause of his skin problem. Such infections are often encountered in people with a suppressed immune system, as in HIV.

We found poor carbohydrate metabolism on his urinalysis which also showed up in the palpation, a problem with the absorption of carbohydrates into the cells, and an inability to utilize the carbohydrates he was ingesting. There was heavy calcium content noted in the urine and an acid pH, usually representing a respiratory problem. He did, in fact, experience asthma and bouts of bronchitis over time. A Vitamin C deficiency showed up on the urinalysis as well as a difficulty digesting sugars and fats. His calcium oxalate and his uric acid were slightly above normal and his calcium phosphate was low, indicating poor carbohydrate metabolism. In general, he did not digest foods well at all.

I immediately prescribed enzymes that contained protease, amylase, lactase, maltase, disaccharidase, and lipase to help him digest sugars, fats, and proteins (pan). I also prescribed an enzyme to support the spleen (spl), one of the body's strongest immune defenses. Situated above the abdomen, the spleen contains two different types of tissue: red pulp and white pulp. White pulp contains lymphoid tissue, and red pulp removes worn-out blood cells from the blood. These lymphatic tissues specialize in different kinds of immune cells and are found in many parts of the body. For example, tonsils, adenoids, and the appendix are made of lymphatic tissue. Lymphatic vessels carry lymph, a clear fluid that bathes the body's tissues and drains out foreign antigens and antibodies to the lymph nodes where they are then eliminated from the body. In addition, I prescribed a respiratory enzyme (rsp), an antifungal enzyme (AllerZyme C), and an enzyme to help the body absorb sugars (srg).

After he started the enzymes, his digestion and elimination improved, and he found that his energy no longer dipped after eating. I always put an immune-suppressed individual on a protease enzyme (AllerZyme V) to help the body fight foreign proteins and antigens, and help the immune system and white blood cells fight infections. Then I began to do some allergy testing.

Richard was allergic to all the basics, including eggs and chicken, calcium, the B vitamins, sugars, iron, minerals, Vitamin A, salt, and chloride. Once I had treated for these allergens, I retested him and found him allergic to quite a few foods including fruit, chocolate, and oils, as well as weeds and shrubs, grasses, phenolics, histamine, pesticides, bacteria, and viruses. We first began to treat for the bacteria, especially the tuberculinum bacteria. He told me his father and grandfather had contracted tuberculosis (TB), and the respiratory reflex I detected may have indicated a genetic tendency to this disease.

Once the tuberculinum bacteria had cleared, I treated him for viruses, including HIV. When I treat people for any kind of viral problem or chronic fatigue, if they do not respond well to the treatment for the specific virus such as Epstein-Barr or HIV, I always treat for the blood. Every time I have done this for chronic fatigue, I have had incredible results, including an immediate change in energy and stamina, a clearer outlook on life, and better sleep habits. There seem to be viruses in the blood that we do not know about but that the body is fighting. When we treat for the blood, it helps clear any viral allergies. After we treated Richard for his blood, he noticed a significant change.

The treatment that caused the most remarkable change in Richard's energy was the treatment for pesticides. We treated him for many different varieties including DDT and Agent Orange. He told me that he had grown up on a farm and had on several occasions helped his father use DDT and other pesticides on the crops. He had anticipated that this might be one of the most powerful treatments. It was.

His primary-care physician had originally given Richard a year to live. But when he started seeing me, he changed so dramatically that instead of making plans to die, Richard and his lover made plans to buy a new house and move out of the city. It has been 2-1/2 years now, and he is doing well. He comes in now and then to reassess the enzymes he takes and to have a urinalysis done to ensure homeostasis is intact. His viral load is good, his energy is much more consistent, and his skin has cleared up as a result of being treated for fungus.

THE IMMUNE SYSTEM

Health practitioners and writers from many different disciplines emphasize the importance and complexity of the immune system and its interconectedness with other parts of the body. In my practice, I mention the immune system hundreds of times daily. This system does not have one central regulating organ like other body systems; for example, the circulatory system has the heart, the respiratory system has the lungs, and the digestive system has the stomach and intestines. The immune system's components are located throughout the body and communicate with one another through the immune cells. The primary function of the immune system is to be sensitive to invaders and to be able to distinguish them from the body's own cells. Anything foreign to the body is a potential enemy, called an antigen. Once the antigen has been sighted, a complex immune response comes into play.

Components of the Immune System

The immune system is composed of the lymphatic vessels, the lymph nodes and the lymph they contain, as well as organs such as the thymus, spleen, and tonsils. It includes white blood cells such as lymphocytes, neutrophils, basophils, eosinophils, and monocytes, as well as specialized white blood cells called macrophages and mast cells. The lymphocytes, the body's scavengers, collect waste products and consume invaders. The lymphocytes consist of T cells and B cells. B cells mature in the bone marrow, whereas T cells are produced by the thymus gland. Lymphocytes are transported in lymphatic fluid through the lymph nodes, small lumps of glandular tissue located along the lymph channels throughout the body. The lymph nodes are most noticeable in the armpits, the groin, the tonsils, the throat, behind the knees and other joints, at the base of the lungs, and in the abdomen.

The thymus, the major gland of the immune system, is composed of two gray lobes that lie just below the thyroid gland and above the heart. The thymus is responsible for many immune system functions including the production of T lymphocytes, which are in charge of cell-mediated immunity. Two basic types of of acquired immunity occur in the body. In B-cell immunity, the body develops circulating antibodies, molecules that are capable of attacking foreign agents. In T-cell immunity—also known as cell-mediated immunity because the immune mechanisms are controlled or mediated by white blood cells instead of antibodies—large numbers of activated lymphocytes are formed that are specifically designed to destroy foreign agents. This type of immunity is important in the resistance to infection by parasites, yeasts (Candida), and viruses (herpes, Epstein-Barr, and hepatitis). If an individual is suffering from a chronic infection, it generally indicates their cell-mediated immunity is not functioning as well as it should. Cell-mediated immunity can also help the body protect itself against cancer and other autoimmune disorders such as rheumatoid arthritis and allergies.

The thymus gland releases hormones, such as thymosin, thymopoeitin, and serum thymic factor which regulate other immune functions. When the levels of these hormones are low, a profile associated with depressed immunity, there is increased susceptibility to infection. Thymus hormones are often low in elderly individuals, particularly those who are prone to infection and cancer.

Enzymes are active participants in the immune system and T-cell mediated activity. For example, protease can help break down viruses and other infectants and thereby strengthen the immune system. If patients are allergic to their own thymus gland or if the gland is not functioning properly, NAET can be used to treat them for the gland or its hormones. A noticeable improvement is often achieved overnight which can then be reinforced with thymus extract supplements.

The lymph, along with the lymphatic vessels and lymph nodes, comprises one sixth of the entire body by weight and is the substance that fills the spaces between the cells. Lymphatic vessels, which run parallel to the circulatory system, drain waste products from tissues and transport lymph to the lymph nodes where the fluid is filtered. The cells most responsible for filtering the lymph, called macrophages, are the guardians of the immune system that destroy bacteria, viruses, and other infectants. The lymph nodes also contain B lymphocytes which produce antibodies in response to infectants.

The spleen, which is the largest mass of lymphatic tissue in the body at about seven ounces, lies in the upper left abdomen behind the lower ribs. Its functions include producing white blood cells which can engulf and destroy bacteria and cellular debris, destroying worn out blood cells and platelets, and serving as a blood reservoir. Like the thymus, the spleen releases many potent substances that enhance immune system function.

Other white blood cells include: the neutrophils which engulf infectants like bacteria and dead matter such as tumor cells, and are especially important in preventing bacterial infection; the eosinophils and basophils which are involved in allergic conditions by secreting histamines and other compounds that break down antigen-antibody complexes; and the monocytes, the large white blood cells that clear up debris after infection. Macrophages, which are called monocytes before they fully mature, are located in the liver, spleen, and lymph nodes. They function as the body's first line of defense, engulfing foreign particles including bacteria and cellular debris. And there are mast cells, discussed in the allergy section, which take up residence along the blood vessels and release histamine and other prostaglandins, substances involved in allergic reactions.

Function of the Immune System

Among the lymphocytes, the T cells (short for thymus lymphocytes) orchestrate many different immune functions, especially cell-mediated immunity. There are several different types of T cells: the helper T cells help other white blood cells to function; the suppressor T cells inhibit white blood cell function; and the cytotoxic T cells attack and destroy foreign tissue, cancer cells, and virus-infected cells. The ratio of helper T cells to suppressor T cells is usually a determinant of immune function. If the ratio is too low, there is an immune deficiency; if the ratio is too high, there is the possibility of autoimmune disorders like rheumatoid arthritis and lupus. Both high- and low-T cell ratios have been found in chronic fatigue problems.

The B cells are responsible for producing antibodies which are large protein molecules that bind to antigens, other foreign molecules like bacteria and viruses, other organisms, parasites, and tumor cells. Antibodies make it possible for phagocytes and the other engulfing parts of the immune system to attack these substances and eliminate them from the body. The cytotoxic cells are given that name because of their ability to destroy cells that have become cancerous or infected with viruses. They are the body's first line of defense against cancer development.

When the immune system is not functioning properly, a number of problems may develop, some of which are apparent, others that are more subtle. More and more researchers and health practitioners are acknowledging the role of immune dysfunction in many unexplained illnesses. When the immune system responds appropriately and quickly, we are able to resist infections. When the response is inadequate, the result is illness from a common virus to a more serious autoimmune problem such as rhuematoid arthritis, lupus, or even cancer.

Causes of Immune System Dysfunction

The underlying cause of immune system dysfunction is poor digestion and allergies. When the body doesn't digest food properly, the undigested food is absorbed into the bloodstream, and the immune system targets it as a foreign invader and starts attacking it. This antigen-antibody response creates circulating immune complexes (CICs), which can inhibit certain immune system backup mechanisms from functioning and ultimately cause autoimmune problems. In autoimmune disorders, such as MS, rheumatoid arthritis, thyroiditis, lupus, and chronic fatigue, the immune system has lost its ability to distinguish between "self" and "not self," and the body starts attacking its own tissues as if they were antigens. When the CICs lodge in different parts of the body, the immune system attempts to destroy them, and in so doing, destroys its own healthy cells.

The incidence of autoimmune disorders is thought to be higher in women, possibly because of hormonal influence and hormonal allergies. When the immune system is suppressed, called immunosuppression, enemy cells such as viruses can reproduce actively in the body and create a fertile environment for the accumulation of other infectants. As the disruptive agents become stronger, symptoms increase. If the body cannot destroy them, they will ultimately destroy the body.

As mentioned earlier, the body's first line of defense, the macrophages, eliminate foreign bodies, pathogenic microorganisms, nonfunctioning cells, waste materials, and toxins from the body. This process is of extreme importance. Unfortunately, the chronic ingestion of drugs, chemotherapuetic agents, medications, and antibiotics, as well as environmental toxins, stress, and allergens, can inhibit macrophage activity. When the macrophages are inhibited, the residues, antigens, and metabolic wastes accumulate in the body and can cause chronic illness. In particular, the inhibition of the macrophages may mobilize other parts of the immune system to attack the CICs, leading, as we discussed earlier, to an autoimmune response. Enzyme therapy can interrupt the formation of these pathogenic immune complexes and activate the macrophages. And the treatment of allergies with NAET can prevent the accumulation of allergens and the CICs that form in response to them.

There are many different immune system disorders, including some that do not even have names. In the rest of this section I will discuss the most common ones and how I test for and treat them. All of these chronic ailments are caused by the autoimmune response of a compromised immune system, as I described earlier. Perhaps the best known, and also the most complicated and probably the most debilitating, is chronic fatigue syndrome, also known as chronic fatigue immune dysfunction syndrome, or CFIDS.

As I mentioned earlier, the immune system is made up of circulating components that are capable of acting at sites far removed from their original source. The thymus gland, the bone marrow, and the lymph nodes are all major immune system centers, and the brain is known to transmit electrical and chemical signals along the nerves to stimulate immune responses to infection. When bacteria, fungi, viruses, dead tissue, or cancer cells are located in the body, the immune system is alerted and disposes of these materials. Most immune cells originate in the bone marrow, which is a soft, spongy material located in the core of the major bones.

Probably the best known of the immune system cells is the macrophage. The guardian of the immune system and its first line of defense, this large cell scavenges for dead matter, viruses, and bacteria. Macrophages develop from stem cells in the bone marrow and in their infancy are called monocytes. When monocytes are released into the blood, they migrate to the different tissues, then mature into macrophages. There they have the crucial function of distinguishing between "self" and "not self," between the body's own cells, and intrusive microorganisms. How they do this, however, is still largely unknown.

The greatest accumulation of macrophages, also known as kupffer cells, is in the liver, where they play an active role in helping the organ clear viruses from the blood. When the liver is disrupted, the immune system is disrupted as well, causing the various symptoms of autoimmune disorders. Macrophages also accumulate in tissues that are injured or inflamed and seek out infectious substances or irritants. For example, when they encounter a bacteria or a fungus, they surround the substance and secrete an enzyme that destroys it.

Like the macrophages, the neutrophils, another immune system component, have a large appetite for foreign matter. Instead of congregating in the spleen and liver as the macrophages do, they remain in the blood where they are far more numerous than macrophages. Their principal role is to attack and destroy antigen-antibody complexes, or CICs. At the same time, they send out chemicals that trigger inflammation and summon other defensive cells to act upon the inflammation which can trigger an autoimmune reaction.

Eosinophils tend to show up at sites of allergic reactions and parasite infections. They secrete histamine, an immune mediator, and other enzymes which causes tissue inflammation and protects the cell tissue from other immune elements such as inflammatory chemicals released by the neutrophils. They can also devour the allergen that caused the original allergic reaction.

The surface of the basophil cell is coated with special antibodies called IgE. If a foreign antigen bumps against a basophil that carries an antibody to that particular antigen, the antigen will become bound to the basophil. This is the antigen-antibody response which can trigger the release of the allergic mediator histamine that causes blood vessels to dilate and allows neutriphils and eosinophils to reach the trouble spot very rapidly. The mast cells are identical to the basophils except that they are located in the tissues and not in the blood. They also secrete histamine and immune mediators which cause inflammation and other allergic symptoms.

Both B and T cells are produced in the bone marrow, although T cells develop in the thymus gland. At any given time, the thymus is preparing tens of millions of T cells. The T cells have a number of different functions, including recognizing the different antigens that appear in the body. The leader of all the T cells is called the helper T cell, or T^4 lymphocyte. This lymphocyte carries no antibody weaponry but instead directs other T cells. According to recent evidence, when a macrophage attacks a bacteria, it simultaneously secretes an immune mediator called interleukin-1 which excites the T_4 cell. Interleuken-1 communicates with the brain, instructing it to raise the body's temperature, thereby causing a fever that further stimulates the immune system. The T_4 cell releases interluken-2 which stimulates other T cells to grow and divide and also stimulates the T_8 lymphocyte. The T_8 cell, known as the "killer T cell," dissolves the bacterial cell wall, then moves on. Without a cell wall, the components of the cell become separated from each other and pass into the bloodstream. The macrophages then come in and clean up the debris.

Antibodies, which are proteins made by lymphocytes, match the different antigens that enter the body. They melt holes in these cells and bind to them, forming antigen-antibody complexes that are large enough for neutrophils and macrophages to locate and destroy. At the same time, the T_4 lymphocyte produces a substance called interferon which regulates the extent and speed of these activities. Interferons are produced by a variety of other cells in response to the presence of a virus. The T_4 simply keeps the process going, and the macrophages clean up the debris, including antigen-antibody complexes.

If the antigen-antibody complexes grow too large, however, the macrophages cannot destroy them, and they attach to different tissue cells, creating inflammation and causing autoimmune reactions. Enzymes, especially protease or proteolytic enzymes, are instrumental in fighting antigens and preventing the production of CICs. Good digestion is paramount because it prevents undigested food particles from entering the bloodstream. In addition, interferons stimulate B cell antibody production, enhance the production of T_8 killer cells, and slow the growth of the body's own cells in the infected area to limit the number of new cells available for infection and to impede the formation of tumors.

This is how the battle proceeds. Once it has penetrated the body, the virus attacks cells and tissues. Many of the viruses are trapped and consumed by macrophages which secrete interluken-1, activating the helper T cells and alerting them to the invasion. Once activated, the helper T cells begin to multiply and release interluken-2, which in turn stimulates the production of more helper T cells as well as killer T cells. As their numbers increase, the helper T cells release a substance called B-cell growth factor which stimulates the production of B cells and in turn, produces immune mediators such as IgE, IgA, IgM, IgB, and IgE. The antibodies bind to the viruses and create large complexes (CICs) that are easy prey for the macrophages. The body cells that have been infested with the viruses are attacked by the killer T cells which sacrifice themselves before they can turn into other viruses. The macrophages devour both the viruses and their antibodies. If they are not destroyed, the CICs can become bigger and bigger and lodge in an organ such as the kidney or colon, and joints, and cause an autoimmune reaction which creates the immune disorders described in this book.

5 GENETIC AND ENVIRONMENTAL CAUSES OF IMMUNE DISORDERS

I resent
having my T-cells defined
in military terms.
I refuse to carry an arsenal
inside my bones.
I am a pacifist.
I believe
in the moon.

—from "The Language of War or
T-Cell Immunology, 1A

Carol

Carol, 41, came to see me complaining of constant fatigue which had begun about two years before with a severe flu and swollen glands. Since that time, she had noticed that she was much more susceptible to colds and flus. She had tried a variety of different treatments, including herbs, juice cleansers, and Chinese medicine, all of which helped but had not restored her energy of two years before. She knew she was allergic to beans and suspected she was allergic to spicy foods and meats, which she craved. She had been asthmatic as a child, and when she got a cold as an adult, she often developed a wheeze. She also experienced insomnia and digestive difficulties, including bloating.

A complete abdominal diagnostic evaluation showed a low thyroid and a mineral deficiency. As a result, I had her do an axillary basal body temperature test and a blood test for thyroid antibodies and TSH (thyroid stimulating hormone, produced by the pituitary). Besides discovering low thyroid, I found a positive respiratory reflex, common in asthmatics. (She also happened to be a smoker.) In addition, I found liver toxicity and some reflexes related to yeast and fungus. Because of her digestive problems, she was suspicious of parasites and hoped I would look into that as well. I found a calcium deficiency, low adrenals, and a positive reflex in the lower right and left quadrants, which usually represents colon problems such as an inability to absorb certain foods like proteins and complex carbohydrates. This reflex is sometimes indicative of irritable bowel or ulcerative colitis, but in her case it was probably based on allergies or poor digestion.

On the nonfasting part of the palpation, which represented how she digested foods, I found a problem digesting sugars and proteins, so I prescribed an enzyme for sugars and protein (hcl) as well as a respiratory enzyme (AllerZyme A) and an enzyme for liver toxicity (lvr). As we cleared certain allergies, I decided to prescribe enzymes for calcium (para), adrenal (adr), and enzymes for the colon, depending on subsequent allergy testing and how she responded to the allergy elimination.

On the blood test, there was evidence of an elevated triglyceride level and a low TSH, sometimes representative of low thyroid. Her basal temperature reading averaged 97.6 which was slightly below normal. After looking at her symptoms and history, including depression, fatigue, insomnia, digestive problems, some constipation, hair loss, headaches, sensitivity to cold, and allergies, I prescribed a thyroid enzyme (AllerZyme thy) for two to three months. Within four days she noticed improvement in her energy level.

We did thorough allergy testing and found her allergic to all the basic allergens including eggs and chicken, calcium, Vitamin C (which explained some of the fatigue), other vitamins (including B_1, B_2, and B_3), sugars, minerals (including magnesium and phosphorus), some trace elements, and salt. I also found she was allergic to many hormones including adrenaline, estrogen, progesterone, testosterone, thyroglobulin, T_2, T_3, T_4, many foods, viruses (Epstein-Barr), parasites (*blastocystis hominis*), antibiotics, vaccines, and nail chemicals. As a manicurist for many years, she had expressed concern about the toxicity of the hair and nail chemicals to which she had been exposed.

We treated for eggs, chicken, and tetracycline, calcium (which needed to be treated in combination with seratonin and emotions), Vitamin C, all the B vitamins, all the sugars, Vitamin A, minerals, and salt. After the basics, I added a Vitamin C enzyme (opt), and I had her continue the liver enzyme for liver toxicity. I also recommended the sugar intolerant diet included in this book with a slight modification in the amount of protein because of her difficulty in digesting it.

Careful evaluation also revealed that she was infected with a total of 13 parasites, more than most patients. In addition to the allergy treatment for parasites, I gave Carol a variety of enzymes (AllerZyme P) to help her body eliminate them, which is what I generally do in such cases. Among the parasites we cleared were *blastocystis hominis, enamoeba histolytica, entamoeba coli, endolimax nana, fasciolopsis buski, opistorchiasis felineus, echinococcus granulosus*, and a few other round worms. We needed to treat her four times to desensitize her to these parasites. It is important to understand that NAET helps to desensitize to the parasites, and enzyme therapy helps to rid them from the system. Unless the allergy is cleared, the enzyme or other medication will not be effective, and the parasite may remain in the body indefinitely and wreak havoc on the immune system. In combination with the parasitic enzyme, I also recommended an acidophilus enzyme supplement (sml) to help restore the beneficial flora to the intestines.

When we were finished, Carol reported that she had never felt so energized before in her life. Her insomnia had cleared, her digestion had improved, and her bloating had disappeared. She had spent quite a bit of time with animals over the years, and she had traveled to Mexico often, where she had had several bouts of dysentery but had never been treated correctly.

After we treated Carol for hormones, she was able to reduce her natural thyroid enzyme almost immediately. Treatment for Epstein-Barr and herpes VI yielded further improvement. In fact, since we had begun working together, she had not gotten sick. Then she did a liver cleanse, something I prescribe for most patients about a month after they have cleared parasites and bacteria. I recommend doing a cleanse once or twice a year.

After she had cleared the basics and parasites, I retested her and found that she had cleared all of her foods except some nuts and seeds, coffee, chocolate, food additives, and food coloring. When we treated for these, her health improved even further. It has been a year since we began treatment, and Carol's health continues to be extraordinary.

GENETICS

I have had good results in treating the familial tendency toward immune disorders with NAET (refer to the DNA and RNA section in Chapter 10). If we work with DNA or RNA as well as deal with the causes of immune disorders, there is a strong possibility that we can prevent the genetic transmission of immune disorders in the future.

INFECTANTS

Infectants are at the root of immune disorders. As a result, most of my clinical research in recent years has been in the area of infectants as allergens. Allergies to these infectants including bacteria, viruses, fungi, and parasites are common and can be debilitating.

In my practice, I have found a high incidence of this bacterial allergy in immune disorders and have had success treating it with NAET and enzyme therapy. Dr. Hahn, M.D., Director of the Dean Foundation for Health Research and Education in Madison, Wisconsin, contends that, despite doubts expressed by some experts, there is a growing body of evidence that bacterial allergies do exist.

I also believe that many of the antibiotics and other drugs used to treat infectants only drive them deeper into the system, mask the symptoms, weaken the immune system, and toxify the body, especially the liver. When a person is not allergic or hypersensitive to an organism, the organism can be easily eliminated by the immune system or, in extreme cases, with antibiotics. An infectant that is an allergen can stay in the body and surface when the immune system is weak or overloaded. The overload might occur because of an overabundance of allergies, emotional stress, or a toxic system. This reemergence can produce cycles of chronic bronchitis, chronic ear infections, and chronic sinus infections.

An allergy to an infectant can be treated with NAET and enzyme therapy, thereby ending the cycle of infection. People with immune disorders tend to store many bacteria and viruses in their systems as allergens that create excessive mucus, coughing, wheezing, sore throats, tightness in the chest, and difficulty breathing. I have found NAET to be dramatically successful in both children and adults for treating infections of viruses including flu and herpes, bacteria, parasites, and fungi including Candida.

Individuals can be successfully treated with their own saliva at the first sign of infection such as a runny nose, a cough, a slight fever, or tightness of the chest. This technique is particularly effective if they have already been cleared for many infectants. Keep in mind, however, that new infectants are always showing up. I discovered this treatment when a colleague became ill with a cough, fever, and runny nose. I called Dr. Nambudripad and asked for treatment suggestions so my friend would have more energy and stamina. She recommended that I treat him for his own saliva. To my amazement he began to improve, and after the second treatment was much better.

This incident began a research project in my practice and at home. As soon as one of my family members sneezed, coughed, or experienced any symptoms, I had them spit into a glass and did a muscle test on the saliva. If they showed any weakness I treated them with NAET. Invariably they improved immediately and their symptoms disappeared. Treating with NAET when symptoms first arise can cause an instantaneous reversal of symptoms and prevent an asthma attack or further progression of an infection.

Self-Treatment

Since immediate treatment is essential, I hold classes to teach people how to do this treatment on themselves or their family members at the first sign of symptoms. The symptomatic person holds a glass vial or jar containing the saliva, is given acupressure on the points beginning on the back and others indicated in the diagram beginning with the right hand and progressing around the body clockwise three times, then ending with the right hand. Light pressure is applied in a circular motion for seven seconds at each point (refer to Figure 5–1). After treatment for saliva, one should refrain from putting his or her fingers in the mouth or touching another's saliva (25 hours for children and adults, and 6 hours for children under the age of eight).

Performed at the onset of symptoms and every two to three hours thereafter, this treatment stimulates the body's immune mediators to fight the virus or bacteria and generally leads to an elimination of symptoms within twenty-four hours. Certain enzymes (trauma, opt; see Resource Guide for enzymes) with natural antibiotic properties can also be helpful in bolstering the immune system,

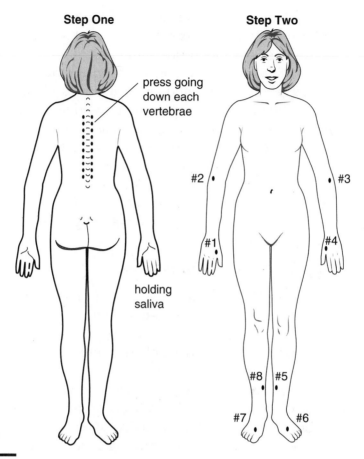

Figure 5–1 Self-treatment for runny nose, sore throat, fever, cold, viruses, and the flu at first onset of symptoms. This treatment can also be used for combinations of the above symptoms or emergencies.

and other allergens may also be included in the NAET treatment if they are suspected of causing a susceptibility to infection.

When treating chronic illnesses, it is important to check the saliva at the first signs of infection as well as treating all other possible infectants to prevent further allergies. I always perform another muscle test fifteen minutes after each treatment to ensure it was successful.

To help strengthen one's immunity, I often treat individuals with their saliva on every visit (they hold both the allergen being treated on that visit and their saliva sample) in case they have been exposed to some new infectant. Many patients bring in their saliva samples and ask to be tested because they know how effective this treatment is. Some of my patients used to become ill with some virus or bacteria every other week and were on antibiotics intermittently for years. After we began testing and treating for their saliva, they no longer became ill.

Antigen-Antibody Complexes

We have also found that infectants can link up with other allergens—food, environmental factors, inhalants, and even other infectants—by means of the antigen-antibody complexes. Exposure to linked allergens can result in chronic infections.

For example, a bacterial allergy in an asthmatic can be linked with a chocolate allergy, forming an antigen-antibody complex. When an individual eats chocolate, an infectious reaction results, causing fever, excess mucus, bloating, sweating at night, sinus infections, ear infections, and runny nose.

These antigen-antibody complexes, made up of T and B cells from the bone marrow, invade tissues or organs of the body and latch themselves onto the tissue cells. When the immune system tries to destroy these complexes, it destroys its own tissue cells (autoimmune or autoaggressive reaction). If the complexes inhabit the bronchial or lung tissue, inflammation and autoaggressive reactions occur. These reactions cause a destruction of tissue and trigger chronic asthma attacks. If the complexes lodge themselves in synovial fluid in the bone, they can cause arthritis or colitis in the colon. Infertility, chronic fatigue, migraines, Alzheimer's disease, and senility can also be caused by this autoimmune phenomenon.

After seeing how well these treatments worked, I began to research and experiment in my practice by clearing all bacteria, viruses, parasites, and fungi in patients suffering from chronic health problems such as candidiasis, asthma, chronic fatigue, chronic sinusitis, chronic ear infections, bronchitis, fibromyalgia, arthritis, and eczema. With the help of muscle testing and other techniques, I began to treat chronically ill people with NAET for these infectant allergens with excellent results.

Bacterial Allergies

I have found that people suffering from chronic bacterial allergies often suffer from arthritis and those with bacterial and parasitic allergies suffer from chronic gastrointestinal (GI) problems. People who have ulcers or gastritis are sometimes suspected of having Heliobacter pylori, a bacterium that seems to play a part in duodenal ulcers. It is also suspected of being involved in allergies and allergic reactions such as hay fever. Chronic viral allergies can result in chronic infections such as Epstein-Barr, mononucleosis, and herpes and people with infective allergies tend to have more frequent chronic fatigue.

Allergies to Parasites

Allergies to parasites such as malaria or Giardia can challenge and compromise an immune system. These parasites may live in the body for fifteen or twenty years and can be carried by children as well as adults. Asthmatics can have allergies to parasites that lodge in the lungs. CFIDS sufferers can have allergies to parasites that lodge in the bowel and nervous system. Children should be taught to wash their hands after touching animals because animals carry many parasites that can be passed on to humans.

Fungal Allergies

Fungal allergies are another group that can cause chronic illness. Fungi include Candida, aflatoxin, Aspergillis, and many others. I rarely see an individual who does not have large amounts of fungi in their system, including Candida. Candida is a systemic fungal infection that manifests itself in different parts of the body. It is sometimes found in the bronchi or lungs of asthmatics and can be a cause of emphysema. Candida is treated with NAET, enzymes, and a ten-day diet. Candida and Fungus are discussed at great length in the section on Fungus and Candida.

Allergies to Vaccines or Immunizations

I include allergies to vaccines in the category of infectants because I have seen they can be a troublesome trigger for chronic immune disorders. For example, people with chronic joint and nervous system problems do well when treated with NAET for polio. I have also treated many children suffering from side effects of the diphtheria-pertussis-tetanus (DPT) vaccine. When the DPT vaccine is given to people who are allergic to it, it can cause chronic immune suppression and can be involved in immune reactions. Children with these allergic reactions might develop headaches, digestive problems, asthma, or chronic ear infections and research has shown vaccines being used on autistic patients. I always teach parents how to use muscle testing to check their children for an allergic response to the vaccines before the children are inoculated. NAET can successfully treat for allergies to the vaccines, rendering the vaccination harmless.

Several studies have been done in the United States and abroad on anaphylactic reaction to the measles-mumps-rubella (MMR) vaccine to determine if the reaction is caused by an egg allergy. A recent study reported that 222 children with severe egg allergy were safely immunized, and the majority of the handful of children who had an anaphylactic reaction to the vaccine did not have a history of egg allergy. Researchers suspect that something else in the vaccine is causing the reaction. Perhaps the children are allergic to the vaccine itself, which is why muscle testing is recommended.

I receive questions from parents every week as to whether or not they should immunize their children. I always tell them I believe it is a personal decision that each parent has to make after careful study and research. There is so much written about it that I refer them to various sources and avoid giving my opinion. I do say that I would like to test the children for vaccines before they are immunized to avoid adverse reactions. I have seen adverse reactions to both the MMR and the DPT vaccines that can cause long-term health problems, especially for asthmatics.

Flu Vaccines

Adults should think about vaccinations also. Every year many Americans receive the flu vaccine. When people ask me if they should get the vaccination, I tell them I do not have an opinion either way, but I do ask them to be tested and treated with NAET to ensure they are not allergic to the vaccine before they use it. If people are allergic to the vaccine, they can suffer many side effects such as the flu, depression, sleeping problems, other central nervous system effects, muscle aches, fever, and flu-like symptoms. When we treat them for the flu virus with NAET, they rarely get the flu—and if they do, they only get a mild case.

The flu vaccine is produced from eggs and activated particles of influenza viruses. For this reason, people with a strong egg allergy could react severely and should consider alternatives. Unfortunately, many people are not aware of their egg allergies. One man with multiple food allergies did not know he was allergic to eggs. He had a flu vaccination and was sick for days. I finally treated him for his egg allergy and many of the symptoms cleared up. Now he is tested for the vaccine before he receives it.

If people are given a vaccine to which they are allergic, it will not be eliminated from the system and can contribute to autoimmune problems. The immune system forms antigen-antibody complexes with the vaccine which, in turn, creates more toxicity than the liver and the other organs of elimination can handle.

INGESTANTS

The following section contains discussions of some common ingestants to which people are allergic.

Drugs and Supplements

Drugs and supplements such as vitamins can also cause problems. Aspirin, for example, is a common trigger for asthmatics. An asthmatic person told me today that she was at a party recently and got a headache. Someone gave her an Excedrin® and she immediately began wheezing and had to use her inhaler. Chemical dyes such as tartrazine are used in some foods and drugs and can also cause reactions.

When new patients with chronic fatigue, fibromyalgia, and thyroiditis come to see me, I always make sure they bring any drugs they are taking, including antidepressants such as Prozac®, Zoloft®, and Wellbutrin®, and synthetic hormones such as Synthroid®. Many people are allergic to these drugs because they contain synthetic chemicals that are not produced naturally by the body. I treat for drug allergies with NAET. Frequently, drug allergies need to be treated again and again and checked every few months, perhaps because the companies change some of the materials or a new prescription is not the same as the last. This is particularly true of generic brands.

AMALGAMS

Modern silver amalgam is mixed with mercury. It has been used as a tooth restoring material for over 180 years, and accounts for seventy-five to eighty percent of all tooth restorations. Worldwide, hundreds of metric tons of mercury are placed in teeth each year. Some of this material makes its way into sewage and refuse systems.

Mercury is highly toxic to the human body and seems to vaporize continuously from dental fillings. The process is intensified by chewing, toothbrushing, and drinking hot liquids. After chewing or toothbrushing, it takes almost ninety minutes for the rate of vaporization to return to the previous rate. This process puts an individual on a roller coaster of mercury vapor exposure each day that peaks at breakfast, lunch, mid-afternoon coffee or tea, evening meals, and bedtime snacks. The larger the number of fillings and the larger the chewing surface, the greater the mercury exposure. It is estimated that the average individual with eight biting surfaces of silver amalgams is exposed to large amounts of mercury daily.

The release of mercury may be stimulated by other factors as well. One study placed amalgam in synthetic saliva and exposed it to a computer monitor for six hours. The amalgam was found to release two to five times as much mercury as that not exposed to a monitor. This may account for an increase in allergic reactions to electricity and some of the adverse health effects of exposure to computer monitors.

In Sweden, some researchers believe that the way to treat electrical allergies is to replace all amalgam with nonmetallic fillings. Despite autopsies showing that mercury levels in brain and kidney tissue are higher in people with mercury fillings, many dentists in the United States have resisted the conclusion that mercury is a health hazard. I have talked to many dentists, however, who say that amalgams should be replaced because as a person gets older, the mercury released causes more and more problems. If a person replaces mercury fillings, it is important to make sure he or she is not allergic to mercury because removal of the fillings will release mercury into the system and a reaction could cause serious health problems. More problems may result when silver fillings are replaced with gold because many people are allergic to gold as well. The best thing to do is to check all new filling material for allergic reactions.

One researcher claims that mercury is more toxic than lead, cadmium, or arsenic. He argues that no exposure to mercury can be considered harmless. One average size amalgam filling can release enough mercury to exceed the United States Environmental Protection Agency's (EPA) adult index standard for nondietary mercury for more than one hundred years. Mercury from amalgam passes rapidly into the system and accumulates in body tissues in the brain, kidneys, liver, fetus, and in breast milk. The amount of mercury in these tissues correlates to the number of amalgam fillings.

Mercury suppresses the immune system and causes antibiotic resistance at doses below amalgam exposure levels. Mercury can contribute to cardiovascular depression, kidney failure, reproductive disorders, and depression. I have seen mercury fillings cause allergic reactions, chronic sinusitis, fibromyalgia, chronic pain, and depression. With long-term exposure they are also a factor in ear infections, memory problems, ADD, hypersensitivity, fatigue, and other chronic health problems, all of which respond to NAET treatment for mercury. Because mercury is passed to fetuses and through breast milk, I also check children for mercury, even if they do not have fillings. Possible signs of mercury exposure in children are asthma, attention deficit problems, hyperactivity, and behavioral problems.

Other dental materials can cause problems as well. Cariophyllus or carnation oil, used to disinfect pulpitis, can be very damaging to kidneys. Phosphate cements, used to fill root canals, are toxic to the dentist as well as to the patient. Zincum Oxydatum, used for filling root canals and gum dressings, is also toxic, and acrylate, autoprylate, polyester, and vinylpolymerisate nonhardening thermoplastic can be irritating to the GI tract.

I have also noticed that dentists are adversely affected by mercury vapors. In one study, dentists and control subjects who had not suffered occupational exposure to mercury were tested on motor speed, visual scanning, visual motor coordination and concentration, verbal and visual memory, and visual motor coordination speed. The dentists scored thirteen and nine-tenths percent worse than the control subjects. They scored ten percent lower on trail making, digits span, logical memory, delayed recall, and on Bender Distal Time Test Scores. It would seem that mercury is harmful to both dentists and their patients.

An article from the International Dental Amalgam Mercury Syndrome (DAMS) Newsletter by Stephen O'Dell, D.D.S., sums up the mercury problem:

> There is a limit that we can tolerate and beyond that limit we reach the threshold of our body's ability to maintain health.

> Mercury is one of the worst environmental poisons. It is a strong protoplasmic poison that penetrates all living cells of the body.

> Toxic metals like mercury and lead are very difficult for our systems to eliminate. They affect the liver, the heart, the digestive system, the kidneys, the gallbladder, thyroid, pituitary, parathyroid, the hormone producing organs, etc. . . .

> With heat and chewing the mercury leaches out of the filling and is absorbed into the body. The roots of absorption are through the tooth pulp, the surrounding tissue, the sinus, the lungs, and the digestive system.

Mercury is cytotoxic and in the intestinal tract kills normal bacteria. The normal bacteria that survive become mercury tolerant but lose their normal function. The result is a lack of intestinal function and yeast-like symptoms. In many cases yeast infections and yeast-like symptoms go hand in hand with mercury poisoning.

INHALANTS

The following categories contain examples of allergens that enter the body through inhalation.

Dust

One of the worst indoor allergens is house and office dust. There are many components of dust that provoke allergic reactions but the most important is dust mites. A dust mite is a microscopic insect-like creature related to the spider that lives in mattresses, pillows, blankets, carpets, upholstered furniture, and curtains and thrives in humid and warm conditions and at low altitudes. Its diet consists of shed scales of human skin. Female mites can lay twenty-five to fifty eggs and a new generation is produced every three weeks. Mattresses and other household items contain large numbers of living and dead mites. The waste products of these creatures are the main allergen in house dust and the one that causes the most problems for asthmatics. Each mite produces about twenty waste particles each day and these particles can continue to produce allergic reactions including runny nose, sneezing, watery eyes, coughing, and wheezing long after the mite is dead.

Dust mite allergy can be especially bad in homes where the indoor humidity is high or in houses located at low altitude. Carpeting laid over concrete tends to harbor dust mites.

House dust can also be produced indoors from fibers, plant and animal material in the home such as feathers,

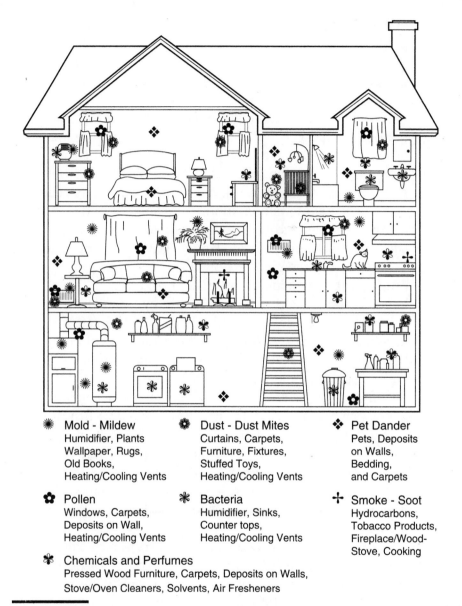

* Mold - Mildew
Humidifier, Plants
Wallpaper, Rugs,
Old Books,
Heating/Cooling Vents

Dust - Dust Mites
Curtains, Carpets,
Furniture, Fixtures,
Stuffed Toys,
Heating/Cooling Vents

Pet Dander
Pets, Deposits
on Walls,
Bedding,
and Carpets

Pollen
Windows, Carpets,
Deposits on Wall,
Heating/Cooling Vents

Bacteria
Humidifier, Sinks,
Counter tops,
Heating/Cooling Vents

Smoke - Soot
Hydrocarbons,
Tobacco Products,
Fireplace/Wood-
Stove, Cooking

Chemicals and Perfumes
Pressed Wood Furniture, Carpets, Deposits on Walls,
Stove/Oven Cleaners, Solvents, Air Fresheners

Figure 5–2   Household Sources of Allergens

cotton, wool, jute, hemp, or animal hairs. Less appealing
components of house dust include human skin scales, ani-

mal dander and saliva, molds, and cockroach drop-
pings.

Pets

A common source of allergens is domestic pets. I constantly treat people for allergies to animals and animal
dander, including reactions to leather. Cat dander is the
most potent, and controlling the dander can be difficult.
A cat carries 60 to 130 milligrams of allergen on its coat
and sheds it at the rate of about .1 milligram per day. As
a result, carpets and upholstered furniture can accumulate large quantities of cat dander. Cat hair is not the
trigger for an allergic reaction. Rather it is the allergy
produced by proteins in the dander and saliva. The allergens become airborne as microscopic particles that
are inhaled into the nose. Although individual cats may
produce more or less allergen, there is no relationship
between the pet's hair length and allergen production,
and no such thing as a nonallergenic breed.

Individuals with animal allergies can react to proteins from the animal's dander, urine, or saliva that are
spread throughout the house. The urine of small animals
such as gerbils and mice also can produce allergic reactions. Removal of the animal may be the most effective
control measure, but the results will not be immediate.
Allergens can remain in a house for months after the animal is removed.

Cat allergen can even be found in homes where
cats have never lived and in office buildings or public
places where animals are not allowed. This is because
cat allergen is particularly sticky and is carried on
clothing from places with cats to other locations. It is
almost impossible not to be exposed to some level of
cat allergen. Because more allergen is present in locations with cats, an allergic individual is more apt to
have rapid onset of symptoms there. The amounts of

airborne particles can be reduced by opening windows, using exhaust fans, and employing efficient air cleaners.

Carpets, upholstered furniture, and mattresses will hold cat allergen even after a cat is removed or banished from the bedroom. It can take up to twenty weeks for allergen levels in carpets to decrease to the level found in homes without cats and up to five years in mattresses. Since cat allergen can also be found on vertical surfaces, walls should be cleaned as well when attempting to decrease allergen levels.

Carol was a patient with severe eczema, chronic fatigue, and severe animal allergies, especially to cats. In her work environment she reacted dramatically to the cat dander carried on the clothes of coworkers who owned cats. It was the only allergen she could imagine that would cause such severe reactions. Her itching and fatigue were so severe that they almost disabled her.

After her basic allergies were cleared with NAET, her eczema subsided. Two days ago we treated her for cats and dogs, and to her own and her coworkers' amazement, she is allergy and symptom free. She can now continue working without disabilities

Feathers

Feathers can produce a variety of reactions. Many people sleep with down pillows and comforters, unaware that feathers may cause sinus problems and headaches. One woman who came to me suffered from sinus problems most of her life. We treated her with NAET for feathers. After twenty-five hours I retested her. Her runny nose and other sinus symptoms were completely gone.

Synthetic Fibers

Synthetic fiber bedding is also a source of inhalant allergens.

Although feather pillows are a wonderful nesting place for house dust mites, it may not be advisable to replace them with synthetic fiber pillows. It is possible that problems with synthetic fibers are caused by a low-level release of gasses. Synthetic fibers are generally made of plastics such as polyester derived from petroleum and may tend to release irritating organic compounds over a long period of time. Many patients who come to me have as many problems with their synthetic fiber pillows as with feather pillows. I muscle test them for each pillow and recommend that they use the kind of pillow they do not react to or be treated with NAET for one or both kinds.

Cooked Foods

Allergens can be contained in the steam from cooking foods. I have even noticed that some people cannot stand to be in close proximity to food to which they are allergic. One time I treated a young boy for sugar and suddenly noticed that his mother was about to pass out. "You know," she said, "sometimes even being near foods I might be allergic to I feel symptoms." She was feeling faint as a reaction to the sugar her son was holding.

Research has been done by boiling shrimp and analyzing the steam. The researchers found shrimp allergens in the steam and concluded that inhaling such steam may cause allergic reactions in sensitive individuals.

Smoke and Chemicals

Other inhalants include smoke, smog, pollutants, chalk, perfumes, carpet pad fumes, and formaldehyde. Formaldehyde is found in new clothes, clothing labels, rugs, polyurethane foam, perfumes, refinishing materials, plywood, particle board, counter tops, electronic equipment, deodorants, chlorine, and certain foods. Outdoors its primary source is the combustion of gasoline and diesel fuel; indoors it is contained in cigarette smoke, carpets, and furniture. Toxic pollutants can be given off by a number of building products such as wood glue, paint (acrylic, latex, and oil), paint thinner, and turpentine. Household products that emit fumes include chlorine and other laundry detergents, as well as heating and cooking fuels such as diesel, natural gas, propane, and butane. Freon, contained in air-conditioning systems and refrigerators, and hydrocarbons, which are chemical compounds released by the combustion of coal, oil, and gas are problems for people with immune disorders.

Smoke includes tobacco smoke and wood smoke. Cigarette smoke is one of the most disagreeable and potentially dangerous indoor pollutants. It is made up of a complex mixture of gasses and particles that contain a variety of chemicals including synthetic compounds added to the cigarette by the tobacco companies. Indoor tobacco smoking substantially increases levels of carbon monoxide, formaldehyde, nitrogen dioxide, acrolein, hydrocarbons, hydrogen cyanide, and many other substances.

Wood burning stoves used in cold, oxygen-poor conditions result in the release of large amounts of carbon monoxide and other inhaled chemicals and particles. Increased use of wood as a heating fuel has raised many concerns about indoor contamination.

Molds

Molds are microscopic fungi made up of clusters of filaments. Unable to produce their own food from sunlight and air, they live on plant, fabric, or animal matter that they decompose for their nourishment. Molds are some of the most widespread living organisms with tens of thousands of different varieties. Bread mold may be the most familiar. Some molds produce penicillin or other antibiotics or are necessary for agriculture. Others produce potent toxins or are major sources of plant disease. Many molds reproduce by releasing spores into the air that settle on organic matter and grow into new mold clusters. These airborne mold spores are far more numerous than pollen grains and can cause allergic symptoms when inhaled.

Molds are found in most indoor and outdoor environments and on food. Their distribution varies from region to region. Unlike pollens, molds do not have a limited season although their growth is encouraged by warmth and high humidity. As a result, they are more prevalent during humid seasons. Outside, molds are present in the air unless there is a cover of snow on the ground. They are most prevalent in shady damp areas, on decaying leaves and other vegetation, and where plant materials have been disturbed. The highest fungal levels are in temperate zones, near oceans, and in areas with the least snow cover.

In North America, grain crops are particularly susceptible to smuts and rusts. Farm workers exposed to these fungi often have many allergic symptoms. Exposure is greatly increased by activities such as thrashing, baling, and combining that release spores. People doing yard work can spread spores by cutting grass or clearing dry brush. Peak levels of the spores of fungi such as Alternaria and Cladosporium are reached on hot, breezy, rain-free days. At night and during rainfall a very different array of fungi is found. They are Ascomycetes, fleshy types called basidiomycetes, and yeast, which require high humidity and splashing water droplets to become airborne.

Some molds are produced in humid areas of the house such as bathrooms and basements, whereas others enter from outside. Houses are never completely free of mold, and exposure is high in areas where plant material has been stored or processed. Molds include mildew and rust, also allergens. Molds also exist in our diet in such foods as blue cheese along with mushrooms, the other member of the fungi group.

Molds are highly irritating to many individuals with immune disorders. In fact, I have never seen one of these individuals who is not affected by them. Molds can cause a stuffy or runny nose, sinusitis, nasal polyps, eczema, bloating, chronic fatigue, headache, depression, and many other problems. NAET treatment for mold and mold spores can cause dramatic improvement in people with chronic health problems such as chronic fatigue and poor digestion. One woman I treated suffered arthritic pain in her back every time she sat on a particular piece of furniture. It turned out she was reacting to mold in the furniture. Chiropractors who find themselves working on the same area over and over would do well to consider that the problem might be caused by an allergy.

Pollens

Pollens, the final group of the inhalants, has a more widespread effect than we previously suspected. For example, I have long surmised that some fruit allergies are really caused by an allergy to the pollen of the fruit tree. Discussed more fully in the case history section, I have successfully treated allergies to fruit by treating for tree pollen. The reverse is not true, however; treating for fruit does not cure allergies to the pollen.

Pollens cannot be avoided but the amounts dispersed vary throughout the year. Tree pollens cause problems in the early spring, grass pollens strike in late spring and early summer, and weed pollens cause flare-ups in late summer. Seasonal patterns vary in different regions of the United States and it is important to know the pattern in your area. For example, ragweed is at its highest level in the east coast and midwest regions from mid-August to late October. In temperate climates such as

California, pollens are present year round. Weather and time of day also have an effect on asthma symptoms.

Ragweed, for example, releases pollen in the early morning. It has been estimated that up to seventy-five percent of seasonal hay fever in the eastern United States is caused by ragweed. There are seventeen different species, and each plant produces up to one billion pollen grains that can be carried five hundred miles by wind.

Pollen is produced by weeds, shrubs, grasses, flowers, and trees. When treating an individual, I always consider all these possibilities. I remember treating one little boy who suffered a headache whenever he went out to play. We treated for flowers, weeds, and shrubs with some improvement but treating him for grasses made all the difference. We recheck periodically because new kinds of pollens can show up and cause problems.

ENVIRONMENTAL ALLERGENS

In this section I discuss allergens found in the environment. They are classified into two categories: indoor allergens and outdoor allergens.

Indoor Allergens

Indoor pollution is a serious problem with at least five hundred harmful chemicals reported in many buildings. This pollution can come from fumes from room dividers, telephone cables, paint, and carpeting. The worst offender is formaldehyde discussed earlier in the inhalant section. Some sensitive individuals react as soon as they walk into a department store because of the formaldehyde found in new clothing.

Volatile organic compounds (VOCs) are found in many household products including dry-cleaned clothing, paint solvents, cleaning products, wood preservatives, aerosol sprays, air fresheners, stored fuels, hobby supplies, disinfectants, repellents, and automotive products.

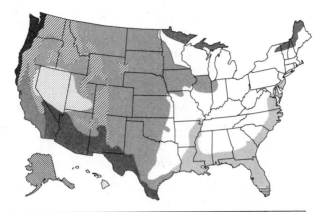

Region	Season	Region	Season
Great Basin		*Great Plains*	
TREES: Juniper, Elm, Poplar, Willow, Sycamore, Box Elder.	February-May	TREES: Mountain Cedar, Poplar, Juniper, Ash, Oak, Elm, Willow, Hackberry, Sycamore, Hickory, Pecan Mulberry, Osage Orange	January-June
WEEDS: Sage, Goosefoot, Amaranth, Ragweed	Mid June-September		
California Lowlands		WEEDS: Sorrel, Dock, Hemp, Goosefoot, Amaranth, Ragweed, Marsh, Elder, Sage.	May-Mid October
TREES: Mulberry, Alder, Ash, Willow, Walnut, Collonwood (Poplar), Elm, Sycamore, Oak, Birch, Olive.	February-May		
		Southeastern Coastal	
WEEDS: Sage, Goosefoot, Amaranth, Ragweed.	Mid May-November	TREES: Red Cedar, Hackberry, Elm, Willow, Poplar, Aspen, Bald Cypress, Bayberry, Wax Turtle, Ash, Birch, Hickory, Pecan, Paper Mulberry, Sycamore, Oak, Walnut, Mulberry.	Mid January-June
Northwestern Coastal			
TREES: Incense Cedar, Ash, Hazelnut, Willow, Alder, Birch, Box Elder, Aspen Poplar, Elm, Maple, Oak, Walnut.	January-June		
		WEEDS: Red (Sheep) Sorrel, Plantain, Nettle, Sage, Goosefoot, Amaranth, Ragweed, Marsh, Elder.	Mid May-October
WEEDS: Plantain, Red Sorrel, Goosefoot, Amaranth, Ragweed	Mid April-October		
		Southern Florida	
Western Mountain		TREES: Oak, Bald Cypress, Elm Maple, Bayberry, Wax Turtle, Australian Pine, Hickory, Pecan, Mulberry.	January-June
TREES: Mountain Cedar, Elm, Juniper, Alder, Maple, Ash, Oak, Aspen, Poplar, Birch, Walnut.	January-July		
WEEDS: Ragweed, Sage, Goosefoot, Amaranth.	July-November	WEEDS: Ragweed, Marsh Elder Sorrel, Dock, Goosefoot, Amaranth.	April-November
Eastern Agricultural		*Southwestern Desert*	
TREES: Red Cedar, Hazelnut, Elm, Alder, Aspen, Poplar, Box Elder, Maple, Birch, Bayberry, Wax Turtle, Ash, Sweet Gum, Paper Mulberry, Willow, Beech, Sycamore, Oak, Hackberry, Walnut, Mulberry (Red), Hickory.	Mid February-July	TREES: Mountain Cedar, Elm, Arizona Cypress, Ash, Poplar, Mulberry, Olive.	January-June
		WEEDS: Sugar Beet, Ragweed, Gossefoot, Amaranth, Sage.	March- Mid May, July-November
WEEDS: Red (Sheep) Sorrel, Plantain, Nettle, Hemp, Sage, Goosefoot, Amaranth, Ragweed, Marsh, Elder.	Mid May-October	*Alaska*	
		TREES:	May-August
		Hawaii	
Northern Woodland		TREES:	January-Mid July
TREES: Hazelnut, Aspen, Poplar, Alder, Birch, Willow.	April-Mid July	WEEDS:	April-September

Figure 5–3 Pollen Chart to Identify the pollen seasons in your area.
(For more information on pollen, contact the Asthma and Allergy Foundation of America.)

Some chemicals appear to penetrate nasal membranes and cause congestion, runny nose, tearing eyes, and, in asthmatics, wheezing and coughing.

Asbestos is a major health hazard that was used from 1945 to 1975 in ceiling materials, synthetic tiles, acoustical wall coatings, stove guards, and as insulation on hot water heaters. It is a dangerous allergen to many and a major trigger for asthmatics.

Indoor chemical sensitivities are becoming more prevalent because there is less ventilation in tight, energy efficient houses and buildings. Media attention has led to increased public awareness of this problem in recent years. Poor indoor air quality in buildings has been associated with a variety of syndromes or groups of symptoms loosely known as building related illness or **sick building syndrome**. These terms are applied when one or more occupants in a building develop certain recognized symptoms that are apparently related to some indoor pollutant. Many of these illnesses involve hypersensitivity of the lungs and respiratory system. In one illness, called hypersensitivity pneumonitis, organic dust can create complex immune system reactions and symptoms including mucus membrane irritation, coughing, chest tightness, headache, and fatigue. People with these illnesses are diagnosed as having multiple chemical sensitivities (MCSs) or environmental illness (EI).

Chemical sensitivities can be triggered through the use of, or exposure to, cosmetics, perfumes, hair spray, hair products, chlorine and other cleaning products, and detergents. A common offender is dichlorobenzene, found in moth balls, insect spray, disinfectants, and solvents. Cooking on a gas stove can also be hazardous to your health. A study of over one thousand British women found that those who cooked with gas were more likely to suffer wheezing, breathlessness, and hay fever—and two and a half times more likely to suffer asthma attacks—during the previous year than women who did not cook with gas.

Your car can be filled with pollutants from plastics and carpets to leather preservatives.

The house and car are not the only hazardous areas. Many Americans suffer from chronic fatigue caused by breathing some kind of irritant at work. One article reported that five to fifteen percent of all asthma cases are caused by on-the-job irritants. According to an anonymous author, the most common agents on the job are isocyanates, chemicals used in the manufacture of foam for chairs and car seats and in spray paint and glue. Other common workplace irritants are latex, molds, animal dander, grain dust, and wood dust. A recent report of a 12-member panel of the American College of Chest Physicians estimates that five percent of workers exposed to isocyanates will develop asthma.

Outdoor Allergens

In combination with drug therapy, food allergies, and other allergies discussed in this book, environmental allergies resulting from outdoor pollutants, chemicals, and toxins are compromising our immune systems and causing severe health problems. The pollutants may not be the direct cause of disease but allergic reactions to pollutants can cause the immune system to link antibody complexes to these substances. An immune system faced with an overabundance of these compromising substances might simply not be capable either of dealing effectively with major diseases such as cancer or with **free radicals** that damage the body's tissue.

Since the Clean Air Act went into effect in the fall of 1995, Methyl-Tertiary-Butyl Ether (MTBE) has been added to gasoline to reduce the amount of carbon monoxide emissions. Unfortunately, this fuel additive is responsible for increased bronchial and lung problems as well as skin rashes and symptoms of disorientation. Most of the public is unaware that some scientists fear MTBE produces elevated levels of formaldehyde. The EPA contends that MTBE is not harmful to the environment or to health but increasing evidence suggests it can exacerbate or cause asthma.

The propellants used in metered dose inhalants for asthmatics contain **chlorofluorocarbons** (**CFCs**), chemical agents that when released into the air become part of the chemical brew that can damage the Earth's ozone layer. These CFCs are also found in air-conditioning, hair sprays, cleaning solvents, and other products that rely on propellants.

Other atmospheric environmental pollutants include car exhaust, gas and diesel fuel exhaust, acid nitricum and Acid Sulfurosum (sulfurous acid from coal-fired plants and gasoline exhaust), and asbestos dust generated from automotive brakes in sufficient quantities to be measurable. Fumes, exhaust gases, and pesticides contain ethylene oxide, car exhaust contains cadmium sulfuricum and chromium oxydatum, a by-product of burning jet fuels, and paint (latex, oil, acrylic) contains plumbum metallicum. Fertilizers sometimes contain Calcium cyanamide (calcium nitrate) that is also found in foods, and Potassium nitrate (K-saltpeter); superphosphate; and Thomasmeal, a pre-emergent bud inhibitor.

Radon is a naturally occurring environmental toxin, the by-product of uranium 238. It is formed in soil and rock and can accumulate in enclosed places. Risks to individuals are evaluated according to the intensity of the radiation and the length of exposure to the toxin. Radon absorption occurs through inhalation and drinking ground water. Levels are highest during the warm months of the year and are higher in lower parts of an enclosed space. There is an increased incidence of lung cancer among miners working in a high radon environment and among members of residential households with excessive levels of radon.

Many people are also sensitive to naturally occurring radiation. For example, I used to get a bad headache every time I was in the sun, even if I wore a hat or other head covering. Since I have been treated for a sensitivity to radiation with NAET, I have no problem in the sun. Natural radiation levels fluctuate and are highest during changes in weather. Some people feel sick whenever it starts to rain or the weather changes in some way. Individuals with Candida, chronic fatigue, and fibromyalgia especially tend to be worse during a change of weather but treating for radiation with NAET can change this situation.

Carbon dioxide may also cause an allergic reaction in some individuals, leading to a buildup of the gas in the bodily fluids. This allergy is especially apparent when people climb to higher altitudes and takeoff or land in airplanes but it can also be provoked by drinking carbonated water. I have seen people suffer migraines as a result of this allergy. In order to attain normalcy of the respiratory gases, people have to breathe more forcefully. This can lead to dyspnea (labored respirations) associated with the inability to breathe enough to satisfy the demand for air. The allergic reaction to carbon dioxide is referred to as "air hunger." Since many are also allergic to adrenaline, this fear makes the symptoms even worse as adrenaline levels rise.

Outdoor pollution can result from natural causes (the eruption of volcanoes, dust storms, forest fires) or from man-made causes (vehicle exhaust, fossil fuel combustion, or petroleum refining). General air pollution and smog affects us all. There is substantial scientific evidence linking specific air pollutants to an increase in illnesses, especially in children. Sulfur dioxide can cause bronchial spasms, hives, GI disorders, inflammation of the walls of the blood vessels (vasculitis), and related disorders. Temporary or perhaps permanent bronchial hypersensitivity has been connected to inhaling ozone, and long-term exposure to nitrogen dioxide has been associated with the increased occurrence of respiratory illness. As mentioned earlier, the greatest exposure to airborne pollution occurs inside homes, offices, and other nonindustrial buildings.

Common symptoms associated with environmental allergens include respiratory problems, chronic dizziness, headaches, burning eyes, aching throat, and loss of energy. These symptoms are often mistaken for viral infections such as colds and the flu.

ATMOSPHERIC CONDITIONS

Atmospheric changes can have dramatic effects on individuals, especially when the temperature falls and the humidity increases. Even jumping into cold water, eating something cold, or inhaling cold air can be irritating.

INJECTANTS

This last category deals with allergens that enter the body by injection or puncturing of the skin.

Insects

Stinging insects include the bee, yellow jacket, wasp, and two types of hornets: yellow and white-faced. All of these can cause allergic reactions. There are four basic levels of reaction: (1) a small local reaction; (2) a large local reaction; (3) urticaria, or hives that is not life threatening; and (4) a life-threatening reaction such as swollen throat tissues that block breathing, an asthma attack, or dizziness and fainting. When the throat closes off, a venom amino therapy injection containing actual venom may be necessary. Such injections are successful eighty to one hundred percent of the time.

The best ways to deal with stinging insects are to avoid them and take precautions: wear shoes when walking through grass; do not stand around trash receptacles; limit the use of perfumes; and do not wear bright-colored clothing in areas around insects.

We have had wonderful results treating insect allergies with NAET. Once patients have been treated they should no longer react to being stung by that insect.

One young girl was brought in by her mother because she had apparently been stung by a bee. She had a rash, her arm was swollen, and she was in a great deal of pain. We found that she had been stung by a wasp and we treated for the allergy. Before she left the office, all symptoms of the sting, including the rash, had completely disappeared. I have witnessed similar results with bites from mosquitoes, bees, spiders, and ticks.

One woman patient who was bitten by a tick brought the creature with her when she came to be treated for a reaction to the bite. By the time she left the office, all reactions to the bite were gone.

6 | METABOLIC CAUSES OF IMMUNE DISORDERS

And don't even think about
going down the detergent aisle
in the grocery store
or you'll be off in the
o   z   o   n   e
. . . which might not be so bad
if you don't mind the idea of
Death by Pine Sol.
              —from "Case Study of Cognitive Dysfunction
                         in 3.5 Million CFIDS Patients"

Linda

Linda, a 35-year-old school teacher who was referred to me by the mother of one of her students, complained of mild to moderate asthma with frequent cases of bronchitis and coughing throughout the year. She also had problems with extreme weight gain, bloating and abdominal swelling, chronic fatigue, and difficulty handling stress. Six years before, she had been diagnosed with Epstein-Barr virus. Because she came from a distance, it was not easy for her to get to my office on a regular basis, but she was hopeful that I might be able to help her. She had very little strength and needed all she could summon to deal with her students.

I began by performing an abdominal diagnostic exam, a palpation exam, and a urinalysis. The palpation exam is an acute summary or evaluation that gives me a good idea of what is happening at the present time, whereas a urinalysis gives me an assessment of what has happened on a long-term basis. We do both a fasting and a nonfasting test. Fasting helps me detect an inflammation or a severe enzyme deficiency.

The first thing I noted was a possible thyroid imbalance, and I instructed her to do a basal axillary temperature test to determine whether she was hypothyroid. I also found a positive respiratory reflex, which is common with asthmatics, as well as a positive kidney reflex, which is usually representative of a kidney problem, a low back problem, or a congested lymph system. Since the lymph feeds into the kidney, backed up lymphatic channels can overload the organ, especially when the body is not digesting foods well and there is a build up of toxicity. This may then manifest as severe fatigue and depression.

Linda evidenced a positive reflex in the lower right quadrant with fasting (for at least two hours), which usually indicates a calcium deficiency and possibly an allergy to calcium (including milk), and an inability to absorb calcium. She also showed signs of low adrenals, which is often the case with people suffering from chronic fatigue, as well as irritable bowel which showed up in the lower right and lower left quadrants, and an inability to absorb simple carbohydrates.

On the nonfasting examination, I found that she had trouble digesting proteins and fats and difficulty absorbing sugars. On the 24-hour urinalysis, a high sediment index, especially in uric acid and calcium oxalates, suggested significant difficulty digesting proteins and fats, perhaps because she was eating too many of them. This was corroborated by high toxicity as indicated on the urinalyis evaluation. She also showed low calcium, potassium, and magnesium and a very low overall pH of 5.66. Her Vitamin C was normal, which suggested that she was not allergic to it.

After performing the urinalysis palpation, I prescribed an enzyme that helps digest protein and fat (hcl), and a kidney enzyme (kdy) that acts as a mild diuretic and detoxifyer. I also prescribed a spleen enzyme (spl) to boost the immune system, something I often do with immune depressed people like AIDS or chronic fatigue patients who tend to get sick frequently. The enzymes and herbs in this formula help the body's immune system fight off infections until we can effectively treat the allergies that weakened the immune system in the first place.

When I tested her, I found that she was allergic to all the basic allergens, especially Vitamin A and betocarotene, eggs, chicken, B vitamins, minerals, and sugars. She was even allergic to Vitamin C, although she showed no deficiency. We cleared the basic allergies, but her symptoms didn't improve, which was especially frustrating for her because she traveled so far to see me. On retesting, I discovered that several sugars had not cleared, and I taught her how to treat herself for them at home.

Those self-treatments helped her reduce her craving for sugar, which for her was quite an accomplishment. For example, one day she ate the following: for breakfast, a blueberry bagel and instant lemonade; for lunch, apple sauce and chocolate cake; and for dinner, shredded wheat cereal and milk, followed by ice cream and a persimmon. Although she acknowledged that her diet was virtually devoid of any nutritional value, she said she really did not care and did not intend to change it. After the self-treatments for sugars, her diet did not improve but she craved the sugars less and felt a little more hopeful about the treatment.

As I do with all patients, I mentioned to Linda that it might take some time to detoxify, balance, and strengthen the body once certain allergies had been cleared. Sometimes after an especially powerful or important treatment, I recommend that we take some time off to let the person regenerate. Then we can retest and begin another course of treatment.

After we finished the basics, Linda took a break from treatment. When she came back sometime later, I retested her. Many foods to which she had been intolerant had now cleared, and I began to treat for other items I thought were important: herbs, spices, and hormones, including adrenal, estrogen, testosterone, T_2, T_3, and T_4. Because her temperature was still quite low (96.5), I prescribed a thyroid enzyme (AllerZyme thy). Then I treated her for a few other foods.

When she returned recently, she reported that she had never felt as good before in her life. She was happy to get up in the morning, her diet had improved, she had plenty of energy, she was focused, and she enjoyed her students. She referred three of her friends to me and told me that she is so committed to this work that she would appear on any talk show with me.

By clearing the basic allergies, which took about a month, we cleared most of her food intolerances, and her health was restored. When she returned a month later, she was like a new person. You can not underestimate the importance of these basics, especially with people who suffer from chronic fatigue, because their problems are usually rooted in food allergies. At some point, we will clear her of the Epstein-Barr virus, some of the fungi, and some of the other contactants and inhalants that are contributing to her asthma.

FOOD ALLERGIES

Food allergies are the most obvious of all recognized allergies and most frequently the cause of all chronic immune disorders. At some time we all have felt a number of varied symptoms from eating foods we could not tolerate or to which we were allergic. Asthmatics can experience this at every meal. Individuals with immune disorders can experience fatigue, nausea, fogginess, muscle aches, bloating, and depression. NAET is the only successful, permanent answer to ending these food allergies.

Walk into an elementary school, sit in a classroom, and observe the number of children coughing. Their energy declines or they feel bloated and ill, complaining of headache, abdominal pain, and fatigue. My daughter, who is in the second grade, came home the other day and said "Mom, so many kids in my class are coughing, they are all allergic to some foods." I said "absolutely!" It is a result of their immune systems being unable to fight off the bacteria and viruses they are inhaling, ingesting, and contacting. Food allergies are key allergens to treat for individuals with immune disorders.

Sugars and Carbohydrates

I was grateful when Dr. Barry Sears' book *Enter the Zone* appeared with its intelligent discussion of sugars and carbohydrates. I have felt for a long time that people eat far too much sugar, particularly those who are sugar intolerant or allergic. Here is what Sears had to say about carbohydrates:

> Unfortunately, many people don't really know what a carbohydrate is. Most people will say carbohydrates are sweets and pasta. Ask them what a vegetable or fruit is, and they'll probably reply that it's a vegetable or fruit—as if that were a food type all its own, a food type that they can eat in unlimited amounts without gaining weight.

> Well, this may come as a surprise, but all the above—sweets and pasta, vegetables and fruits— are carbohydrates. Carbohydrates are merely different forms of simple sugars linked together in polymers something like edible plastic.

> Of course, we all need a certain amount of carbohydrates in our diet. The body requires a continual intake of carbohydrates to feed the brain which uses glucose (a form of sugar) as its primary energy source. In fact, the brain is a virtual glucose hog, gobbling more than two-thirds of the circulating carbohydrates in the bloodstream while you are at rest. To feed this glucose hog, the body continually takes carbohydrates and converts them to glucose.

> It's actually a bit more complicated than that. Any carbohydrates not immediately used by the

body will be stored in the form of glycogen (a long string of glucose molecules linked together). The body has two storage sites for glycogen: the liver and the muscles. The glycogen stored in the muscles is inaccessible to the brain. Only the glycogen stored in the liver can be broken down and sent back to the bloodstream to maintain adequate blood sugar levels for proper brain function.

The liver's capacity to store carbohydrates in the form of glycogen is very limited and can be easily depleted within ten to twelve hours. So the liver's glycogen reserves must be maintained on a continual basis. That's why we eat carbohydrates.

Now what happens when you eat too much carbohydrate? Here is Dr. Sears' answer:

Whether it is being stored in the liver or the muscles, the total storage capacity of the body for carbohydrate is really quite limited. If you're an average person, you can store about three hundred to four hundred grams of carbohydrate in your muscles, but you can't get at that carbohydrate. In the liver, where carbohydrates are accessible for glucose conversion, you can store only about sixty to ninety grams. This is equivalent to about two cups of cooked pasta or three typical candy bars, and it represents your total reserve capacity to keep the brain working properly.

Once the glycogen levels are filled in both the liver and the muscles, excess carbohydrate has just one fate: to be converted into fat and stored in the adipose, that is fatty tissue. In a nutshell, even though carbohydrates themselves are fat-free, excess carbohydrates end up as excess fat.

Finally, he talks about insulin:

Any meal or snack high in carbohydrates will generate a rapid rise of glucose. To adjust for this rapid rise, the pancreas secretes the hormone insulin into the bloodstream. Insulin then lowers the levels of blood glucose.

All well and good. The problem is that insulin is essentially a storage hormone, evolved to put aside excess carbohydrate calories in the form of fat in case of future famine. So the insulin that's stimulated by excess carbohydrates aggressively promotes the accumulation of body fat.

In other words, when we eat too much carbohydrate, we are essentially sending a hormonal message, via insulin, to the body (actually to the adipose cells). The message: "store fat."

Hold on, it gets even worse. Not only do increased insulin levels tell the body to store carbohydrates as fat, they also tell it not to release any stored fat. This makes it impossible for you to use your own stored body fat for energy. So the excess carbohydrates in your diet not only make you fat, they make sure you stay fat. It's a double whammy and it can be lethal.

To put it another way, too much carbohydrate means too much insulin."

People generally eat too many carbohydrates. This causes stress on the hormonal system and throws the body out of balance. For anyone with allergies or an immune system under stress, sugar can put a stress on the immune system. Sugar allergies are a common cause of a buildup of mucus. Carbohydrates and sugars consist of fructose (found in fruit), lactose (found in dairy products), glucose, and maltose (found in grains, pasta, breads, cereals, and vegetables).

I have often seen children's immune systems destroyed by excessive amounts of carbohydrates and sugar. These children burn themselves out more quickly, their energy fades during a particular time of the day, they lack prolonged focus and attention, and they constantly crave carbohydrates and sugar. For children with a chronic cough, I remove sugar from their diets and much of the coughing stops right away. Treating with NAET for an allergy to sugar diminishes both the craving and the cough.

Sugar is also one of the primary foods that is linked to infectants, especially bacteria and fungi. Eating excessive amounts of sugar can create an allergic reaction that brings to the surface a linked infectant. This starts a cycle of ear, sinus, or bronchial infections. In children, this can result in repeated school absences.

It is also important to clear and desensitize allergies to sugar. We recommend that protein, with its rich supply of amino acids, be eaten with carbohydrates to balance it, but many people are allergic to amino acids as well. People who are allergic to one or all of the amino acids do not absorb or digest them properly and cannot utilize them. This results in a craving for sugar because the body is not able to absorb sugar without the necessary amino acids. Fifty percent of our protein is converted to sugars, another reason that an allergy to amino acids may increase sugar craving. Because the brain requires a constant supply of glucose, it is important to check for, and clear allergies to, amino acids and proteins as well as to sugars.

When large amounts of sugars are eaten, B vitamins and minerals, especially potassium, are depleted. People who have allergies to B vitamins do not get enough because the body is unable to absorb and use them. For these people, it is important to clear the B vitamin allergy with NAET before the sugar allergy is cleared. Otherwise, their already low levels of B vitamins may be further depleted. B vitamin deficiency can cause depression, mental fatigue, low energy, and exhaustion.

Sugar is also responsible for bloating in many people and is strongly linked to fungal infections. I have found that people who are allergic to B vitamins and sugar are especially likely to have fungal infections.

The craving for carbohydrates and sugars is always a result of B vitamin problems. When people tell me they crave complex carbohydrates, I always look for B vitamin allergies and sugar allergies. When people crave sugars I look for the amino acid allergies as well as the B vitamin allergies.

Fats

Fats must be well digested in order for the body to utilize the fatty acids necessary for the health of the nervous system. Fatty acids help to control neurotransmitters and assist in the manufacture and secretion of vital hormones in the thyroid, adrenal, and pituitary glands. They also act as antioxidants and inhibit the secretion of acid in the stomach. Clearing sensitivities to fats can be very beneficial to individuals with chronic immune disorders.

Dairy Products

An allergy to dairy products such as milk, yogurt, and cheese is one of the most common and widely recognized form of food allergies. I have found that dairy product sensitivities often can be cleared by clearing sensitivities to calcium and lactose. Sometimes, the dairy product itself has to be treated. With a combination of NAET treatment and enzyme therapy, dairy intolerance or allergy can be eliminated.

One of the most common complaints of dairy product allergy is the production of excess mucus. All of us have had this kind of experience at some time or other: the need to clear our throats after eating a certain food. I remember one woman who constantly had mucus in her throat, especially after she ate dairy products. After we treated her with NAET, she no longer had the problem with any food, including dairy foods. She was surprised because, being in the health field, she believed that dairy products were always mucus producers. Before working with this method I had the same idea and was equally surprised by our results.

Every food is unique and has its own electromagnetic energy field. A person might have a reaction to yogurt, for example, but not to milk. There are many ingredients in the food that may be causing the problem such as **phenolics**, (discussed later in this chapter), sugars, calcium, and B vitamins. For this reason it is necessary to test each member of a food group separately to ensure that eating the particular food will not cause symptoms.

Eggs

Eggs and chicken are the first foods we treat for in our practice. My daughter has always had mucus in her throat: in fact, she had to clear her throat almost immediately after she was born. This became more apparent as she grew older, and by age three she began to comment about it. She also craved eggs. When I treated her for eggs using NAET, her craving disappeared and she no longer needed to clear her throat after eating them. Now if she has mucus after eating a food, she know she needs to be checked and treated. She has turned into a detective to discover her own allergens.

Soy Products

The soybean is an excellent source of protein but it is also frequently an allergen. Many mothers tell me they take their children off milk early and put them on rice and soy milks. The mothers mean well but this practice can result in children with chronic upper respiratory infections caused by allergies to soy.

Soy is now used to make milk, cheese, nuts, flour, and vegetarian "meat," with new products coming out all the time. Lecithin is a soy product often used in candy to prevent drying and to help emulsify the fats. Clearing lecithin often clears a chocolate sensitivity. Soy is also used in many other foods. Soy flour is used in hard candies, fudge, nut candies, and caramels. Some bakeries use soy milk instead of cow's milk in recipes. Soy products are used in custards and coffee substitutes as well as other household products such as varnish, paints, enamels, printing ink, massage creams, celluloid, paper finishes, cloth, nitroglycerin, some dog food, adhesives, soap, fertilizer, automobile parts, textiles, and lubricating oil (for a complete list refer to Part VI). Ford Motor Company uses soybeans to make plastics for window frames, steering wheels, and other automotive parts. They even use soy to make a rubber substitute and an upholstery fabric. As soy becomes more common in the environment, it is important that sensitive people be treated for it.

Grains

Corn is a major grain allergen. Dr. Nambudripad believes it is the most common allergy today. Many foods contain corn in the form of cornstarch and corn syrup. Most prepared foods contain cornstarch such as Chinese food, baking powder, and toothpaste. Additionally, it is the binding product in most pills and vitamins including aspirin, Tylenol®, and other kinds of drugs. Corn syrup is a common sweetener found in many soft drinks. Corn is found in food mixes, canned foods, and foods cooked in corn oil and corn silk is used in many cosmetics and makeup products.

In Chapter 9, I describe how successful we have been clearing wheat allergy by treating for maltose and the B vitamins. Foods that contain wheat are so numerous that I have listed them in Part VI.

Barley, oats, and rye can also be allergens. We have had success treating them by treating for gluten and gliadin.

Fruits

Any fruit can be a potential allergen. I have seen people allergic to all types including apples, bananas, grapes, pears, and melons. The more acid fruits such as pineapples, strawberries, and kiwi, and the more sugary fruits such as papaya and mangos also cause allergic reactions in some individuals. Many children drink a lot of apple juice that can be mucus forming. The chemicals that are sprayed on fruit can also be a problem.

Treating for Vitamin C and sugars often clears these fruit allergies as well as treatment for phenolics, salicylates, and acid, all common ingredients in fruits.

Peanuts

Peanuts are a widely used food and a common food allergen. The incidence of peanut allergy has increased in the last decade, perhaps because of the increased use of peanut products and of peanut butter as a source of protein. Research indicates that many lactating mothers use peanut butter to supplement their protein intake while breast feeding. Because peanut allergen is secreted in breast milk, this can create a sensitivity in an at-risk child.

Reactions from peanuts include mucus formation, asthma attacks, and anaphylactic shock. I have treated adults and children successfully for all of these reactions. Other nuts that can cause problems are cashews, pecans, and walnuts.

Nightshades

Eggplants, potatoes, tomatoes, and peppers are all members of the nightshade family. Any of them can be serious allergens. I have seen the nightshades act as irritants for arthritics or others with joint pain. Sometimes what is diagnosed as arthritis is actually an allergy to one of these foods. Studies have indicated that an allergy to eggplant is linked to a certain grass and other allergies such as ragweed, birch, or animal dander.

Vegetables

Most vegetables are potential allergens. Onions and peppers are sometimes a problem as well as yams, cucumbers, and carrots. I have seen people develop a migraine immediately after eating a carrot. Sometimes treating for Vitamin A will clear a sensitivity to carrots without having to clear the carrots themselves. Before being treated for Vitamin A, I used to get a headache and nausea whenever I ate carrots but not anymore.

Dried beans can also be a problem, especially garbanzo, kidney, and pinto beans.

Fish, Seafood, and Meat

Fish and seafood can cause severe reactions. One of the first cases I treated with NAET involved a woman whose throat closed off when she ate prawns. After the treatment I was still skeptical and I called Dr. Nambudripad. I asked her, "Do you really think this treatment will work, because this woman could die?" She assured me there should be no problem if I treated the woman and made sure she stayed away from seafood for twenty-five hours. After the treatment, the woman's daughter called me up to express her concern that her mother might get seriously ill or die if she tried to eat shellfish or prawns again. Although I said that I was confident, I added that the patient should not be too far from an emergency room when she tried it, just in case. The woman has been eating prawns and shellfish for years now without any problems.

Turkey, chicken, and pheasant are common allergens although I have found chicken to be the most common. A turkey sensitivity is sometimes a reaction to the **neurotransmitter** serotonin which occurs naturally in turkey. Serotonin allergy can produce feelings of depression, tiredness, and mental fogginess.

Chocolate, Caffeine, and Coffee

Chocolate and caffeine are common allergens. Children should be checked for a chocolate allergy because they tend to eat it so often. A craving for chocolate usually indicates an allergy to it. In addition to obvious sources like coffee and tea, caffeine is also a hidden ingredient in some soft drinks and over-the-counter medications such as Excedrin® and other aspirin-based products. Both the allergy to caffeine and the allergy to chocolate that tends to result in fatigue, joint pain, and depression.

Salt and Spices

Salt has been found to be a common allergen for thyroiditis and fibromyalgia.

Most of these individuals have allergies to spices. Garlic is a common allergen although it is regarded by many to be a healthy food. I have seen asthmatics who begin wheezing after eating excessive amounts of garlic. It can also cause indigestion, bloating, and headaches. Vanilla and artificial sweeteners are also allergens to some people.

Combinations of Food Groups

Even after they have been cleared for the foods they are eating, many individuals feel symptoms such as fatigue and bloating after eating a meal which suggests they are possibly allergic to combinations of foods. To eliminate these episodes, I have them describe several typical meals then treat them with NAET for the combinations. I also recommend they set aside a portion of each meal so they can treat themselves if they notice symptoms after eating.

Fluoride

Fluoride is found naturally in certain foods and added to the water supply in many areas. Recent studies show an increase of certain chronic health problems with exposure to fluoride. Although much has been written about the benefits of fluoride, people should educate themselves about the possible dangers as well.

Food Additives

Many food additives can cause problems for individuals who are sensitive to food. These include sulfites, MSG, hydrolyzed vegetable protein, sodium nitrate, and sodium nitrite. The sulfites in particular are potentially deadly. I have seen several cases of children who had serious reactions after eating in fast food restaurants. Most food additives are listed on prepared foods. Small amounts do not need to be mentioned, however, so sensitive people eat them without being aware. Preservatives such as butylated hydroxyanisole (BHA) and butylated hydroxytoluene (BHT) used in packaging may cause reactions in sensitive people who eat the food contained in that packaging.

MSG has been used for many years as a flavor enhancer for a variety of foods prepared at home and in restaurants. Manufactured by a fermentation process using starch, beet sugar, and cane sugar or molasses, it is the sodium salt of glutamic acid, an amino acid, that is found naturally in our bodies. Glutamic acid makes up a large part of the proteins found in foods such as cheese, meat, peas, mushrooms, and milk.

The FDA has studied many of the reportedly adverse effects of MSG and unfortunately still considers it a safe ingredient. I disagree. I treat many people who are allergic to MSG and find that it causes particular problems such as bloating, joint pain, and migraines.

Any packaged food with MSG must list this ingredient on the label. Other food ingredients that contain glutamate include hydrolyzed vegetable proteins, autolyzed yeast, extract flavorings, natural flavorings, and potassium glutamate. Hydrolyzed vegetable protein contains five to twenty percent glutamate and is used in place of MSG as a flavor enhancer in many foods such as canned tuna, dried soup mixes, canned vegetables, and processed meats. People who are allergic to MSG can be allergic to other glutamate products as well. Be aware that MSG and the other glutamates do not have to be listed as ingredients if they are a component of an ingredient that is listed such as hydrolyzed vegetable protein. This can have serious consequences for people who are allergic and have no way of knowing they are eating these additives.

It is important to check labels. You can look for MSG in dips, soup mixes, stews, gravies, sauces, prepared meats, poultry, fish, and vegetables. Some restaurants that claim they do not use MSG use commercial sauces or spice mixes without realizing they contain MSG or one of the glutamates. Because it is difficult to avoid them completely, it is best to treat for them if a person is allergic. I have had excellent results in treating for sensitivities to MSG, hydrolyzed vegetable proteins and other glutamates, and food additives. If an individual is not allergic to them, the body will eliminate them quickly and easily.

Gums, such as Acacia, karaya, xanthan, and tragacanth gums are other kinds of additives that can cause problems. They are found in many foods including yogurt, candy bars, cottage cheese, soft drinks, soy sauce, barbecue sauce, macaroni and cheese, and ready-made foods.

Other additives include acidum Sorbicum (sorbic acid found in canned meats), acidum Benzoicum (a food preservative), Diphenyl (a preservative for oranges), and

Hexamethylenetetramine (a preservative in canned fruit). Sodium pyrophosphoricum gives the red color to meat, especially processed meats. Sodium o-phenylphenolate, Sodium Sulfurosum, sorbic acid, Urethanum (used in wine manufacturing), and Carbamide (inhibits potato sprouting) can all produce reactions.

Another major additive group is the salicylates. Salicylates are food preservatives that are used, among other places, in the manufacture of aspirin. Many individuals have problems with salicylate foods although they appear to build up in the system before provoking a reaction.

Salicylate is both a food additive and an ingredient that appears naturally in many foods. Salicylate food may be tolerated on a four-day rotation diet but not if eaten every day. Most sensitive individuals do not react every time the food is eaten unless it is consumed in excessive amounts. Salicylates are found in a variety of fruits, including apples, apricots, blackberries, boysenberries, cantaloupe, cherries, cranberries, currents, dates, guava, grapes, loganberries, orange pineapple, plum, dark red raspberries, frozen strawberries, gooseberries, and currants. They are also found in vegetables such as chicory, chili peppers, endive, mushrooms, sweet and green peppers, radishes, tomato paste, tomato sauce, zucchini, almonds, peanuts, water chestnuts, bay leaves, basil, caraway, champagne, chili flakes, chili powder, ginger root, mint, nutmeg, cloves, green olives, white pepper, peppermint, port, tea bags, herbal teas, vanilla flavoring, and wine vinegar. A variety of crackers, some cereals, cake mixes, muffins, biscuits, cakes, coffee, pastries, tobacco, mayonnaise, ketchup, Jell-O® and gelatin, candies, gum, and corned beef contain them as well.

Food coloring is another important category of additives. I discuss some case histories involving food coloring in a later section. Many candies, jelly beans for example, contain large amounts of coloring. Even foods sold in natural food stores may contain artificial coloring, so beware! Reactions to food coloring can be serious, from severe constriction of air passageways to coughing, runny nose, and fever.

Pesticides are also food additives and are particularly serious because they are everywhere. Even banned pesticides such as DDT still exist in residues in the soil and in people's bodies. I have worked with people who register a sensitivity to DDT. I remember treating one man who was HIV positive and suffered from severe fatigue and a depressed immune system. One of the breakthroughs in our treatment occurred when I treated him for pesticides to which he was highly allergic. He told me that he grew up on a farm and helped his father spray the plants and trees with pesticides. (A list of different pesticides appears in Part VI.)

We should eat foods that are free of pesticides but they are so pervasive in the environment that they are very difficult to avoid. For this reason, we should treat for sensitivities to them.

Alcohol

Alcoholic beverages such as beer, wine, and liquor cause difficulties for many people and alcohol is the root of the problem. I treat first for B vitamins and sugars, then for alcohol. Our clinic has successfully treated several alcoholics for their addiction to alcohol, and with the help of other therapies, have successfully recovered. Often the craving for alcohol is a craving for sugar and the B vitamins that have been depleted by alcohol consumption. It is a vicious circle because alcohol depletes many B vitamins and minerals.

Alcohol is not just a problem for those who drink alcoholic beverages. It is produced in the body by anyone who consumes large amounts of fruits and sugars. Alcohol was a difficult allergy for me to clear. Although I did not drink it often, I ate lots of fruit, and I was showing signs of becoming addicted. After I was treated for alcohol and sugars, the craving diminished. I also noticed that when I did drink alcohol I no longer had headaches, depression, or the other symptoms I used to experience.

Alcohol tends to aggravate or sustain yeast and other fungal infections. Therefore, it is important to eliminate alcohol cravings when treating for fungi.

Wines contain other ingredients that can be problematic as well: sulfites, which I have already discussed, and histamines, which I will talk about later in this chapter. Alcoholic beverages made from grains are problematic for anyone allergic to them. Because beer and wine are both made with yeast, they cause problems for anyone with fungal allergies. Other ingredients in beer may also cause difficulties.

Water

Surprisingly enough, some people react to their drinking water. One woman told me she thought she was allergic to the bottled spring water she used. Every time she drank it, she coughed. When I tested her, I found she was indeed allergic. When she stopped drinking it, her cough went away and her mucus production diminished significantly. Some people seem to be allergic to their tap water, others to their bottled water. The reaction may be to something in the water such as fluoride or other minerals, or to the plastic in which the water is bottled.

Phenolics

Phenolics are derivatives of benzene used to give flavor and color to foods and to help preserve them. They also occur naturally in some foods. Once phenolics enter the bloodstream, they are broken down in the liver and excreted into the intestines in bile or eliminated in the urine. Cow's milk naturally contains high levels of phenolics and often provokes a reaction. There are said to be fourteen different phenolics in milk, and people treated for cow's milk, which might normally desensitize them to milk, may continue to react to phenolics until treated for them. Tomatoes and soybean products are also high in phenolics.

Some of the phenolics that individuals with immune disorders react to most often are acetaldehyde (also called ethanol), alanine, androsterone, apiol, beta alanine, butyric acid, caffeic acid, carnitine, coumarin, ferrous fumerate, glutamine, 5-hydroxytryptophan, hypericin, lactic acid, malvin, menadione, nicotine, oxalic acid, phytic acid, piperine, proline, threonine, uric acid, indole, and skatol. Each of these is described in more detail in the following section.

Acetaldehyde, commonly found with Candidiasis, is found in car exhaust, perfumes , rubber, wood, apples, broccoli, cheese, grapes, grapefruit, grape juice, grapes, chicken, beef, pineapples, pears, peaches, oranges, and in the oxidation of propane and butane. It is produced during the metabolic cycle of Candida albicans in the intestinal tract. It is formed by the decarboxylation of pyruvate and is reduced to ethanol by anaerobic fermentation. It is used in the manufacture of rubber, gelatin, perfumes, and in synthetic fruits, berries, butter, chocolate, apple, ice cream, gelatin desserts, and chewing gum.

Alanine is a nonessential amino acid and is a phenolic found with candidiasis. Its sources are chicken, turkey, pork, cottage cheese, and ricotta cheese. It can be converted by the liver to form glucose that is utilized by the body and is released by muscles for energy. It is associated with metabolism of tryptophan.

Androsterone is a male hormone made from cholesterol and is found in both sexes, It is a phenolic that is commonly found with immune system disorders. It is derived from pregnenolone and progesterone via testosterone by the adrenal cortex. It can increase sexual libido, basal metabolic rate, and renal transport of sodium and potassium.

Apiol, is very often found in individuals with CFIDS. Its source is pollen, vegetables, parsley, and fennel. It is also involved with musculoskeletal problems such as fibromayalgia.

Beta alanine is a non essential amino acid. It is also found in individuals with candidiasis. It is a metabolite of candida albicans. It forms part of the molecule of pantothenic acid in living organisms as well as in the laboratory. High levels of this amino acid can be an indicator of bowel toxicity because it can be recognized in the intestine.

Butyric acid is implicated in fibromayalgia and arthritic conditions. It is a saturated fatty acid. Its sources are present in butter and found in grapes, strawberries, apples, and rose oil. It is produced as a byproduct in hydrocarbon synthesis. It is commercially used in making candies, liquors, soda water syrup, butterscotch, caramel, fruit and nut flavoring, agent for gum, and ice cream and ices.

Caffeic acid is indicated with chronic fatigue, arthritis, lethargy, and mental confusion.

Its sources are asparagus, yam, potato, tomato, and tobacco. It has been isolated from green and roasted coffee, and it is found in decomposition of certain tannins.

Carnitine is a non essential amino acid and is indicated with muscle weakness and fibromayalgia. It is a constituent of striated muscle and liver. It is in avocado, breast milk, adrenal glands, and isolated from meat. Carnitine is stored in skeletal muscle. Ascorbic acid, niacin, and iron are necessary for synthesis of carnitine. There is a greater loss of carnitine in urine of muscular dystrophy. It also provides energy for sperm motility.

Coumarin is indicated with candida infections. It is found in wheat, rice, barley, corn, soy, cheese, beef, eggs, many plants, sweet clover, and commercially used for perfumes, deodorant soaps suntan lotion and flavoring for tobacco, and butter.

Ferrous fumerate is also indicated in candida infections and is used in antianemia preparations.

Gallic acid is indicated with CFIDS and is found in food coloring, cream of tartar, maple syrup, beer tea, and may have some antiviral activity.

Glutamine is a non essential amino acid and indicated with CFIDS and multiple sclerosis. It is found in sugar beets, carrots, radishes, and celery root. It is vital for energy and highly concentrated in the brain. It is a dominant amino acid in cerebral spinal fluid. Manganese is important in the synthesis of glutamine. It is essential for the synthesis of niacin.

5-hydroxytryptophan is a precursor of seratonin and is an antidepressant. Children with Down syndrome improved with the use of this and vitamin B6. Parkinson's patients also improved in mental behavior.

Hypericin is important for fatigue and depression.

Lactic acid is indicated for muscle fatigue, fibromyalgia, rheumatoid arthritis and osteoarthritis . Lactic acid occurs in sour milk, apples, tomato juice, beer, pickles sauerkraut, and wines and is found in muscles after activity. It is prepared commercially by fermentation of whey, cornstarch, potatoes, and molasses. It is involved in muscle contraction, and is increased in muscle and blood after vigorous activity. Epinephrine increases lactic acid in muscle and can cause muscle cramping. It is commercially used in food products, in medicine, and manufacturing cheese. It is found in ointments, and shampoos for scaly dermatitis.

Malvin is indicated with Multiple sclerosis, neuropathy, and depression and is the natural red and blue pigment in fruits and vegetables, such as strawberries, tomatoes, and concord grapes. It is also found in oranges, eggs, chickens, milk, soy foods, and dairy products.

Menadione is indicated in CFIDS, arthritis; colitis, and irritable bowel. It is found in fruits, cauliflower, green leafy vegetables, kelp, alfalfa, soy, and egg yolks. It can be manufactured in intestinal tract with intestinal bacteria. A deficiency can occur in hepato-biliary dysfunction which results in the inability of individuals to produce bile that is needed for absorption of fat soluble vitamins. It is also necessary as vitamin K for function of prothrombin in blood clotting. It is commercially used to prevent souring of milk products and is used as a fungicide.

Nicotine is implicated in those with candida, muscle inflammation and fibromyalgia. It is found in tobacco, beef, potato, tomato, and banana. It is commercially used as by-product in the tobacco industry. It is a vasoconstrictor.

Oxalic acid is indicated with those with fibromyalgia and arthritis. It is present in beet leaves and rhubarb. It ties up calcium and interferes with calcium absorption. It can be poisonous and can cause paralysis of the nervous system. It can lead to increase formation and deposition of oxalates in the kidney. It is commercially used in printing, dyeing, and bleaching fabrics, leathers, and straws. It is used in paper industry and photography. It removes paint, varnish, rust and ink stains.

Phytic acid is indicated in fibromyalgia and is a source in chlorophyll, grains, seeds and plants. It accounts for 86% of phosphorus present in seeds and is liberated by the germination process in wheat, rye, oats, peas, beans, barley, rice, flax seed, soybeans and peanuts. Phytic acid prevents absorption of zinc and trace minerals from the intestinal tract.

Piperine is found with those with candidiasis, and arthritis. It is found in beef, beet sugar, cheese, chicken, eggs, lamb, milk, tuna, turkey, yeast, black pepper, tomato, and potato. It is found in the nightshade family. It is commercially used as a pungent taste to brandy.

Proline is important for CFIDS and is a non essential amino acid. Its sources are wheat, gelatin and gelatin. Collagen is the main source. A deficiency of proline can cause degenerative disease and is common in the elderly. An increase of proline in the blood is seen in alcoholics and an excess of proline is seen in osteoporosis.

Threonine is common in all individuals with fatigue and is found in eggs, skim milk, casein, gelatin, oats. wheat germ, ricotta and cottage cheese, pork, chicken, turkey. Low levels of threonine and glycine are found in depressed patients.

Uric acid is important phenolic for arthritis. It is present in the urine of all carnivorous animals and in cat saliva. The end product of the nitrogenous metabolism of protein, it appears in the urine when the plasma concentration is slightly hither than normal. A high concentration of uric acid in the urine is an indication of poor protein metabolism or excess protein consumption. It may also be an indication of stones or calculi in the kidneys or bladder and may be linked to gout, hepatitis, and leukemia. We look at this level in the twenty-four hour urinalysis we conduct to monitor similation of various proteins. Certain foods can produce high uric acid levels including caffeine, beans, nicotine, meat, spinach, and mushrooms.

The amino acid tryptophan is broken down by bacteria to form indole and skatol. When indole is detectable in feces, it indicates bowel toxicity and fermentation of food by putrefactive bacteria. Indole is found in all complete proteins. When ingested, it penetrates the bowel and moves into the liver where it is converted to alcohol and excreted in the urine. Excessive production of indole can be carcinogenic. It is found in oranges, flowers, green vegetables, perfumes, and, in high levels in dairy products. When I find high levels of indole in laboratory tests and a person suffers from bloating and constipation, I suspect poor protein digestion. Based on indole levels and other markers, I recommend enzymes to help digest protein. Chronic bowel problems are fairly common among all immune disorders, especially CFIDS and Candidiasis.

I have had excellent results treating those with immune disorders for phenolics. Not only does it help reduce immune deficient symptoms but also helps desensitize people to many foods which contain phenolics.

ACID- AND ALKALINE-FORMING FOODS

Acid foods are sour and contain the element hydrogen. The sour taste of oranges and lemons, for example, is due to the acid they contain. Alkalies, or bases, have properties opposite to acids, and they neutralize acids. Our body fluids—blood and extracellular fluid—maintain a constant condition of alkalinity or acidity.

Foods can be acid or alkaline, or they can be acid or alkaline forming. The first category refers to how much acid or alkaline the foods contain. The second refers to the condition the foods cause in the body after being metabolized. Protein, for example, is an acid-forming food because acid is the by-product of its metabolism. The same is true of grains. Fruits and most vegetables oxidize when broken down and are considered alkaline-forming foods.

Some common acid- and alkaline-forming foods are:

ACID FORMING	ALKALINE FORMING
eggs	salt
grains	vegetables
meat	fruit
fish	wine
sugar	
nuts	
beans	

Individuals with colitis are commonly allergic to acid-forming foods and they tend to become more metabolically acidic (acidotic). This acidity causes sluggishness and bloating. It also causes gastritis, or reflux, which irritates the mucous membranes of the stomach, duodenum, or esophagus, a condition commonly known as "heartburn." This condition can even be the precursor to an ulcer.

This reaction is due to an allergy to the acids. Sugars, the major allergens for most immune disorders, are high in acid. An allergy can be detected with my normal muscle response testing procedure and treatment with NAET and enzymes. I have found antacid enzymes (stm) taken at night are very helpful.

Sometimes acid stomach irritation will mimic a hiatal hernia. This condition is especially prevalent among the elderly. There are chiropractic manipulation techniques I teach patients that help them manage this condition (refer to Hiatal Hernia Manipulation in Part VI, page 402 in *Winning the War Against Asthma and Allergies*).

POOR DIGESTION

The by-products of poor digestion can cause allergic reactions. Any undigested food—whether protein, carbohydrate, fat, or fiber—is absorbed into the bloodstream and regarded by the immune system as an allergen. In diagnosing and treating for allergens in our clinic, digestion is a key factor. We make sure that digestion is optimal because after clearing many allergies, we do not want people to walk out and develop more of them. I stress good digestion and talk about it with everyone who comes to see me. I make sure they chew their food well and recommend predigestive enzymes to help predigest their food. In my own experience, I found that using enzymes helped me reduce the reaction to foods to which I was allergic. Until all the foods are cleared with NAET, this can be a lifesaver and prevent them from developing new allergies.

VITAMIN AND MINERAL DEFICIENCIES

Vitamins are important supplements but many people are allergic to the vitamins they need to take. People tend to be deficient in the vitamins they are allergic to because their bodies are unable to absorb and use them. The vitamin allergies I have found most common in immune disorders are to Vitamin C, all the B vitamins, Vitamin A, Vitamin F (fatty acids), and Vitamin E.

Vitamin C

We all know that Vitamin C has a wide range of applications in the treatment and prevention of many diseases. Studies have shown it to be important to the health of the immune system and many books have been written about its benefits and the effects of Vitamin C deficiency. It is necessary for healthy skin, connective tissue, and gums. It is the most widely taken vitamin supplement.

As a chiropractor, I know that Vitamin C is vital to combating disease and healing muscle damage. It can also prevent the loss of other vitamins in the body such as A, E, and some of the B vitamins. Vitamin C has been shown to help protect the bronchial airways and lungs from the effects of environmental toxins such as cold temperatures, pollens, smog, fumes, and chemicals. It is also said to protect against viral and bacterial infections, such as colds and the flu, and to protect against radiation. Vitamin C is the primary **antioxidant** vitamin, preventing oxidation from damaging tissue and there is a high concentration of Vitamin C in white blood cells, especially lymphocytes. During infection, Vitamin C is depleted. Vitamin C has been shown to benefit many different immune functions including enhancing white blood cells to help fight infection. It also increases antibody response, and is a natural antiviral compound.

Clearly, the proper absorption and use of Vitamin C is an essential one and needs to be tested for an allergy to it. As suggested earlier, an allergy to C may be causing many of the symptoms the person is trying to treat by taking the vitamin in the first place. For example, chronic sore throats may be caused by an allergy to Vitamin C and taking the vitamin only makes the symptoms worse. After treatment for the allergy, the sore throat will disappear and Vitamin C can be taken freely without the recurrence of symptoms.

People spend large amounts of money on vitamins recommended by health food stores, doctors, and other practitioners that may not be doing them any good. If people are allergic to a vitamin they will not be able to absorb and utilize it, no matter how much they take. Once an allergy to Vitamin C has been treated, people begin to absorb it from their food. They also are able to better utilize the nutrients from their food without having to take excessive supplements.

Food sources for Vitamin C are tomatoes, citrus fruits, broccoli, strawberries, peppers, leafy greens, and potatoes. I do both laboratory testing and muscle response testing to determine the best dosage for each individual. For those who are not allergic, Vitamin C is harmless. It may increase toxicity, however, in those who are allergic and are not treated for the allergy.

B Vitamins

The B vitamin complex also presents problems to sensitive people. The complex is made up of at least eleven types of vitamins essential for the proper nourishment and functioning of our bodies. Almost everyone, however, is deficient in one or more B vitamins because it is difficult to get enough through normal diet, especially when there is a high consumption of processed foods. Excessive sugar intake can also deplete B vitamins. By reducing the body's reserve of B vitamins, sugar actually decreases the energy available. High levels of caffeine deplete Vitamin B, especially the natural relaxant inositol, as do alcohol, stress, illness, and physical activity. We need a fresh supply of B complex vitamins every day because the body does not store them. Any excess is washed out through the kidneys or through perspiration.

The B vitamins include:

- B_1, thiamin
- B_2, riboflavin
- B_3, niacin or niacinamide
- B_5, pantothenic acid
- B_6, pyridoxine or pyridoxal-5-phosphate
- B_{12}, cobalamin or cyanocobalamin
- folic acid or folicin
- biotin
- inositol
- choline
- para-aminobenzoic acid (PABA)

These eleven vitamins are synergistic which means they work as a team to perform all their vital individual functions properly, and are more potent taken together than separately. Therefore, many nutritionists recommend taking a B vitamin complex rather than single vitamins. For proper metabolism of the B vitamins the body must also maintain adequate levels of other nutrients such as iron and coenzymes. Thiamin, riboflavin, and niacin all bind to enzymes to help them do their job. None of these vitamins could function as effectively without their coenzymes. When treating for B vitamin allergies, it is important to check all the vitamins, related nutrients, and coenzymes for sensitivity.

The primary function of B vitamins is to convert carbohydrates, fats, and proteins into energy the body can use. They are vital to the proper functioning of the nervous system, production of red blood cells, maintenance of muscle tone in the GI tract, and the health of skin, hair, eyes, mouth, and liver. A high potency vitamin B complex helps in recovering from debilitating illness, alcoholism, or excessive use of medication by reducing the effects of stress and supporting the adrenal glands. Vitamin B supplementation is recommended for heavy coffee drinkers, women who take birth control pills, and people with high carbohydrate diets.

B_1, Thiamin B_1, or thiamine, aids in the digestion of carbohydrates, stabilizes the appetite, promotes growth and good muscle tone, inhibits pain, and assists in the normal functioning of the nervous system, muscles, and heart. Thiamin helps the body release energy from carbohydrates during metabolism. People who expend more energy and have high caloric intake need more thiamin than those who eat fewer calories. It can be depleted by excessive consumption of alcoholic beverages. A person deficient in B_1 might experience a loss of appetite and weight, feelings of weakness and fatigue, paralysis, nervousness, irritability, insomnia, unfamiliar aches and pains, depression, heart difficulties, and constipation or gastrointestinal problems. A thiamin deficiency can also cause the disease beriberi that results in weakness, nervous tingling of the body, and poor coordination.

Grain products including bread, cereals, pasta, and rice are good sources of thiamin. Others are meat (especially pork, poultry, and fish), fruits, vegetables, and sunflower seeds. Pasta, most instant and ready-to-eat cereals, and most breads made from refined flour are enriched with vitamins to replace the nutrients lost in processing, including thiamin.

B_2, Riboflavin   Vitamin B_2, or riboflavin, is necessary for the metabolism of carbohydrates, fats, and protein. B_2 also promotes general health by maintaining cell respiration, aid-ing in the formation of antibodies and red blood cells, ensuring good vision, relieving eye fatigue, and maintaining healthy nails and hair. The body's need for riboflavin may increase during periods of healing and pregnancy and in conditions such as asthma. A person deficient in B_2 might experience sluggishness, itching, and burning or bloodshot eyes, sores or cracks in and around the mouth and lips, purplish or inflamed tongue and mouth, dermatitis, oily skin, slowed growth, trembling, digestive problems, and respiratory problems.

Breads, cereals and other grain products, milk and milk products, meat, poultry, and fish are all good sources of riboflavin. Pasta and most breads made from refined flours are enriched with riboflavin because riboflavin is another of the nutrients lost in processing. To retain riboflavin during storage and cooking, food should be stored in containers through which light cannot pass, vegetables should be cooked in minimal amounts of water, and meat should be roasted or broiled.

B₃, Niacin   Vitamin B_3, niacin or niacinamide, helps to improve circulation and reduce the blood's cholesterol level. B_3 also assists in maintaining nervous system tissue, respiration, and fat synthesis. It aids in metabolizing protein, sugar and fat, helps to reduce high blood pressure, increases energy through the proper use of food, produces acid, metabolizes sex hormones, activates histamines, prevents pellagra (a disease characterized by diarrhea and dermatitis), and maintains healthy skin, tongue, and digestion. The body requires more niacin in periods of stress, acute illness, and low tryptophan intake.

B_3 is a good example of how a vitamin can be as effective as a drug in combating disease. Niacin, much less expensive than prescription medication, is successfully used to lower levels of harmful cholesterol **low-density lipoprotein (LDL)** and raise levels of good cholesterol **high-density lipoprotein (HDL)**.

A person deficient in B_3 might experience gastrointestinal disturbance, loss of appetite, indigestion, bad breath, canker sores, skin disorders or rashes, muscular weakness, fatigue, insomnia, vague aches and pains, headaches, nervousness, memory loss, irritability, or depression. It can also result in respiratory problems including asthma, chronic bronchitis, or pellagra.

Niacin is formed in the body from tryptophan, an essential amino acid found in meat, poultry, fish, and eggs. If a diet includes these foods, an individual will have less need for niacin from other sources. Good sources are meat, poultry, fish (especially tuna), bread, cereals and other grain products such as wheat bran, vegetables such as mushrooms or asparagus, and peanuts. Pasta and breads made from refined flours are usually fortified with niacin. Loss of niacin from foods due to preparation and storage is slight but vegetables should be cooked in a minimal amount of water, and meat should be roasted or broiled to retain the nutrient.

B_5, Pantothenic Acid B_5, pantothenic acid, participates in the release of energy from carbohydrates, fats, and proteins, aids in the utilization of vitamins, and improves the body's resistance to stress. It helps build cells, aids in the development of the nervous system and the immune system, maintains healthy skin, supports the adrenal glands in the production of cortisone in times of stress, fights infection by building antibodies, detoxifies the body, stimulates growth, and utilizes Vitamin D.

B_5 deficiencies can cause muscle cramping, painful and burning feet, skin abnormalities, retarded growth, dizzy spells, weakness, depression, decreased resistance to infection, restlessness, digestive disturbances, stomach stress, vomiting, and asthma.

B_6, Pyridoxine B_6, pyridoxine or pyridoxal-5-phosphate, is necessary for the synthesis and breakdown of

DNA, RNA, and amino acids, the building blocks of protein, and is required by the central nervous system for normal functioning of the brain. B_6 also aids in the metabolism of fat and carbohydrates, the formation of antibodies, and the removal of excess fluid and discomfort during menstrual periods. It aids hemoglobin in its function, promotes healthy skin, reduces muscle spasms, leg cramps, and stiffness of hands, helps prevent nausea, and promotes the balance of sodium and phosphorus in the body.

Conditions that respond to B_6 therapy include carpal tunnel syndrome, joint pain, homocystinuria, sensitivity to bright light, sensitivity to MSG, burning or tingling in the extremities, the inability to recall dreams, and imbalances of the liver. Because Vitamin B_6 is used by the body to break down protein, the more protein one eats, the more Vitamin B_6 one needs. Deficiencies can produce skin eruptions of dermatitis, loss of muscular control or muscle weakness, arm and leg cramps, fatigue, nervousness, irritability, insomnia, slow learning, water retention, anemia, mouth disorders, and hair loss.

Good sources of B_6 are meat, poultry, fish, fruits, vegetables, and grain products. Most ready-to-eat and instant cereals are fortified with B_6. To retain B_6 during cooking, serve fruits raw, cook foods in minimal amounts of water for the shortest time possible, and roast or broil meat and poultry.

B_{12}, Cobalamin B_{12}, cobalamin or cynocobalamin, is required for the formation and regeneration of red blood cells to help prevent anemia. B_{12} is also necessary for building genetic material, metabolizing carbohydrates, fat, and protein, increasing energy, and maintaining a healthy nervous system and muscles. It is important for promotion of DNA synthesis in childhood growth, cell longevity, memory improvement, maintenance of the appetite and digestive system, and strengthening of the immune system. It aids in the absorption of iron and calcium and helps prevent inflammation. It also assists in folate metabolism and in the synthesis of DNA and is essential to produce insulation for nerve fibers. B_{12} aids in the conversion of fat to lean muscle tissue. For this reason many athletes, such as weight lifters take B_{12} as a safe, competitive, and legal alternative to steroid hormones. A B_{12} folate complex can be used as a tonic to assist in the conversion of iron to hemoglobin, to help normalize hormonal production, and to improve short-term memory in the elderly. B_{12} is even considered an antiaging nutrient and an agent for increasing sperm count.

There is some controversy today about the best way to get enough B_{12} in our diets. Some claim that B_{12} is only acquired naturally by eating meat, eggs, and milk products, but vegetarians and vegans claim they have found numerous nonanimal sources of this vital nutrient including edible seaweed such as hijiki and wakame, certain mushrooms, sourdough bread, tofu, tempeh, miso, barley malt syrup, parsley, beer, cider, wine, and margarine. Some nutritionists disagree, saying that the only source of B_{12} available to vegetarians is fortified nutritional yeast, fortified breakfast cereals, soy milk, and other soy products.

Supplements that contain spirulina or nori can interfere with B_{12} absorption. Some experts also advise against taking multivitamin products because these preparations may contain products that interfere with the breakdown of B_{12}. By preventing the absorption of B_{12}, they help to create the deficiency they are supposed to correct.

B_{12} can be produced by bacterial activity in the body's own small intestines, mouth, teeth, gums, nasal passages, and around the tonsils, tongue and upper bronchial tree. Because B_{12} is often found in soil, freshly picked raw, unwashed vegetables, especially root vegetables, may have B_{12} on their surfaces. To retain the B_{12} in meat or fish, they should be roasted or broiled.

A person deficient in B_{12} could experience pernicious (life-threatening) anemia, degeneration of the spinal cord and nerves, poor appetite, stunted growth in children, nervousness, depression, lack of balance, neuritis, or brain damage. Symptoms of anemia include a pale yellow, sallow complexion, a shiny or red, sore tongue, weakness and fatigue progressing to paralysis, numbness or tingling in hands and feet, gradual deterioration of motor coordination, moodiness, poor memory and confusion, delirium, delusion, hallucinations, and psychotic states. Paralysis and possible death may occur with the deterioration of myelin sheaths and the failure of DNA production.

A B_{12} deficiency, especially among the elderly, may occur even though the person's diet contains enough B_{12} because other substances needed for B_{12} absorption are lacking. For example, the stomach manufactures an "intrinsic factor" that must bond with B_{12} before the body can absorb it. Other substances needed for absorption include iron, folic acid, and a factor manufactured in the stomach that can be blocked by intestinal parasites. Microorganisms in the stomach can compete for the B_{12} and toxins can block absorption. Enzyme deficiencies, liver or kidney disease, and atrophic gastritis can interfere with the utilization of B_{12}.

B_{12} can be further depleted by disease, **hypothyroidism**, and an allergy to lactose. Consumption of foods such as meat and animal products, refined sugars, carbohydrates, drugs, chemicals, caffeine, alcoholic beverages, tobacco, mega doses of Vitamin C, egg albumen, egg yoke, and allergies to any of those can all use up the body's storage of B_{12}.

Sufficient levels of B_{12} are considered especially crucial for women during pregnancy and lactation. The most nutrient-dense source of B_{12} is organ meat such as the heart, liver, and kidney. Clams, oysters, beef, pork, eggs, and milk are also good sources of B_{12}.

Folic Acid   Folic acid (folate or folicin) helps the body form red blood cells and aids in the formation of genetic material within every body cell. Folic acid also works with Vitamin B_{12} in synthesizing DNA and RNA, essential for the growth and reproduction of all body cells. It is useful in amino acid conversion, breakdown and assimilation of protein, stimulation of appetite, the maintenance of a healthy intestinal tract, and nucleonic acid formation. Folic acid may reverse certain anemias, reduce the risk of cervical dysplasia, and lower the likelihood of heart attack. It becomes even more essential during times of growth and cell reproduction, especially during pregnancy, when folic acid seems to be in short supply. It protects the body against neural tube defects in unborn babies and other midline birth anomalies.

Folic acid deficiency during pregnancy can cause the disease spina bifida in the child which can be permanently crippling. Recently it was discovered that folic acid reduces the risk of premature birth. Deficiency can result in megaloblastic anemia in which red blood cells fail to divide properly and become large and abnormal, causing a shortage of red blood cells. Other symptoms of folic acid deficiency are GI disorders, prematurely gray hair, pale tongue, and Vitamin B_{12} deficiency.

Good sources of folic acid include fruits and vegetables, especially citrus fruits, tomatoes, foliage, cooked spinach, lettuce, broccoli, grain products, and organ meats. To retain folic acid, fruits and vegetables should be served raw, if possible, or steamed or simmered in a minimal amount of water. Store vegetables in the refrigerator.

Biotin   Biotin helps to strengthen the immune system, aids in the utilization of protein, folic acid, pantothenic acid, and Vitamin B_{12}, aids in cell growth, fatty acid production, and synthesis, helps in the formation of DNA and RNA, and helps produce healthy hair.

Anyone allergic to this B vitamin is not properly absorbing it or the other B vitamins. An allergy to biotin produces a deficiency in all the B vitamins. A biotin deficiency leads to drowsiness, extreme exhaustion, depression, loss of appetite, muscle pain, and gray skin color.

Inositol   Inositol, found in every cell of the body, is necessary for the growth of muscle cells and the formation of lecithin. It aids in the breakdown of fats, helps reduce blood cholesterol, and helps prevent thinning hair. Inositol is also an antioxidant free radical scavenger and is known as "nature's tranquilizer" for the calming effect it often has. A deficiency may result in hair loss, eczema, constipation, migraines, and high-blood cholesterol.

Choline   Choline is very important in controlling fat and cholesterol buildup in the body, preventing fat from accumulating in the liver, and facilitating the movement of fats in the cells and throughout the bloodstream. It also helps regulate the kidneys, liver, gallbladder, and is important to the health of myelin sheaths that cover the nerve fibers, and to nerve transmission. Choline is known to help improve memory, support brain chemistry, and is an essential component of acetylcholine, an important neurotransmitter.

A deficiency may result in cirrhosis and fatty degeneration of the liver, hardening of the arteries, heart problems, high blood pressure, and hemorrhaging kidneys. Choline should be taken with the other B vitamins for optimal effectiveness.

Para-Aminobenzoic Acid (PABA)   Para-aminobenzoic acid (PABA) is a component of folic acid as well as an antioxidant and membrane stabilizer. It helps to prevent red blood cells from bursting and lysosomal membranes from breaking and releasing tissue-damaging enzymes. PABA helps to produce folic acid and aids in the formation of red blood cells and the assimilation of pantothenic acid. It produces healthy skin and skin pigmentation, helps return gray hair to its natural color, and screens the skin from sun exposure. A PABA deficiency causes extreme fatigue, irritability, depression, nervousness, eczema, constipation, digestive disorders, headaches, and premature gray hair.

Allergies to B vitamins are among the most important to treat with NAET because many foods have high B vitamin content. Eating vitamin-rich food and taking supplements can do more harm than good to B vitamin sensitive people. For individuals with immune disorders the most common problems are with Vitamin B_2 (riboflavin), B_3, B_5, B_6 (pyridoxine), and B_{12} (cobalamin). Other B vitamins, or all of them, can cause difficulties. With these individuals, I test each of the B vitamins separately.

Possible symptoms of B vitamin deficiency are mood swings, behavioral problems, cold sores, herpes, extreme fatigue, severe bloating, malnutrition, chronic sinus congestion, and chronic yeast infection. Chronic yeast infections always involve B vitamin allergies and deficiencies, and treating for B vitamins can sometimes clear the infections before the yeast is treated. I have seen miraculous results with all kinds of symptoms from clearing only one of the B vitamins. These are so important that I sometimes have patients treat themselves at home for several days or a few times in one day, using the acupressure points shown in the Self-Treatment Section of Chapter 5 (p. 66) and some chiropractic reflex points.

Vitamin E

Vitamin E is a fat soluble antioxidant that protects cells from free radical damage and neutralizes the damaging effects of ozone. Because many individuals with immune disorders tend to worsen after ozone exposure, this can be a key nutrient for them.

Vitamin A

Vitamin A comes in two forms: betacarotene, found in a wide variety of fruits and vegetables; and Vitamin A itself, found in liver, eggs, cod liver oil, butter, and dairy products. Recent research suggests that betacarotene, known to be a precursor to Vitamin A, boosts the immune system and prevent arteries from clogging. Betacarotene and Vitamin A are both fat soluble vitamins. Vitamin A is important for good eyesight, healthy skin, a healthy intestinal tract, and as protection against pollutants. It is important in strengthening the immune system and protecting against infection. High doses of Vitamin A can help fight viral infections and are effective in combatting illnesses and treating wounds.

Excessive consumption of alcohol and the liver damage that results depletes Vitamin A. When the liver is impaired, the body is not able to metabolize Vitamin A and several other nutrients. Smoking also depletes Vitamin A in the respiratory tract. When treating a patient for smoking, it is important to treat for Vitamin A allergy and deficiency as well.

Because Vitamin A is retained in the body, it is important not to take excessively high doses that can build up to a toxic level. An allergy check should always be done before taking supplements.

I have treated many people, especially children, for Vitamin A. This allergy is significant in children who have chronic coughs, chronic infections involving the respiratory system, and asthma. Treating their Vitamin A allergy with NAET and giving them liquid Vitamin A with betacarotene has been helpful.

Food sources of Vitamin A include eggs, butter, fish, oils, and milk. Betacarotene is found in deep green vegetables such as spinach, broccoli, sweet potatoes, carrots, squash (especially winter squash), grapefruit, mangos, and apricots. These foods also contain large amounts of Vitamin C and other antioxidants. People with hypothyroidism have trouble converting betacarotene to Vitamin A and require regular intake of Vitamin A through food or supplements.

Vitamin F (Fatty Acids)

Essential fatty acids help build cell membranes, support the nervous system, and boost the immune system to help ward off disease. Fat also helps slow the release of sugar into the bloodstream and is especially important for those who are hypoglycemic or diabetic. Fat is needed for absorption of Vitamins A, D, K, and betacarotene.

Of all the fats we consume only two are essential. They are the omega-6 fatty acid (linolenic) and the omega-3 fatty acid (alpha linolenic). Eating junk food, including fat-free health store junk food, depletes the body's store of essential fatty acids. Fried foods, margarine, and vegetable shortening cause oils to become rancid and should be avoided.

Omega-6 can be found in all vegetable oils and most grains and beans. Omega-3 is found in flax seed, flax oil, fresh walnuts, walnut oil, pumpkin seeds, soy, and canola oils. It is important to buy oils that are not refined or rancid and to avoid buying oils sold in light glass bottles in supermarkets (look for the dark green bottles instead).

Because good fat metabolism is a key to proper use of essential fatty acids, I use enzyme therapy to ensure absorption of the good fatty acids from the regular diet. This works well in combination with NAET treatment for any allergy to fatty acids or the foods containing them.

Minerals

Minerals that may cause sensitivities include silver, gold, copper, vanadium, potassium, sulfur, copper, chromium, and magnesium. A deficiency of magnesium, an important mineral for those with immune disorders, is characterized by mental confusion, irritability, problems with muscle and nerve contraction, muscle cramps, insomnia, and loss of appetite. Magnesium is involved with energy production and cellular replication. One man with chronic Candida and chronic sinus infections came to see me. After treating for the first few basic allergens, I tested him for minerals and found an allergy to magnesium. When I treated him for this allergy and gave him supplements of 1,000–1500 milligrams per day, he had far fewer symptoms with infrequent reactions. For infants and children, I supplement their diets with a liquid magnesium that is tolerated at about one teaspoon per twenty pounds of body weight. As with other supplements, I test the individual to find out how much supplement is needed. Foods that are high in magnesium include seafood, whole grains, dark green vegetables, molasses, nuts, and bone meal. As it turns out, immune disorder sufferers are allergic to magnesium and respond well to treatment for it.

Antioxidants

Antioxidants are known as free radical scavengers because they remove dangerous free radical particles from the tissues, strengthen the immune system, build up tissues, and regenerate the body. They are particularly important for anyone with a chronic illness. The basic antioxidants are Vitamins C and E, the B vitamins, fatty acids, and beta-carotene. New antioxidants are being discovered all the time including zinc, copper, selenium, N-acetylcystine (NAC), glutamine, and choline. I test and treat for each one of these because they are so important. Once people are cleared of sensitivities to antioxidants, they should be able to derive them easily from eating a good diet because antioxidants are plentiful in many foods.

One antioxidant worth discussing in greater detail is NAC, an amino acid and building block for glutathione, one of the most powerful free radical scavengers in the body. Glutathione helps the liver detoxify medications and is particularly helpful for those on large amounts of medication. Their immune systems have been compromised. They need help in detoxifying their immune system and building up their energy and stamina.

Selenium, a trace mineral, is another building block of glutathione and is important for detoxification. Selenium also helps Vitamin E prevent free radical damage.

Ginkgo is a traditional herb in Chinese medicine that can also be helpful to CFIDS.

ENZYME DEFICIENCIES

Through muscle testing, the palpation exam, and urinalysis I use for enzyme evaluation, I have found that many individuals with immune disorders are extremely deficient in amylase (refer to Chapter 13 for a more in-depth discussion). Because amylase is an important anti-inflammatory, people who are deficient cannot fight properly against environmental pollutants and allergens. In combination with other enzymes, amylase is important in digesting carbohydrates. I have found that this deficiency is often linked to an allergy to amylase and to the enzyme amylopsin. Treating the allergies and then supplementing with the enzymes can be very helpful.

Protease is another enzyme that is critical in treatment. It is important for digesting protein and as a natural antibiotic, anti-infectant, and anti-inflammatory agent. It can help fight pathogens, repair tissue damage, regenerate tissue, remove tissue debris, and break down foreign bodies that might be identified as allergens or pathogens by the immune system.

Much of the vulnerability to infections is because of a deficiency of protease. I always test for it and then supplement with it in high doses once the allergy (trauma) is cleared. Since those who are allergic to protease may experience upper gastrointestinal problems or pre-ulcerous gastritis, treating this allergy often resolves such problems.

Cortisone, a synthetic version of cortisol, is commonly used as an anti-inflammatory for chronic conditions such as Multiple Sclerosis (MS) and rheumatoid arthritis. People who are allergic to their own cortisol also may be allergic to cortisone, causing serious reactions. A study done on seventy-six patients treated with cortisone showed that cortisone therapy tended to cause an inability to digest carbohydrates that may have resulted from a deficiency of amylase. Cortisone can also causes a worsening of gastroduodenal ulcers, bleeding, and even perforation of the intestinal lining. Women over fifty tend to have reflux and gastritis and cortisone therapy can worsen these conditions.

Gastric problems can be helped with several enzymes including papain from papaya, lipase, and protease. Because people who have problems digesting proteins may be sensitive to protease, it can be helpful to treat for cortisone, protease, and food allergens.

Cortisone therapy also lessens the resistance of patients to infection that results in fever, malaise, chronic bronchitis, and sinusitis. Many individuals who have been on prednisone and cortical steroids or hydrocortisone therapy for some time are deficient in protease, a natural anti-inflammatory. Supplementing with protease helps them fight infections and deal with inflammation naturally. The enzyme inhibits inflammation without suppressing amino acids, as steroids do, and improves blood circulation and nutrition of the tissue.

Many people with chronic health problems such as fatigue, asthma, and rheumatoid arthritis do extremely well with enzyme therapy. The most noticeable results are with asthmatics who have problems with chronic infections. They generally come in with recurring bronchitis, always on antibiotics, never looking well, and never having enough energy. After enzyme therapy they are able to fight infections without using antibiotics and have far fewer asthma episodes than with steroid therapy. They are happier, feel and look better, and do not age as quickly.

One asthmatic patient of mine was traveling with a friend who showed signs of infection. The patient treated herself for her saliva with NAET using the acupressure points she had learned and increased her protease and antioxidant intake. She was able to resist the infection without using antibiotics which she had been unable to do before.

METABOLIC IMBALANCES

One of the primary causes of metabolic imbalance is the toxicity resulting from the body's inability to rid itself of metabolic waste products. This condition is worsened by incomplete oxidation in the tissues, poor nutrition, and the resulting chronic disease. The liver, the organ primarily responsible for the elimination of toxins, is severely stressed by prolonged treatment with cortisone, antibiotics, and other medications. Other organs responsible for detoxification include the skin, intestines, kidneys, and lungs.

Good blood and lymphatic circulation is also important for detoxification. The blood supplies oxygen and nutrients to the cells and cleanses, transports, and disposes of metabolic waste through excretion by means of the intestines, kidneys, lungs, and skin. In the lymphatic system, macrophages, the body's first line of defense against infection, travel around, eating up foreign substances and breaking them down into smaller, nontoxic components. Well-functioning macrophages are essential to the effective elimination of pathogens, metabolic waste, and toxins.

In a healthy immune system, the antibodies and lymphocytes are present in the blood and lymph and immediately recognize foreign cells such as bacteria, viruses, fungi, and toxic waste. They bind with these substances to form immune complexes that can be degraded and eaten up by the macrophages. When a small number of immune complexes are present, the macrophages can easily consume them before they do harm. But when an overabundance of immune complexes are present or the macrophages are inhibited by medications and metabolic waste, these complexes affix themselves to body tissue. This calls the secondary backup immune defenses into play that cause autoimmune inflammation and, ultimately, chronic degenerative disorders such as chronic fatigue, fibromyalgia, rheumatoid arthritis, thyroid disease, and colitis.

These immune complex diseases do not occur as long as macrophages retain their ability to function properly. Many metabolic toxins and addictive substances such as cocaine, morphine, steroids, and cortisone inhibit macrophage activity and thus contribute to immune complex disease. Certain enzyme mixtures are effective in removing and preventing immune complexes and keeping macrophage activity intact. Treatment of chronic degenerative disorders caused by circulating immune complexes with enzymes and NAET can result in improvement in appetite, reduction in depression, and decrease in inflammation.

To correct metabolic imbalances in individuals with immune disorders, it is important to facilitate the excretion and elimination of metabolic waste and toxins from the body. Those with Candida are often constipated, experience chronic loose stools, or fluctuate between the two. They may also suffer bloating and malabsorption. These problems are usually caused by sugar and starch intolerance and poor digestion. I use enzymes to treat this condition rather than more invasive therapies such as enemas or colonics.

In addition to facilitating proper intestinal elimination, I also ensure the kidneys are working properly. They can be stimulated by increasing liquid intake, using herbs such as horsetail and goldenrod, and prescribing enzymes for optimal kidney detoxification. The herbs are mild diuretics that stimulate kidney function. Exercise and diet are also important, as is the process of clearing food allergies and avoiding highly toxic food such as alcohol, caffeine, and excess salt.

The skin is an important organ of elimination and skin brushing is one method of helping the skin detoxify.

Using a firm, hard vegetable brush, brush your skin vigorously for five minutes before you take a shower in the
morning. Foods that can clog or toxify the skin are food
allergens found in dairy products and highly fatty foods.
Foods that help the skin with elimination are those high
in enzymes and Vitamins A and E such as wheat germ oil
and betacarotene.

The liver, the principle organ of detoxification, eliminates inhaled and ingested substances, toxic compounds,
and drug by-products from the gastrointestinal organs. Allopathic physicians assess liver function with blood tests or a
blood panel that evaluates the combination of liver enzymes appearing in the serum when hepatic tissue damage
occurs. Many of these blood tests, however, only show abnormalities when there is liver injury or other physiological
problems. Unfortunately, they do not detect toxification. To
accurately detect dysfunction, we must inspect other areas
for evaluation and diagnosis. There are certain laboratories
that do assess liver dysfunction through a specialized "challenge test" to the liver. The test assesses an individual's
functional capacity or hepatic detoxification ability. One
laboratory doing this type of liver function test is Great
Smokies Diagnostic Laboratory in North Carolina (refer to
Miscellaneous Resources in Part VI).

Many factors contribute to liver toxification such as
drug reactions, pesticides, hormones, inhaled toxic substances, food allergies, and genetic disposition. Genetically
determined enzyme processes may vary and influence the
individual's ability to detoxify. For example, risk for smoking induced cancer and other health problems depend in
part on one's genetic detoxification system. Individuals
who cannot adequately detoxify the hydrocarbons in cigarette smoke have increased risks for smoking induced cancers. Exposure to fat soluble toxins, pesticides, and alcohol
may also increase the risk of liver damage by depleting important antioxidants and increasing oxidant induced damage. Oxygen free radicals play a significant role in the

promotion and progression of liver diseases. Metabolites from gut bacteria as well as substances such as sulfites, naturally occurring compounds in foods that are used as food additives, can deter liver detoxification and contribute to liver damage.

By decreasing allergic response and improving digestion and immune function, NAET and enzyme therapy can help spare the liver unnecessary toxification.

In addition, there are many good liver detoxification programs utilizing supplements and nutrients such as the amino acids, Vitamin B_5 (pantothenic acid), certain hepatic coenzymes, glutathione, and sulfates to rid the liver of drugs, food additives, environmental pollutants, and steroid hormones. Recent studies have shown that people with chronic fatigue, fibromyalgia, multiple chemical sensitivities, and asthma suffer metabolic toxicity and imbalance and, therefore, benefit from such programs.

Liver and bowel detoxification programs are begun after the ten basic allergies and the infectant allergies are cleared. They usually last for two to three weeks, sometimes longer if necessary. For intensified detoxification, I complement the program with enzymes and dietary recommendations.

7 | LITTLE-KNOWN CAUSES OF IMMUNE DISORDERS

Oops, sorry, starting to fade again.
Beware the Ides of Marshmallows,
MSG and cottonseed oil.
—from "Case Study of Cognitive Dysfunction
in 3.5 Million CFIDS Patients"

Jonathan

Jonathan, a 47-year-old with HIV, changed more quickly and dramatically than any other patient I have ever seen. In relatively good health, he was referred by a friend whose migraines had responded well to NAET. A smoker, Jonathan knew how stressful the combination of smoking and HIV was for his immune system, and he wanted to keep his immune system strong. He also hoped I might be able to help him stop smoking.

He did remodeling work for a living and found that he developed a rash when he was exposed to dust and certain chemicals. As a child, he had been diagnosed with colitis, and he still had some minor problems digesting food. He also knew that he was allergic to corn. Although he had had HIV for 10 years, he was almost symptom free. The fact that his body had adapted well to the virus suggested that his immune system was unusually strong. He was not taking any medication for HIV, but he was on all kinds of vitamins, including one to combat yeast because he suspected that the rashes were related to yeast.

A urinalysis indicated that Jonathan was quite healthy. The only thing that stood out was a slightly acidic pH and a very low calcium phosphate, usually related to sugar digestion. Everything else was normal. On his abdominal diagnostic exam, the only thing I noticed was a problem absorbing and digesting sugars. I prescribed an enzyme to help digest sugars (pan) and some other standard enzymes for HIV or chronic fatigue (AllerZyme V), as well as a spleen enzyme (spl) and protease to help fight antigens, bacteria, and viruses (trauma). Then I did some allergy testing and found that he was allergic to quite a few things. As I mentioned earlier, the test shows intolerances as well as allergies, and these usually disappear when the the basic allergies clear. He was allergic to dairy, milk, some grains, beans, nuts, seeds, eggs, food additives, food coloring, vegetables, minerals, hormones, sugars, salt, yeast, coffee, chocolate, caffeine, some trace elements, fruits, and some viruses including HIV.

I treated him with NAET for the basics, consisting of eggs and chicken, calcium, Vitamin C, all the B vitamins, sugars, and salt. Then I did a retest to see what was left. Much to my amazement, the only allergens we still needed to treat were the HIV and Epstein-Barr viruses, DDT, and dairy. The change was remarkable. I have never worked with anyone who cleared so many things by clearing the basics. His digestion was vastly improved, his low back pain had subsided, and he had much more energy. But the smoking was still a problem.

Next, we treated him for the blood and for the HIV virus, alone and in combination with DNA-RNA. Then I treated with many other combinations as needed. When we treated for dairy and for corn, Jonathan noticed another shift in his energy. Then we did DDT. Two days later, he called me up to tell me that the most amazing thing had happened. He had lost his desire to smoke. Apparently cigarettes contain some DDT, and he had developed an addiction to it. It has been two years now, and he has not smoked since. Jonathan made remarkable progress for someone with HIV, and he continues to do well.

In Chapters 5 and 6, I covered some of the most obvious causes of immune disorders. In this chapter I provide both practitioners and patients with insights into some of the less obvious causes of immune disorders. Some of the least researched allergens found in immune disorders are included in this chapter. These allergens were uncovered because of persistent study and research. Patients gave me the tools and their suffering gave me the motivation to find answers that would end their struggles. Sometimes the results were dramatic: in a matter of twenty-four hours their lives were profoundly changed. Many of these results surprised me and gave me the drive to further explore potentially new areas of allergies.

CONTACTANTS

Latex

One of the most common but largely unrecognized **contactants** is latex. Over the past five years latex has been used more frequently in a variety of professions. More than 100,000 health-care workers such as dentists, doctors, nurses, and laboratory technicians are exposed to latex on the job. People with high exposure to latex and a history of allergies are at risk for an allergic reaction as well as people who have frequent surgical procedures. Dermatitis and rashes may be irritated by latex exposure. Studies in the United States and Great Britain have found that the body produces specific antibodies to high levels of latex. Latex is used in hospitals and medical practices for such items as anesthetic tubing and ventilation bags.

The American College of Allergy, Asthma, and Immunology (ACAAI) has called for the protection of health-care workers and consumers who are said to use over seven million metric tons of latex every year in such items as balloons, condoms, tires, waist bands, rubber toys, bottle nipples, and pacifiers. The ACAAI wants immediate implementation of FDA regulations that would require labeling of latex, banning the "hypoallergenic" label on some latex gloves, and regulating maximum amounts of extractable allergen in latex products. The organization also recommends improved testing for the allergy, the identification of nonallergenic forms of latex, "latex safe" zones in workplaces, and research into the cause of latex allergies.

NAET offers an alternative approach. I have treated many people successfully for serious latex allergies. Many of them were able to continue using latex in their jobs for their protection and the protection of their clients. One patient was a nurse practitioner who had to wear latex all the time which exacerbated her fibromyalgia and fatigue. Since her treatment with NAET, she has been able to wear latex on the job without any problems. Many dentists I see also wear latex gloves all day. Most sensitive people who wear latex for prolonged periods of time will develop an allergy to it. NAET can provide a way to deal with this new and growing problem.

Formaldehyde

Some contactants also identified as inhalants include formaldehyde, hair spray, bug sprays, clothing labels, nail chemicals, and hair chemicals. Formaldehyde is extremely widespread. It is found in new fabrics, the dye on clothing tags, pressed wood, Wite•Out®, plastics, finishing materials, leather goods, decaffeinated coffee, ice cream, embalming fluid, plaster, concrete, antiperspirant, antiseptics in mouth washes, germicidal and detergent soap, hair products, aerosol deodorant, tanning agents, and the like.

Although formaldehyde is used in the formation of slow-release nitrogen fertilizer, it can also be responsible for plant disease. Because it kills bacteria, fungi, mold, and yeast it is used to disinfect equipment used in fermentation processes and in the manufacture of antibiotics. It is used in the synthesis of explosives as well as the synthesis of Vitamin A and to improve the activity of Vitamin E preparations. Formaldehyde improves the strength and water-resistance of paper products and is a preservative and accelerator for photographic developing solutions. It is sometimes used in the manufacture of both synthetic and natural fabrics, making them crease-resistant, wrinkle-resistant, crush-proof, water-repellent, dye-fast, flame-resistant, water-resistant, shrink-proof, moth-proof, and elastic.

Chemicals

Many other chemicals act as contact allergens and more are found to be problems every year. The following is a list of contact chemicals used in a wide variety of cleaning, makeup, and fabric products that I have found to be particularly problematic for those with immune disorders:

- acetone in nail polish remover
- methanol
- benzyl alcohol
- ethylene oxide
- butter yellow
- estradiol benzoate-8
- Congo red
- sulfa-urea
- carbon tetrachloride used for dry cleaning
- trichloroethylene
- chromium oxide
- benzinum crudum
- mangan peroxydatum
- plumbum bromatum
- plumbum sulfuricum

- polyester

- dimethyl terephthalate

- ethylene glycol

- isopropyl glycol found in many cosmetics and deodorant sprays

- paraffinum

- laundry detergent

- hydrazine sulfate

- toluene

- xylene

- asbestos

- tipa white

- benzanthracene

- cyclohexanol

- amyl alcohol

Fabrics and Dyes

It is important to treat individuals for fabrics because any fabric, natural or synthetic, can cause symptoms. I have treated people for reactions to cotton, linen, silk, wool, rayon, nylon, acetate, acrylic, polyester, jute, and kapok. One woman always wore linen. Whenever I did NAET treatments, I could never get a strong muscle response in the testing. It turned out she was allergic to linen and wearing it weakened her. Another woman was allergic to virtually every fabric. We had to treat her lying almost naked, making sure that there was no fabric near her hand when we were muscle testing. Leather can also be a problem, particularly for those allergic to animal dander or tannic acid. A tannic acid allergy can also cause a reaction to tea. I have seen miraculous results from treating for fabrics, sometimes within the first twenty-four hours. One person's smelling and tasting abilities were restored. Another's long-term eczema subsided and yet another client felt more focused and energetic. Itching, dry skin, and chronic ailments can all decrease dramatically or disappear. Treating for the dyes in fabrics is also important in desensitizing people to clothing, wallpaper, mattresses, bedding, and towels.

Several years ago I bought my daughter a bed sheet decorated with Disney characters. Every time she slept on it she would get stuffed up and cough. I found that she was allergic to the dyes in the fabric as well as to the polyester fabric itself. Once she was cleared for these allergens she could sleep on the sheet without any problems. Some of the most important fabric dyes to treat are:

- aniline, the blue-black dye used in newsprint
- anthracene, used in the manufacture of most dye products and fixed with formaldehyde
- anthraquinone, a commercial vat dye
- benzene, used in dye manufacturing
- bromine, used in organic dyes
- chromium oxydatum, a dye used in tannin and in the ink on dollar bills.

Wood

Wood resin is another contactant that should be checked if a person has a lot of exposure to it. I have seen people allergic to wood in musical instruments (a violin bow, piano keys, the wood of a harp) as well as the finishing of the wood itself. Dr. Nambudripad tells of treating one asthmatic for an allergy to bamboo (cane) furniture with very positive results.

Daily Contactants

Contactants also include common household products such as cosmetics, soaps, skin creams, detergents, metal polishes, hair dyes, rubber gloves, acrylic nails, nail polish and remover, metals (silver, nickel, and gold) in jewelry or flatware, gasoline products, celluloid, flowers, and bulbs. Many people are also allergic to computers, computer keyboards, telephones, vinyl chairs, plastic or carton containers, and other disposable products. I have seen women allergic to their panty hose, and people allergic to toilet paper and paper towels. Silicone, found in glass doors, breast implants, and the newest organic fabrics causes allergic reactions in some people. Then there are the less obvious occupational allergens which fall into the contactant group. For example, printers are often allergic to a fine lacquer spray used for drying ink to keep it from smudging.

Allergy to an Individual's Energy Field

Literally anything or anyone, no matter how benign or unlikely, can be an allergen. Surprisingly, we can even be allergic to people: our spouses, children, or parents. I found it hard to believe at first that a mother could be allergic to her own child, or vice versa, or that a man could be allergic to his spouse. It does, however, happen. I have treated many siblings, mothers, and fathers for allergies to their loved ones, and each time there have been dramatic changes. It may be easier to understand when we consider that everything and everyone has its own electromagnetic energy field. One cannot underestimate how severe an allergy can be to another person or the symptoms it can cause. I have seen symptoms such as irritability, constant bitterness, anger, fear, and an inability to be affectionate all respond to treatment. Sometimes being a good detective can transform people's lives and relationships.

Miscellaneous Contactants

Other contactants include plant oils found in plants such as poison oak, poison ivy, asparagus fern, and eucalyptus. Synthetic contactants include adhesive tape, cement, paper products, crude oil, plastics, newsprint, and photocopy paper and materials. I have also treated many people who were allergic to the plastic or other materials in their eyeglasses or contact lenses.

HISTAMINE

Histamine, actually a phenolic, is a very important allergen that plays a major role in all allergy reactions. Histamine is a major neurotransmitter in the brain, particularly in the hippocampus, and throughout the nervous system. It can also stimulate the secretion of hydrochloric acid in the stomach. Studies indicate that about twenty percent of schizophrenics have high levels of histamine whereas rheumatoid arthritics and Parkinson's patients have low levels.

All allergic individuals have high levels of IgE antibodies. When an allergen such as dust reacts with an IgE antibody, an allergen-antibody reaction takes place and the individual experiences an allergic reaction. IgE antibodies attach to mast cells and basophiles, causing them to rupture and release histamine. Increased levels of histamine cause the dilation of blood vessels and the contraction of smooth muscle cells. A number of different abnormal symptoms occur, depending on the type of tissue in which the histamine is released. An allergy to histamine greatly intensifies reactions to other allergens.

A sensitivity to histamine can cause depression, fatigue, hay fever, hyperactivity, hypertension, night sweats, premenstrual syndrome (PMS), sinusitis, stomach pain, and vertigo. Histamine is found in wine, beer, oysters, perch, salmon, scallops, shrimp, trout, tuna fish, cod fish, flounder, halibut, haddock, lobster, black bass, catfish, crab meat, yeast mix, human milk, cow and goat milk, cocoa, mutton, ham, chicken, and turkey.

GLANDS AND HORMONES

Many positive results have been obtained by treating individuals with immune disorders for adrenal and thyroid hormones as well as for the glands themselves. If people are allergic or sensitive to their own hormones, they develop a deficiency because they cannot properly absorb them into their tissues. I also have good success increasing energy and restoring good respiratory function by treating for epinephrine, norepinephrine, and adrenaline.

Adrenal Glands

The adrenal glands lie above the kidneys and are composed of the adrenal medulla and the adrenal cortex. The adrenal medulla secretes adrenaline and norepinephrine and the adrenal cortex secretes corticoid steroids, glycol corticoids, and androgens.

When tissue is damaged by trauma, infection, allergy, or by some other means, it becomes inflamed. In some circumstances the inflammation is more damaging than the trauma or infection itself. The body naturally produces cortisol to reduce all aspects of the inflammatory process by blocking the inflammatory response. It is very important that the adrenal glands function normally and are able to secrete cortisol in a natural form. If artificial sources such as cortisone, prednisone, methylprednisone, or dexamethasone are taken for prolonged periods to remedy a shortage of cortisol, they actually shrink the adrenal glands which, in turn, produce less cortisol. These artificial sources of cortisol also suppress the immune system. This suppression causes reduced numbers of **lymphocytes**, T cells, and antibodies that not only increases the incidence of allergies, but also makes a person more susceptible to infections and chronic health problems.

In my practice, every allergic individual is tested and treated for their own adrenal hormones. Individuals always report positive improvement in their health after this treatment. They feel more energetic and are less sensitive to their surroundings.

Thyroid Gland

The thyroid, a gland located immediately below the larynx in front of the trachea (windpipe), secretes the hormones thyroxine (ninety percent) and triiodothyronine (ten percent), respectively referred to as T_4 and T_3, that increase the individual's metabolic rate. The thyroid stimulates all aspects of carbohydrate metabolism and enhances the metabolism of fats. Both the heart rate and blood volume can be influenced by the thyroid. Because most thyroxine is eventually converted to T_3 in the liver and other tissues of the body, a healthy liver is essential for thyroid production and function. The thyroid also secretes calcitonin, an important hormone for calcium metabolism. When the rate of thyroid hormone production increases, most endocrine gland secretions increase as well including the production of adrenal corticoid.

Unfortunately, many people are allergic to their own thyroid gland or thyroid hormones. Because this problem might or might not show up in a blood test, I use the thyroid basal metabolic rate axillary test to evaluate thyroid function. The test measures the metabolic rate by using a thermometer in the armpit immediately after waking up in the morning and before getting out of bed. The temperature is taken for ten minutes. A temperature of 97.7 or below is indicative of low thyroid function (hypothyroidism). Eighty percent of the women I see are hypothyroid, although most are unaware of it. Symptoms include dry skin, cold hands and feet, tiredness, insomnia, eczema, overweight or underweight, sluggishness, hair loss, and poor memory.

If people are secreting enough T_4 but are allergic to their own hormone, they might not be utilizing it and can be as hypothyroid as those with low thyroid function. This may also be the case if there is a problem converting T_4 to T_3 (liver dysfunction). Those individuals show the same symptoms of hypothyroidism but the condition is not likely to show up in blood tests. I have found the basal body temperature test and muscle testing to be accurate in diagnosing both low thyroid function and an allergy to the thyroid and its hormones.

Lymph Glands

One gland that sometimes affects those with immune disorders is the lymph gland. The lymphatic system provides an ancillary route for fluids to flow from the interstitial spaces into the blood. The lymph glands also carry proteins and other metabolites too large to be absorbed directly into the blood away from the tissues. This process is essential for survival. If the lymphatic channels are not working properly, there is a buildup of toxicity in the body and an overload of the lymphatic system.

Salivary Glands

Another problem area is in the salivary glands, important because they are involved in producing mucus and digestive enzymes. The principal glands of salivation are the parotid glands, the submaxillary glands, the sublingual glands, and the buccal glands. Saliva contains two major types of protein secretion: (1) a serous secretion called ptyalin, an enzyme for digesting starches that is found in amylase; and (2) a mucus secretion called mucin for lubrication. The parotid glands secrete the serous type of protein and the submandibular and sublingual glands secrete both the serous type and the mucus type. The buccal glands secrete only mucus.

Parasympathetic nervous pathways, particularly those from the salivary nuclei, regulate the salivary secretions. Salivation can be stimulated or inhibited by impulses arriving in the salivary nuclei from higher centers of the central nervous system. For example, when a person smells or eats favorite foods, salivation occurs. The reaction is even stronger when the person smells food that he or she dislikes. The appetite area of the brain that partially regulates these effects is located in close proximity to the parasympathetic centers of the anterior hypothalamus. It responds to a great extent to signals from the taste and smell areas of our brains.

Salivation also occurs in response to reflexes originating in the stomach and upper intestines, particularly when a very irritating food is swallowed or when a person is nauseated because of some gastrointestinal abnormality. The saliva, when swallowed, helps remove the irritation in the GI tract by neutralizing the offending substances. Salivation can also be affected by the sympathetic nervous system, for example, during "fight or flight"—although less than by the parasympathetic system—and by the blood supply to the salivary glands because secretion requires proper nutrition of the tissue.

When there is a sensitivity or an allergic reaction to the salivary glands, there is either a marked increase or decrease in salivation. I most often see an increase, with increased mucus secretion, creating a breeding ground for bacteria and other pathogens. I had one female patient who was bothered by many allergens and suffered from excessive amounts of mucus and chronic infections, coughing, and wheezing. After I treated her for the thyroid, submandibular, and sublingual glands, in that order, her mucus production diminished, and contributed to fewer infections.

Hormones

Some people are allergic to the female hormones estrogen and progesterone, the male hormone testosterone, and dehydroepiandrosterone (DHEA), an adrenal hormone. I have found reactions to insulin, androgen, and hormones related to the kidneys and their function.

An allergy to progesterone produces symptoms ranging from premenstrual syndrome, breast tenderness, bloating, and depression to irritability prior to the start of a period. People with estrogen sensitivities are more prone to uterine fibroids, ovarian cysts, endometriosis, fibrocystic breasts, painful periods, and migraines at the start and end of periods. Many women are allergic to both hormones. Menopausal symptoms can also be brought on by an allergy to one or both hormones.

Treating for hormone sensitivities can be particularly effective for women who developed chronic fatigue and fibromyalgia later in life.

When I find patients allergic to their hormones, thyroid, or adrenal glands, I treat them with NAET and give them several supplements to take for a period of time to support glandular function. For thyroid, I use high-mineral enzymes containing potassium and magnesium. For the adrenal glands, I supplement with certain B and C enzymes.

Menstrual Period and Pregnancy

Hormones that increase during the premenstrual and menstrual periods and during pregnancy can be involved in immune disorders in women who are allergic to their own hormones. If symptoms increase premenstrually or in pregnancy the trigger is usually progesterone. Postmen-strually there are higher levels of estrogen.

One patient of mine had PMS with migraines, fatigue, and joint pain, increased asthma symptoms, and irritability. When I treated her for progesterone, both her headaches and her other symptoms decreased immediately. We have noticed that treating women for hormones is often effective in dealing with migraines. In men the cause tends to be coffee, caffeine, or chocolate.

Women react to thyroid hormone levels during different points of the menstrual cycle. Treating for allergies to the thyroid and thyroid hormones is often helpful in balancing and regulating the menstrual cycle. After clearing for progesterone, I recommend natural progesterone oils (taken orally) or creams (used topically) made from yams and soybeans to increase progesterone levels. When people are allergic to progesterone they are usually deficient, and supplementation is often necessary.

Adrenal hormones can also be treated with NAET for sensitivities and enzyme therapy for supplementation. These hormones are important to women both pre-menopausally and postmenopausally. The enzymes and NAET treatment are completely safe during pregnancy and can benefit both the woman and her child.

ORGANS

Many people have allergies to their own organs (also thought of as weaknesses in those organs). For example, people may react to glands such as the thyroid, adrenals, parotid, lymph, and thymus or they may be sensitive to the large intestines (colon), spleen, kidney, or liver involved in functions of digestion, elimination, and cleansing. The liver is particularly important to treat with NAET in order to support its function of cleansing and detoxifying the body. This, in turn, keeps the body functioning optimally by supplying scavengers to eat up free radicals.

Emily, a woman in her 40s and suffering from CFIDS, had been undergoing NAET treatments and enzyme therapy for three months. After a course of treatments, she mentioned she was doing quite well but noticed a dramatic change when I treated her for an allergy to her large intestines (colon). I chose to test this organ because in the past, she noticed her energy level changed for the better after I treated her for parasites and bacteria related to the bowel. It prompted me to test and treat, if needed, for her large intestine. One week later, she came to see me with depression, fatigue, and laryngitis. She explained the week's scenario. Things had improved dramatically. Two days ago, however, she felt she was getting sick and considered getting antibiotics. She mentioned she felt nauseous and also looked very pale that day. I said, "Before you do this, let's test you for large intestines to see if you held the treatment or if there is a combination with something else." Not to my surprise, I found an emotional combination. I am always suspicious of this when a person has dramatic symptoms such as severe nausea, wheezing, dizziness, tiredness, and the like. I treated her for two emotional incidences in her life, one of which pertained to her father's death from colon cancer. It was no surprise that such an emotional incident showed up with this treatment. She left that day slightly improved. I talked to her husband the next day, and immediately asked how Suzanne was feeling. He said, "Great! No problem!" I encounter this type of scenario regularly in my practice. Often an organ treatment will have a profound effect on an individual. It is very important to make sure all the emotions have been cleared.

CHIROPRACTIC MISALIGNMENTS AND MYOFASCITIS

When I first began to practice chiropractic care, I treated a young woman who had suffered from depression and exhaustion her whole life. She complained of chronic stiffness and spasms in her upper back and neck. When I examined her, I found some spinal misalignments at the thoracic level (T1–7) with extreme mild fascitis (inflamed soft tissue). Because the nerves from these particular vertebra innervate the spleen, liver, and heart area, I thought that relaxing the muscles in the area, increasing her flexibility, and aligning the vertebra might help her energy and her immune support. I was right. After a series of treatments, her energy improved, her depression lessened, and she no longer required any medication or treatment.

It has been shown that vertebral subluxation in the neck and upper back produces muscle spasms that cause lymphatic congestion. With the lymph system unable to dispose of bacteria, debris, and other foreign materials, toxins accumulate in the area. In many cases, chiropractic adjustments produce immediate relaxation of the neck and back muscles, thereby increasing lymphatic drainage, helping cleanse the body, and improving immunity.

The chiropractic approach to health care is safe and natural and benefits children and adults of all ages. I recommend that all my chronically ill patients undergo chiropractic care at the same time they are being treated for allergy elimination. I see faster results with those patients who use both approaches.

EMOTIONS AND STRESS

Are immune disorders caused or affected by emotions? Absolutely. One female CFIDS I treated was free of symptoms after she divorced her husband. A man's asthma symptoms disappeared when his father died of cancer after a long and painful illness. Another patient stopped having headaches after being treated for sorrow related to an incident with her mother that happened almost thirty years before.

Over the years I have developed a deep respect for our emotions and the power of dramatic events in our lives. Many people suffering from migraines, digestive problems, chronic fatigue, or joint problems should do emotional clearing. Every CFIDS patient I have treated has needed to clear certain emotional blockages in the path to healing and regeneration. Problems or symptom complexes inevitably involve unresolved emotions.

Fortunately, emotional clearing is possible with NAET. NAET unlocks the energy around traumas and helps to clear it from the body so it will not continue to create energy blockages and health problems. Many emotional blockages are easily cleared or worked through during treatment of the basic allergies but some traumas and repressed emotions need to be confronted, felt, and then released from the body and nervous system. These emotions can be connected to food cravings, eating disorders, and environmental factors, as well as to family members, friends, and loved ones. The emotions can be related to love, intimacy, finances, health, physical or emotional abuse, rape, or molestation. They might be rooted in specific incidents such as death of a loved one or divorce. They can also arise from a recurring pattern of events such as fighting at the dinner table, financial stress, marital difficulties, or repeated abuse. Minor, seemingly petty incidents in childhood can create serious allergies or blockages in the energy pathways that act as triggers.

To treat emotional blocks with NAET, we first use muscle or reflex testing to find out how old the patient was when the block first appeared and what other person, if any, was involved: a family member, lover, friend, or business partner. Next we check to see what kind of relationship was involved—intimate, financial, health, business, or spiritual. The last and most important factor is the emotion involved: fear, terror, anger, rage, worry, sorrow, despair, frustration, guilt, abandonment, hopelessness, resentment, disappointment, joy, self-sabotage, rejection, and disgust. Once we have all this information we treat with NAET to clear the obstructions caused by the incidents and emotions identified.

These emotions are often the primary cause of bouts of fatigue and depression. I have seen children with chronic coughs immediately stop coughing after releasing an emotion related to an incident with their mother or father. I have also worked with my daughter and other children on biting their nails. When they released certain emotions related to their parents, the nail biting stopped.

One little girl had a rough time being weaned. Several months after I treated her for allergies to mother's milk and to emotions about nursing, she weaned herself naturally with no emotional upset and no pressure from her parents. A boy who was having trouble with his writing turned out to be afraid of his teacher. When we treated him for his fear, his problems disappeared. And a man with chronic bloating, indigestion, and fatigue was discovered to have unresolved shame in relation to his parents. Within days of being treated, the symptoms disappeared.

Never underestimate the power of emotions or the seriousness of the illnesses they can produce. Many food allergies are the result of emotional experiences with food. If people eat when they are angry, for example, they may develop an allergy to foods eaten at that time. I always tell my patients, "Please don't eat when you're upset, and please don't argue during a meal." Even positive emotions of elation can create allergies. A meal is a sacred event and should be peaceful, similar to meditation. Leave any discussion of intense issues until after the meal is finished.

People often ask me to have lunch with them but I always take a rain check. To avoid creating allergies through emotional situations or discussions during a meal, I prefer to eat at home in a quiet, soothing surrounding. Many of my meals at home as a youngster were emotionally charged. No wonder I had poor digestion and extensive food allergies for most of my life. Now I insist on eating with serenity and awareness, and I recommend that my patients do the same.

I have begun to experiment with referring patients to therapists who use hypnotic techniques such as **eye movement desensitization and reprocessing (EMDR)** to help reveal and release emotional traumas that have an impact on illnesses such as eating disorders and asthma (refer to Part VI for a full explanation of EMDR). I have recommended this technique to patients who seem to have emotional blockages and need help uncovering or processing them. I find that the EMDR technique is sometimes sufficient to release the energy block. At other times I have to treat with NAET as well.

One woman patient with severe food cravings constantly thought about food, ate constantly, and continually gained weight. After she was treated for many of the basic allergies and some of her main food allergies, her cravings dropped off dramatically, but she was still obsessed with food. Nothing we treated seemed to help. There seemed to be many incidents from the past related to her mother, who had been continually ill when my patient was a child. I decided to refer her to a therapist for EMDR and after the treatment, the food cravings decreased significantly. She lost about thirty pounds almost immediately, her energy picked up, and she reported that she felt freer in her everyday life.

Stress is another important factor in the incidence of immune disorders. I believe that if people have good health, a strong immune system, an adequately functioning liver, and good digestion, they will not be physically vulnerable to the stresses they encounter every day of their lives. If, however, they have many hidden allergies, poor digestion, poor eating habits, poor immune function, high levels of immune complexes, and liver toxicity, they will be susceptible to stress that adds just one more strain to an already overburdened system and increases the likelihood of illness. The best way to manage stress and avoid the physical consequences that often ensue is to strengthen the immune system and overall health.

Stress affects people of all ages, including infants, children, and the elderly. Whether the stress comes from being weaned from the breast, learning to write in school, or going through difficult life changes, everyone needs to strengthen the immune system to help the body resist the effects of stress. This is my goal for each individual and I find that enzyme therapy, allergy elimination, proper diet, exercise, and the maintenance of spiritual and mental good health are all important factors.

CHRONIC FATIGUE
IMMUNE DISORDER
SYNDROME (CFIDS)

8

> *Sometimes I wish I could sleep   for two or three years*
> *however long it took   so when I wake   I would wake*
> *fully   open my eyes   from inside a new body*
> *not exhausted before it begins.*
>   —from "Meridians of Longing"

Suzanne

Dr. Ellen Cutler's work with chronic fatigue syndrome is nothing short of miraculous. Thanks to Dr. Cutler's work, I am 100 percent healthy and have my life back.

I am presently 44. I had no health problems until I turned 27. That year, after graduating from law school and starting my first job as a lawyer, I came down with mononucleosis. I experienced typical symptoms—swollen glands and fatigue. The symptoms slowly began to lessen as the months passed, but never fully went away. After six months of feeling tired, I started psychotherapy. My life just was not working. Not only did I not feel well, but I was depressed and did not know why.

Over the next five years (ages 28–32), my overall health slowly declined. Physically, I was chronically tired, came down with a cold or other similar illness every six weeks to two months, and experienced food and other allergies that I had never had before. Psychologically, my depression continued. I discovered in therapy that I had been raised in a highly dysfunctional family. I began coming to terms with the damage I had sustained by having been raised by a mentally ill mother and a sexually abusive father. The healing process was slow and exhausting. My overall lifestyle became quite restricted—I needed to sleep ten hours a day, I could only exercise 15 minutes a day (mostly walking), I had to avoid a myriad of foods to which I was allergic as well as refined sugar, alcohol and caffeine, and I had to avoid stress. To this day, I do not know how I managed to work full time during these years.

I believe I had the equivalent of what the medical establishment now calls chronic fatigue syndrome. However, during this period, no traditional doctors knew what to call my condition and could not offer me any real healing or relief.

During the next five years (ages 33–37), my overall health slowly began to improve. I continued with psychotherapy and found and environmental physician that was helpful. The physician acknowledged that my condition was real, which was a great relief, and found that I had not only been infected with the mono virus, but also the Epstein-Barr virus. I continued to take good care of myself physically and psychologically. I followed the lifestyle restrictions I had implemented in the first five years, and continued to face the truth about my childhood and express all the related feelings. I also began seeing a chiropractor and acupuncturist on a regular basis.

For the next three years (ages 38–41), I felt much better. I had fairly good energy so long as I continued to take good care of myself physically and psychologically. My lifestyle restrictions lessened—I needed only eight hours of sleep, could exercise moderately (one hour a day—running and weight training), and could withstand more stress. I still had to avoid all the foods to which I was allergic as well as refined sugar, alcohol and caffeine, and monitor the stress in my life. I also continued ongoing treatments with my psychotherapist, chiropractor and acupuncturist. I was delighted with my progress.

However, deep inside, I knew I had reached a plateau with my health. I was concerned about my allergies, the status of my immune system, and the effect the aging process would have on my health. I felt there must be a next step out there somewhere, but I was not sure where it was or how to find it. I had tried everything.

Then, one day when I was 41, an acquaintance told me about Dr. Cutler and her work. I decided I had nothing to lose by seeing her but time and money. I remember my first appointment. Dr. Cutler gave me such hope and told me, "Your life will never be the same." She was right and my life changed in ways I could have never imagined.

I have been undergoing treatment with Dr. Cutler for about three years. Through my work with her, I have healed tremendously in all aspects of my life. She began by treating me for the initial ten basic allergens. Once I cleared those, she began treating me for all the foods to which I had an allergy. Once that process was complete, I felt like a different person. It was a gift to be able to eat anything I wanted and not have a reaction. I had been allergic to every ingredient in pizza and had not been able to eat it for over a decade. I went on a pizza eating spree, eating it every day until I could not stand it any longer three months and ten pounds later. After the food groups, Dr. Cutler began treating me for all the parasites, bacteria, fungus and viruses to which I had an allergy. This process was slow and arduous for me, as I was very sensitive to these allergens. Finally, she treated me for my core emotions, which was the last stage in the treatment program. This process was also very slow and arduous for me because of my history.

During my ongoing treatments with Dr. Cutler, I felt as if all that had been holding me down psychologically, physically and spiritually began to lift and the real me began to emerge. I began to see all the ways that I had made choices in my life that I had not made from my authentic self. These choices involved all aspects of my life from work to relationships to living environments. After the first year of treatments, I stopped practicing law and left a dysfunctional relationship. Since then, I have been making other changes on more subtle and esoteric levels, changes I would have never been able to make had it not been for the treatments.

I feel 100% well for the first time in my life. I continue to live a healthy lifestyle—eating well, getting adequate rest, exercising moderately to strenuously, and watching stress—but I do so now not out of necessity and fear of illness, but from a place of choice. I live a healthy life because I want to be and stay healthy.

CFIDS (CHRONIC FATIGUE IMMUNE DYSFUNCTION SYNDROME)

Chronic fatigue is an elusive disease. The symptoms may come and go or linger for years. The cause remains a mystery, although I believe it is rooted in allergies and chronic metabolic imbalances. Some researchers feel it has one cause, while others think it is caused by several factors. Until recently, the medical community as a whole was reluctant to diagnose it as a disease. When it first appeared, very few doctors in the area would even regard it as a problem, and others would send their patients to a psychiatrist for antidepressants.

In 1984 the Centers for Disease Control finally developed a set of diagnostic criteria and gave the disease the name of chronic fatigue syndrome, also known as chronic fatigue immune dysfunction syndrome, or CFIDS. Outside the United States, it is known as myalgic encephalomyelitis. Although the recent attention to this disease is relatively new, the disease itself is not. Reports of similar conditions involving fatigue date as far back as the eighteenth century. A disease called febricula was diagnosed by an English physician among those suffering great fatigue following a fever. "Soldiers heart" or "the effort syndrome" were diagnoses given to soldiers experiencing great fatigue following the stress of war. During World War I, 60,000 British troops were diagnosed with this problem; two thirds were unable to perform, and were subsequently discharged.

During the depression in the United States, "chronic brucellosis" was diagnosed in individuals suffering fatigue thought to be caused by a bacterial infection transmitted by farm animals. During the 1980s, reports in the United States and other countries cited outbreaks of long-term debilitating fatigue whose cause was unknown.

Chronic fatigue is a persistent combination of symptoms that include recurring sore throat, low grade fever, lymph node swelling, headache, muscle and joint pain, emotional stress, intestinal discomfort, depression, and loss of concentration. Less frequent symptoms include severe premenstrual symptoms, stiffness, visual blurring, dizziness, nausea, dry eyes and mouth, chronic diarrhea, cough, lack of appetite, night sweats, sleep disturbances, recurring headaches, irritability, and forgetfulness. Patients often report that they came down with a flu and then never recovered. Fear may accompany the symptoms because they are so persistent and resistant to treatment. Most of the people I have seen with chronic fatigue syndrome say they were active, vibrant individuals until they suddenly got sick, often after a period of sustained stress at work. By the time they seek professional help, they are often so exhausted they cannot get out of bed, they cannot concentrate, and they feel depressed. It is frustrating for them and their families.

It is not clear how many people suffer from the disease, in part because it is often unrecognized and unreported, but it is known to occur throughout the world. More than six million patient visits per year in the United States are made by people suffering from fatigue. Almost everyone I see, even young children and teenagers, reports fatigue. Right now I see an eight-year-old boy with severe chronic fatigue who goes to school but cannot do much else. There are different levels of chronic fatigue, from those who can function with some difficulty to those who are on disability.

It is estimated that two out of a thousand people meet the established criteria for a diagnosis of CFIDS, which is similar to the rate for MS.

Women are two to three times more likely to contract the disease than men, although the percentage of men being inflicted may be rising. The disease seems to be more prevalent among Caucasians and those who are well educated, although one study indicates that it is also widespread but underdiagnosed in lower income and minority ethnic groups. In particular, airline personnel, hospital workers, and teachers have a disproportionate incidence of symptoms, which I explain by the fact that they tend to be exposed more frequently to viruses and other allergens that can cause fatigue. The majority of sufferers can identify the day they first felt the typical flu-like symptoms, headache, runny nose, sore throat, low-grade fever, fatigue, and muscle and joint pain. Again, the difference between these symptoms and the flu is that they do not go away. Many people report feeling sick following emotional stress or during a stressful time in their lives.

Based on what I have already written about the allergy load phenomena, it can be seen that chronic hidden allergies can make the body extremely susceptible to stress. Just a little added emotional or situational stress, combined with the stress of a virus or other infectant, can break down the body's defenses and render it unable to resist the influx of infectants and allergens. The chronic fatigue may be the result of the person's immune system working overtime to maintain homeostasis. NAET works so effectively with CFIDS patients because it helps restore homeostasis by reducing the load of allergies, and enzyme therapy contributes by helping to strengthen the body's resistance.

Some people with CFIDS experience low-grade symptoms all the time, while others experience periodic episodes followed by remissions. Some are bed-ridden for months at a time, and approximately 25 percent of CFIDS patients are housebound, while others are able to function in a curtailed fashion. Most of the people I see, generally women between the ages of 25 and 50, are taken care of by someone else; they cannot make their own meals or drive themselves. In fact, they are often just barely able to come in for their treatments. Typically, CFIDS sufferers tend to relapse after a marked increase in physical activity. Stress or mild exercise may exacerbate the symptoms, and changes in temperature, humidity, barometric pressure, and exposure to sun may cause a decline in functioning.

One distinguishing characteristic of CFIDS, in contrast to normal fatigue, is that adequate rest, exercise, and sleep afford no relief. In fact, CFIDS sufferers may sleep 12 hours or more each night and still be unable to function. Chronic fatigue syndrome differs from ameopathic chronic fatigue, a disease of unknown origin with similar symptoms, in having a defined onset. In many cases, a flu-like illness can also be identified as a precursor. For a diagnosis of chronic fatigue, the symptoms should have persisted for a number of months.

Diagnosing Chronic Fatigue Syndrome

Rather than approaching chronic fatigue syndrome as if it had a single cause, I treat my patients as unique individuals. The problem can have a variety of causes, from food allergies to Candida to the Epstein-Barr virus. In each case, I do a complete analysis and allergy evaluation. Sometimes just eliminating a few allergies can make a world of difference.

When I began working with NAET many years ago, I did not know how to treat chronic fatigue. I simply followed the guidelines provided by Dr. Nambudripad and then did my own research and experimentation. The outcomes were often as surprising to me as they were to my patients. Most people who come to see me have some form of chronic fatigue, whether or not it meets the diagnostic criteria for the disease known as CFIDS. I evaluate each person as an individual and do what is best for them. Often they experience a permanent reversal of symptoms and are able to get on with their lives.

Depression is a common symptom of chronic fatigue, as it is of most chronic health problems. Although dual diagnosis can be tricky, the depression that accompanies chronic fatigue is generally either the result of neurochemical changes brought about by the disease or a response to having the disease itself. Nevertheless, CFIDS-related depression can be just as debilitating as clinical depression.

Sleep disorders are also common in chronic fatigue syndrome. CFIDS sufferers rarely wake up feeling rested. Some sleep excessively, whereas others sleep intermittently. What is common to most chronic fatigue patients is the lack of restful sleep. If the sleep cycle is altered, it can contribute to ongoing health problems and can accentuate feelings of anxiety, depression, and fatigue. Sleeping medications may actually compound this problem.

Many chronic fatigue syndrome patients have problems maintaining their balance. The inner ear is responsible for the body's ability to negotiate itself in a balanced manner, and environmental overstimulation may potentiate balance problems in CFIDS patients. Reading problems, ringing in the ears, impaired walking, lightheadedness, nausea, and fainting may be associated with those problems and may be caused by neurally mediated hypertension which is found in some CFIDS cases.

The course of chronic fatigue syndrome manifests differently in different individuals. Some may be debilitated abruptly, whereas others may experience a slow and insidious onset, in which their energy is sapped gradually over a period of many months. One of the hallmarks of CFIDS is its ability to wax and wane in severity and symptomatology from day to day and even moment to moment. A person might feel fine and energetic during the day, only to find themselves disabled with fatigue and pain in the evening. Resolution of the problematic symptoms may occur as abruptly as they appeared.

According to conventional research, the long-term prognosis for chronic fatigue syndrome patients is difficult to determine. Researchers say that some people may recover in as little as six months to a year, while others may take years. One study suggested that the average duration of the illness is 37 months. In another study only one quarter of the patients showed any improvement after one year. Many patients reported feeling better after one or two years despite experiencing setbacks. Other studies show that only a small number of the study groups fully recovered. Much of the research suggests that people suffering from both CFIDS and depression tend to have poor outcomes. In my experience, however, the combination of NAET, enzyme therapy, and other alternative therapies can bring about a change and even a resolution to this debilitating syndrome.

Other conditions that involve chronic fatigue and which need to be ruled out to ensure proper treatment include depressive disorders, bipolar disorder, and schizophrenia. Although depression may be associated with chronic fatigue syndrome, it is not really the cause of the illness. As I mentioned earlier, depression is commonly associated with many chronic illnesses and with physical or emotional pain.

Another illness to rule out is Lyme disease, which is caused by a tick bite and characterized by flu-like symptoms and fatigue. It is suspected that many people who are diagnosed with Lyme disease actually have chronic fatigue syndrome, and that many people who are diagnosed with chronic fatigue have Lyme disease. Confusion among these disorders and lack of adequate laboratory sanitation suggests that differential diagnosis be made carefully based on the full symptom picture and case history.

Fibromyalgia, which will be discussed later, is another immune disorder that is often confused with chronic fatigue. It is characterized by pain in all the different quadrants and on the 18 trigger points of the body. The symptoms of fibromyalgia and CFIDS overlap considerably: GI symptoms, cognitive dysfunction, mood disorders, headaches, sleep disorders, sensitivity to cold, bloating, anxiety, and morning stiffness. However, the primary symptom of fibromyalgia is joint and muscle pain. The treatments of the two with NAET are generally quite similar.

Like chronic fatigue syndrome, systemic lupus erythematosus is an autoimmune disorder. People with lupus (which means "wolf" in Latin) often have a hyperpigmentation of the skin on their face, which causes a reddish discoloration resembling the markings on the face of a wolf. Early symptoms, such as joint pain and muscle fatigue, may mimic CFIDS. This disease, which occurs most frequently in women, progresses slowly.

Sjogren's syndrome is another autoimmune disease, whose primary symptoms are dry mouth and eyes. Other symptoms may include fever, sore throat, tooth decay, neurocognitive and other central nervous system dysfunction, sleep disturbance, burning throat, and difficulty chewing or swallowing due to the dryness of the mucous membranes. Many of these symptoms resemble those of chronic fatigue. This syndrome, which some researchers speculate is caused by a virus, is diagnosed by a biopsy of the lips and salivary glands. People with Sjogren's often respond well to NAET, particularly when they are treated for viral and bacterial allergies.

Multiple sclerosis (MS), a central nervous system disease, is another autoimmune disorder that typically affects women in their 30s, 40s, and 50s. In MS, the lining of nerve fibers along the spinal cord and brain are separating from the nerves themselves. Early symptoms may resemble CFIDS, but the person gradually loses control of their muscles. I have had good results with MS using NAET and enzyme therapy.

Hypothyroid problems such as Hashimoto's thyroiditis and other disorders cause the person's thyroid gland to underperform. With their basic metabolic function slowed down, these people, typically women, tend to feel depressed and fatigued. Hashimoto's is an autoimmune disease that is quite common in the general population and afflicts some people in the chronic stages of CFIDS. It is the leading cause of hypothyroidism and can emerge after childbirth as a result of endocrine dysfunction and food and hormonal allergies.

Probably 80 percent of the women who come into my office are hypothyroid and have been diagnosed with Hashimoto's or some other form of thryoiditis. The most prominent symptoms include fatigue, cognitive problems, and impaired memory and concentration. Many of these people complain of forgetting things and of feeling "spaced out" and depressed. Other symptoms include cold hands and feet, constipation, muscle cramps, hair loss or damage, especially as a woman gets older and has other hormonal problems, brittle fingernails, puffy face, weight gain, decreased exercise tolerance, joint pain, hoarseness, slow heart rate, decreased libido, irregular menstrual periods, and elevated cholesterol. To assist in proper diagnosis, we generally perform a full thyroid panel and a basal temperature test.

Rheumatoid arthritis is another autoimmune disease whose early symptoms, particularly joint pain and fatigue, can resemble CFIDS. The white blood cells infiltrate the joints and cause inflammation.

Sleep apnea, often accompanied by snoring, is a condition in which a person stops breathing intermittently while sleeping. The problem occurs most commonly in obese people. The interval between breaths may be as long as 30 seconds, and the person will generally awaken when the blood oxygen content reaches a triggering low point. Until the problem is treated, sleep deprivation may occur and lead to fatigue.

Insomnia, the inability to sleep, is a common symptom of chronic fatigue syndrome, although it frequently occurs in other autoimmune disorders and is usually the result of allergies. A person needs to achieve a certain amount of deep sleep each night in order to feel refreshed; otherwise, daytime fatigue is experienced.

Gulf War syndrome, the name of the condition experienced by Gulf War veterans, resembles chronic fatigue and multiple chemical sensitivities. These veterans have been disabled because of exposures to toxic chemicals, pesticides, diesel fuels, jet fuels, and possibly chemical warfare agents,. Other substances to which they may have been exposed include special paint containing cyanide, heavy metals, depleted uranium, and unsanitary conditions. Although I have not worked with any Gulf War vets, I would welcome an opportunity to use NAET and enzyme therapy to boost their immune system and reverse some of their problems.

Post-polio sequelae afflicts almost two million American polio survivors. Fatigue is the most prominent and the most severe symptom, accompanied by muscle weakness, joint pain, difficulty walking and climbing, difficulty with bladder function, headaches, attention deficit, and slow reflexes. Polio is known to cause damage to the spinal cord and to specific areas of the brain, and there is some speculation that chronic fatigue syndrome may be caused by the same enterovirus. Many chronic fatigue patients, MS sufferers, and others afflicted with chronic nervous system disorders, autoimmune disorders, and chronic joint and muscle pain have an allergy to the polio virus and need to be treated with NAET. This allergy can occur in those who were merely vaccinated as well as in those who contracted the virus itself.

Sick building syndrome, which is discussed at great length in my book *Winning the War Against Asthma and Allergies*, is a frequent cause of symptoms in those suffering from chronic fatigue and must be properly diagnosed and treated. This phenomenon occurs in individuals who work in buildings that have few windows and limited ventilation. Symptoms are caused by exposure to the thousands of airborne chemicals and infectants that such buildings harbor, including industrial cleaning solutions, office products such as copier toner and typewriter correction fluid, mold and mildew in air conditioning vents, viruses and bacteria in crowded work environments, and formaldehyde and other chemicals outgassing from carpets and furniture. These substances pass into the bloodstream and trigger a wide variety of allergic reactions, including respiratory problems, headaches, difficulty concentrating or thinking clearly, dizziness, insomnia, and rashes.

First I have these people collect the air in their building, and then I desensitize them to the substances it contains. They may have to be treated every few weeks to ensure that we desensitize them to everything. Of course, this doesn't change the quality of their work environment, but it does support their immune system in protecting them against potential allergens and toxins. Often, chronic fatigue sufferers report that they are fine until they get home or until they sleep in their room, and then they have insomnia or just wake up tired. The problem may be right there in the room, in the form of feathers, dust, mold, outgassing furniture, or cats or other animals. We may need to investigate carefully and do a series of tests before we find it. With women I usually inquire to make sure there are no silicon breast implants involved, since they can cause symptoms similar to chronic fatigue syndrome, environmental illness, and fibromyalgia.

Systemic candidiasis, an overgrowth of yeast in the body, can be the major cause of chronic fatigue in any autoimmune condition. Besides fatigue, it can cause gas, diarrhea, headaches, sore throats, asthma, chronic allergies, irritability, carbohydrate cravings, chemical sensitivities, vaginal infections, eczema, and rashes. Candida can be passed back and forth through skin-to-skin contact. Candidiasis is one of the most important problems I treat for in my practice, and it will be discussed in great depth, together with other fungus infections, in the section on Fungus.

Hepatitis is an inflammation of the liver that can be caused by several viruses and precipitated or exacerbated by drugs and alcohol. Chronic fatigue is a common symptom, and recovery can be a prolonged process. The hepatitis A virus is typically transmitted through food that has been handled by an infected individual. Hepatitis B, caused by a DNA virus, is passed through exposure to blood and other bodily fluids. Immune reactivity to the virus may cause liver damage. Hepatitis C, an RNA virus also transmitted through bodily fluids, can cause severe liver damage and is potentially fatal. Because more and more people are being diagnosed with this virus, it is being closely watched by public health organizations. I am currently treating several hepatitis patients who are responding quite well to NAET. In addition to the virus, some people need to be treated for an allergy to the hepatitis vaccination, which may cause as much of a problem as the disease itself.

Anemia is a low red blood cell count caused by poor nutrition, excessive blood loss, cancer, or other factors. Anemic people do not have enough red blood cells to carry and deliver oxygen to the body's tissues. Therefore, they may become easily fatigued, and their complexion may appear pale. Sometimes such people turn out to be allergic to the iron in supplements they have been taking. Once they clear the allergy and start eating foods high in iron, their chronic fatigue may improve dramatically.

The journey from the onset of the illness to the actual diagnosis of chronic fatigue syndrome can be a long and arduous one, filled with painful misunderstandings and misdiagnoses. Many doctors don't recognize the symptoms. One patient told me she talked to her doctor about chronic fatigue and joint pain, and he told her he suffered from those symptoms every day of his life and had learned to live with them.

There is still no test to diagnose chronic fatigue syndrome. Most people with CFIDS have normal blood tests, or if the test results are abnormal, they are not useful in making a proper diagnosis. Tests do exist that can rule out or eliminate other possible causes of chronic fatigue, which means that CFIDS remains a diagnosis of exclusion, rather than a diagnosis based on certain defining symptoms.

The more patients one sees, the easier it gets to diagnose chronic fatigue. The key is to spend time getting to know your patients and their symptoms and taking a careful family and personal medical history. Questions may include: When did the fatigue begin? Does anything make it worse or better? Is it better during certain times of the day? Does physical activity make it worse? Are there other symptoms such as sore throat or headaches? Has anyone else in your family experienced fatigue? Is your personal/professional life stressful? Any weight gain or loss? Any problem sleeping? Any problem concentrating? I've included a lengthy history in the book for all immune disorders.

Certain baseline tests from which to assess any significant changes in health status include a sed rate, complete blood count, biochemistry profile, and urinalysis, and I use the 24-hour urinalysis evaluation to do a complete nutritional and enzyme assessment. A battery of more specialized tests can detect the presence of viruses, rule out anemia, or measure cellular, immune system, thyroid, and liver function. Other tests can be added depending on the symptoms and circumstances. For example, a patient with a lot of joint pain may be tested for rheumatoid factor or antinuclear antibodies. CFIDS patients should be routinely tested for hepatitis and AIDS, and those who live with cats may be tested for toxoplasmosis, a bacteria carried by cats. People who are overweight can be checked for an underlying thyroid condition on the palpation exam. If they test positive, I recommend blood work and most especially a basal axillary temperature test. Lyme disease should also be ruled out.

A battery of tests to analyze blood chemistry can measure levels of cholesterol, protein, calcium, liver enzymes, iron, electrolytes, uric acid, glucose, and many other substances in the blood. Abnormalities in any of these could suggest scores of potential health problems. A complete red and white blood cell count is important, as is a measure of the sedimentation rate (also known as an ESR), which screens out inflammation and infection. The ESR measures how rapidly red blood cells settle in specialized marked test tubes. In the presence of an infection, the cells will tend to cluster together and thus fall further and more rapidly. An elevated sed rate can indicate a possible infection, an autoimmune disorder, thyroid disease, a connective tissue disorder, or kidney disease, but it is also found in women during pregnancy and menstruation. When I do a routine urinalysis, I test for sugar in the urine, nitrates, ketones, protein, infection, pH (acidity or alkalinity), calcium, specific gravity, sedimentation, dietary stress, absorption of food, bowel toxicity, kidney function, and electrolytes, as well as adrenal and thyroid function. There are a range of other laboratory tests that can be used.

Many patients with unexplained fatigue have elevated antibody levels to the Epstein-Barr virus (EBV), which suggests that they are allergic to the virus and their body cannot deal with it properly. In my experience, EBV is not the sole cause of chronic fatigue, but it can be a piece of the puzzle for a CFIDS sufferer. I regularly treat for EBV and other viruses using NAET and enzyme therapy. (The Resource section of this book contains a list of the common viruses I treat for in cases of chronic fatigue syndrome and other autoimmune disorders.)

The body produces four types of antibodies in response to four different Epstein-Barr virus antigens. The blood levels of these antibodies can tell us whether a person has ever been infected by Epstein-Barr or was recently infected for the first time. A routine Epstein-Barr cytology panel measures IGM antibodies, which appear the first time a person is infected. IGM antibodies are usually undetectable within six months of primary infection. IGG antibodies, which are also measured by an EBV cytology panel, peak within a few weeks and remain detectable for life. Once a person has been infected with the virus, it persists for life, though it generally remains inactive following the initial exposure.

Young adults initially exposed to EBV may develop mononucleosis, which can last for many weeks, with symptoms persisting for months or even permanently. I have treated many young men and women with mono for EBV and have seen quick and full recovery. For example, a 17-year-old boy came to see me feeling tired and run down. He mentioned that his girlfriend had been diagnosed with mono, and he was concerned that he had it as well. Allergy testing revealed that he did indeed have it, but 25 hours after being treated for EBV with NAET and enzymes, he was a new man.

EBV infections in children are said to be asymptomatic, though I disagree. For example, just a few days ago I was treating a 7-year-old girl with a runny nose and cough by treating her saliva, which is an emergency virus treatment described in Chapter 5. However, the treatment was only partially successful: she would clear the virus, her symptoms would diminish, but they would return within a couple of hours. When I muscle-tested her for some other viruses, she turned out to be allergic to EBV. I treated her, and her symptoms disappeared immediately. Anyone can have an allergy to this virus, which may be revealed by higher antibodies on the blood work but will definitely show up on the muscle response test.

NAET and enzyme therapy can prevent any virus from compromising or burdening the immune system. Elevated levels of Epstein-Barr virus antibodies are common in patients with other autoimmune problems, like rheumatoid arthritis, chronic lung disease, MS, or lupus. These people may not have chronic fatigue but instead may experience depression or bloating or severe candidiasis. Elevated levels are also found in older people and women in their third trimester of pregnancy.

Other tests can be performed in the differential diagnosis of chronic fatigue syndrome. One is for the blood level of aldolase, an enzyme that converts sugar to energy in the muscles and can be measured when damage in the muscles or other body tissue is suspected. Adolase levels may rise in certain disorders, for example, mono, muscular dystrophy, and hepatitis. Creatinine phosphokinase (CVK) is an enzyme released into the bloodstream after the heart, brain, or skeletal muscles have been damaged. Hence, this is an important test for those suspected of having had a heart attack, but also for people with possible hypothyroid or muscular dystrophy. EMG is a test commonly used to measure electrical activity in the muscles to determine their function. Although expensive, it can be important in helping to detect stress-related muscle tension, which is a common problem in chronic fatigue patients with neuromuscular problems. In extreme cases a muscle biopsy can be performed on CFIDS patients and may reveal the presence of some viruses, including Epstein-Barr.

When lupus is suspected or there are a number of unexplained symptoms, including skin rash, chest pain, joint pain, or collagen problems, a blood test known as ANA can be done. A higher-than-normal ANA (the level of antinuclear antibodies in the blood) may indicate a viral infection as well as any of several autoimmune diseases. However, it can also be found in relatively healthy individuals, making the test an inconclusive indicator for lupus. Rheumatoid factor is a standard blood test when rheumatoid arthritis is suspected, but higher levels of rheumatoid factor can also show up in lupus, TB, mono, and liver or lung disease.

Although other tests can be utilized to rule out chronic fatigue syndrome or rheumatoid arthritis, often the symptoms alone are sufficient to make a differential diagnosis. Certain specialized immune system tests involve and measure specific immunological functions. For example, lymphocyte phenotyping can detect subtle changes in the levels of the various white blood cells, which can be helpful in differentiating autoimmune disorders. But these tests are quite costly and are not routinely done on CFIDS patients. A blood pressure test called a tilt test may confirm the diagnosis of chronic fatigue caused by low blood pressure. An individual lies on a table tilted upright to a 70-degree angle (head higher than feet) for a prolonged period of time. If the person feels faint, lightheaded, or sick, this indicates a drop in blood pressure, which in turn signifies a reduction in the volume of circulating blood available to the brain.

The Causes of Chronic Fatigue

Immune deficiencies may be genetically based, or they may be acquired as the result of a variety of factors: advancing age, lack of sleep, poor nutrition, surgery,

trauma, certain drugs, emotional traumas, hormonal imbalance, stress, an exposure to various environmental
toxins, and an allergy overload. Even negative emotional
states or traumas can be regarded as allergies since the
body is continually reacting to them, alone or in combination with a certain food or environmental condition.
Negative emotional states or prolonged stress can impair
immunity to a significant degree by causing alterations in
neuroendocrine function, which is the connection between the nervous system, brain, and glandular system.

When the immune system is out of balance, some
parts can become overactive and some underactive. In
fact, as I have already mentioned, immune system dysfunction can just as easily involve an overreaction to relatively benign substances as an inability to defend the
body against attack. Immune abnormalities are part of
the chronic fatigue puzzle, but it is still not clear whether
they constitute a cause or an effect of the illness.

The techniques for measuring immune dysfunction
are still rather primitive and are not altogether useful in
distinguishing one disease from the other. The big question is: What is the basic underlying agent or agents that
cause chronic fatigue syndrome? There are so many con-
tradictions in the literature. There are even, unfortunately
some physicians who will not even recognize chronic fatigue syndrome as a disorder.

One of my chronic fatigue patients, who has been
responding well to NAET, is involved in a CFIDS support group. One of the group members related the story
of going to a physician at one of the HMOs and telling
him she thought she had chronic fatigue syndrome,
based on extensive reading in the medical literature and
an Internet search. The physician replied that he did not
believe in chronic fatigue syndrome. She was stunned:
How could a physician in this day and age ignore all
the evidence and not acknowledge the existence of
CFIDS? Since this wasn't part of her medical care, she

had to read what she could find to make sense of her symptoms.

In my work I believe there are a variety of causes for what we call chronic fatigue. I have witnessed more than one CFIDS sufferer change overnight when they were treated with NAET for Epstein-Barr virus, another get better when they were treated for grains, and yet another for pesticides. I am going to review the various causes that I have encountered in my work over the years. These are the discoveries that excited me and motivated me to write this book on immune disorders.

Most of these causes could also belong to other immune suppressed disorders; therefore, at the end of this section I will explain how I treat for all the immune disorders, including some specifics about each one. For the most part, NAET and enzyme therapy are effective with all the immune disorders.

In my experience, the primary cause of chronic fatigue syndrome is food allergies. Studies have found that 65 percent of CFIDS cases have had food or other types of allergies prior to contracting chronic fatigue. Studies are currently being conducted to determine if CFIDS patients have a more dramatic allergic reaction compared to healthy individuals. There is no one particular food that is the primary cause for all chronic fatigue syndrome patients; any food or foods may be the culprit. Usually people are allergic to the foods they eat most often. Depression and fatigue are two of the most common reactions, as when we feel tired after eating a meal of our favorite foods. Other common symptoms include muscle and joint aches, poor concentration, and nervousness.

The number of people diagnosed with food allergies has increased dramatically in recent years, and I believe food allergies to be a contributing factor in many undiagnosed symptoms and chronic diseases. A recent article in fact in Investors Business Daily states "If you think you may be allergic to anything from milk to shellfish to those ubiquitous bags of peanuts on airlines, your suspicions may not be all in your head." They went on to say that more than five million Americans have food allergies and that food allergies are causing more deaths than allergies to bee stings. "At least 100,000 Americans die from severe allergic reactions to food each year." Genetics plays a major role in causing these allergies; so does poor digestion and stress on the immune system from chemicals in the air, water, and food. Another important factor is the premature weaning of infants and the introduction of solid food. After careful treatment for food allergies with NAET, people with chronic fatigue often take dramatic strides in improving their health.

Many chronic fatigue syndrome patients say their diet is made up primarily of grains, vegetables, and fruits. The primary ingredient of these foods is sugar in one form or another, which is one of the most common allergens. Grains contain maltose, fruit contains fructose, and vegetables contain glucose. Hence, even though these are wholesome foods, they can be irritating to the system if one is allergic to them. If you are eating the foods you are allergic to, you're going to have problems.

A food allergy occurs when there's an adverse reaction to the ingestion of a certain food. The allergy may be to the protein in the food, the starch, the sugars, the acid, the phenolic, the B vitamins, the calcium, or some other nutrient, or it may simply be to the food itself. I generally begin by treating for the basic allergens, as described in the case history section. This often reverses many of the food intolerances and makes it unnecessary to treat for them separately.

Another significant cause that most have heard about is viral, in particular, the Epstein-Barr virus. Viruses are small, protein-covered bundles of genetic material that contain a blueprint for self-reproduction. They can enter, attach to, and invade living cells; antiviral drugs interfere with this process by damaging or destroying the exterior surface of the virus. I believe that NAET treatments have a similar effect.

Unlike bacteria, which are living organisms, viruses are neither alive nor dead. Incapable of reproducing on their own, they require a host organism, whose cells they invade and in which they reproduce themselves. Their only goal is to replicate themselves, not to cause harm, though of course they can wreak havoc when they reproduce. When they invade and attach themselves to cells, they pass on their genes, which in the end causes the cells to keep reproducing them. Their offspring come forth and destroy the previously invaded cell and then seek out new healthy cells. They can hide, combine with other things, mutate, and transform into bacteria.

Although there are thousands of different viruses, I encounter certain ones again and again in my work with immune disorders. There are many that I don't know about, but we have a treatment for viruses in general that covers most of them. Viruses are usually diagnosed based on symptoms, but I do it through muscle testing and other electromagnetic instrumentation. Many viruses can remain in a latent stage in our bodies for long periods of time without reproducing and without causing symptoms. Viral agents that may produce such inactive infections include herpes simplex, herpes zoster, CMV, human herpes virus (HHV-6), and retroviruses. Many viruses are capable of producing chronic illness by alternating dormant and active phases.

In my work I have found that when a person encounters a virus, whether it's herpes, Epstein-Barr, CMV, or a retrovirus or enterovirus, an allergic reaction may occur. When the immune system is weak or compromised and the lymphocytes or white blood cells cannot completely eliminate the pathogen, an antigen-antibody reaction takes place, and antibodies attach to the antigen or virus. The antigen-antibody complex (CIC) that is formed discharges a chemical mediator that causes symptoms. As

I explain elsewhere in this book, these complexes can lodge in certain areas of the body and remain dormant. When the person gets stressed out or the allergy load reaches a critical point, these CICs can become active again, causing autoimmune responses and inflammation.

Many people will be symptom free until they experience excessive stress, like a crisis at work or estrangement from a loved one or exposure to toxic chemicals or medications or even a prolonged period in which they don't get enough sleep or eat the right foods. Then they will develop a familiar set of flulike symptoms: sore throat, swollen glands, abdominal discomfort, fatigue. Some people get these symptoms often, and it can resemble chronic fatigue syndrome. When we locate and treat for the offending virus with NAET, we break the allergen-antibody attachment, and the symptoms disappear and do not recur. The virus stops reproducing, and the body can gradually eliminate it from the system without the symptoms of detoxification. This can be an extremely important treatment for people with chronic fatigue syndrome or any autoimmune disorder.

Certain viruses have been studied for their possible role in CFIDS. For example, adrenoviruses can infect cells and develop very slowly. Herpes viruses, including cold sores, herpes, encephalitis, chicken pox, and shingles, demonstrate a particular ability to remain latent for long periods of times. CMV, which occurs mainly in fetuses and babies, can produce a monolike illness. The Epstein-Barr virus (EBV) is also a herpes virus that virtually everyone has by the time they are 30. Once the virus has infected an individual, it can persist for life, generally remaining inactive following the initial exposure. Those who are allergic to it are the ones who develop symptoms. Young adults initially exposed to it may develop mono, although those with strong immune systems will not. For example, a patient whose son's girlfriend had mono was afraid her son would get it as well. He tested positive for Epstein-Barr, but I treated him, his mother, and his sister with NAET, and he never did come down with the disease.

In addition to the role played by the Epstein-Barr virus in chronic fatigue, it is also possible that we are faced with other new strains of Epstein-Barr and CFIDS. For instance, there's the human herpes virus type 6 (HHV-6), which was initially isolated in 1986. It is a common virus, although infection is often asymptomatic, and like other herpes viruses, it may remain dormant for many years. This virus is frequently found in people with chronic fatigue syndrome.

Other viruses I have found that also play a role in chronic fatigue are the cytomegalovirus (CMV), which is similar to Epstein-Barr, and the Coxsackie virus, which I find to be as much of a factor in chronic fatigue syndrome as EBV. The Coxsackie B6, which is the strain I encounter most commonly, produces severe symptoms when first encountered, including bad sore throats and fatigue. When I treat for it with NAET, I have to be careful to avoid being exposed because it's so contagious.

Other herpes viruses such as herpes simplex I and II have also been implicated, and there is some speculation that CFIDS is another form of polio myelitus or is caused by a non-polio entrovirus. I do occasionally need to treat CFIDS sufferers for the polio virus. Another suspect in CFIDS is a retrovirus, possibly human T lymphotrophic virus type II. Retroviruses contain an enzyme called re-birth transcriptase that can cause complications in other illnesses, such as AIDS and a rare type of leukemia Although there is no definitive research linking CFIDS to a virus, the disease certainly acts like a dormant virus when it comes and goes, as it does for some people. CFIDS patients usually have high levels of antiviral antibodies, which, I believe, reflects their allergies to these viruses.

Viral activity is difficult to measure directly. For one thing, we don't know how many viruses there are, and we are unable to measure the antibodies to many viruses. Since viruses can't be seen, their presence must be determined entirely by symptoms. Once patients have been treated for some of the more common viruses, including those that lie dormant in their bodies, they can do the emergency saliva treatment whenever they start to feel symptoms to help their immune system resist these viruses. For viruses that are more active and more deeply entrenched in the body, however, NAET treatment is necessary first before the saliva treatment will be effective.

Because of the widespread use of vaccinations, including a new rubella vaccine introduced in the late 1970s, there has been some speculation that this vaccine might be the cause of chronic fatigue syndrome. In my experience, any vaccination, whether it is DPT, measles, mumps, or hepatitis, can cause chronic fatigue syndrome in a person who is allergic to it. I always check for vaccinations, especially in children who have more recently received them.

Many people with chronic fatigue syndrome or some other autoimmune disorder have a genetic predisposition as reflected in a weakened immune system, allergies, and other health problems. They may report that they have always felt like there was something in their system that would periodically flare up, causing symptoms of chronic fatigue. In my investigations, I have identified a number of different allergens that can be the culprit or genetic link to the flareups, including certain bacteria, parasites, and viruses, that remain dormant but then become active for periods of time. Many people inherit a sensitivity to certain allergens.

As I mentioned earlier, autoimmune disorders and allergies tend to run in families, and there is a demonstrable link between chronic fatigue, immune disorders, and allergies. Environmental allergies and chemical sensitivities are also common causes of chronic fatigue syndrome, and for some people an exposure to toxic chemicals can precipitate their symptoms. For example, one patient of mine was an artist who worked with various painting materials, and over time it became clear that her chronic fatigue and immune disorders were the result of prolonged exposure to the chemicals in these materials. Other environmental factors that can precipitate chronic fatigue include dry cleaning solvents, air pollution, outgassing furniture and carpeting, adhesives, finishes, and other building materials, and electromagnetic fields.

Americans consume hazardous chemicals in their food, water, and air. Among the toxins we imbibe all the time are food preservatives, flavorings, and colorings, steroids, medicines, antibiotics in meat and poultry, thickening agents, emulsifiers, sulfur dioxide, air pollutants, vinyl chloride in plastics, hazardous industrial solvents, radioactive wastes, mercury in dental amalgams, chromium, lead, cadmium, tin, and aluminum. Government regulations are inadequate to regulate the use of these substances. Witness the use of the additive MBTE in gasoline, which is a severe trigger for asthmatics and has recently been linked to cancer in lab animals. Most people are allergic to at least some of these substances, and when the allergy load reaches critical mass—for example, food allergies are compounded by virus allergies, which are in turn exacerbated by environmental sensitivities—the result can be chronic fatigue syndrome and other immune system disorders.

Each month more new chemicals are added to the existing risk facing Americans. As I discussed earlier, these compounds remain in the body as antigen-antibody complexes, which can cause inflammation and challenge and ultimately weaken the immune system. NAET can help the body eliminate these toxins and support the liver in reducing the allergic response.

Radiation, another suspected factor in chronic fatigue syndrome, is a common allergen among the patients in my practice. For example, people who have chronic herpes are generally sensitive to the sun, and treating for the sun can diminish the outbreaks. Many of the radiation problems among CFIDS sufferers can be traced to low levels of ionizing radiation from nuclear fallout in the environment. Radioactive releases began in the 1940s with above-ground bomb tests as well as radiation from television, radios, and microwave ovens. If you're allergic to radiation and exposed to it for extended periods of time, it can contribute to the allergy load created by environmental toxins and other allergens.

It is amazing to see how many children complain of fatigue. They have difficulty getting up in the morning, and they can't stay awake in class. Although they would not necessarily be diagnosed with CFIDS, they certainly do have a form of chronic fatigue. These children also tend to have the runny nose, cough, and sore throat that are so characteristic of allergies. In addition to food allergies, they are probably reacting to the environmental toxins used in the building materials and cleaning supplies in schools, as well as to the radiation emitted by TVs, microwave ovens, and computers. Another important allergy in kids is the mercury in amalgams, which can be leaked to them in infancy through their mother's milk.

Neuromediated hypotension (NMH) can be a cause of chronic fatigue syndrome in some patients, usually in connection with adrenal problems. These people experience a dramatic drop in their blood pressure when standing upright. NMH is an abnormality in the central nervous system in which the nervous system signals the heart to slow down, thereby causing a decrease in the total volume of circulating blood per minute and a decrease in blood pressure. This results in pooling of blood in the lower limbs, which leaves less blood available to nourish the brain. As a result, the person may feel lightheaded, nauseated, and or faint. One study demonstrated that 96 percent of CFIDS patients had NMH, while only 29 percent of a control group tested positive for it.

Some researchers believe that NMH might be the result of damage caused to the central nervous system by a virus or other infection. However, no conclusive evidence has yet been found. I find that an allergy to the adrenal glands or allergies to certain foods can be important factors in low blood pressure, and these can be remedied through NAET and supplementation.

Another important cause of chronic fatigue is hypothyroidism, which is sometimes overlooked by physicians. Many doctors who fail to see chronic fatigue as a problem also fail to detect chronic low thyroid. Blood tests are not a reliable way to evaluate thyroid function. Before doctors began using blood tests, it was common to use basal body temperature, the temperature of the body at rest. At a recent seminar I attended, a physician reported that 90 percent of the people who came to his office were hypothyroid, but 90 percent of the time the blood did not indicate this. Undiagnosed hypothyroidism is a serious concern, and failure to treat it can cause other health problems over time.

When I suspect hypothyroid as the result of an enzyme evaluation palpation exam and a urinalysis, I recommend doing a basal body axillary (sp) temperature test. Readings below 97.7 are generally accompanied by some or all of the symptoms of low thyroid function, including fatigue, depression, eczema, constipation, headaches, menstrual problems, recurring infections, and sensitivity to cold. High basal body temperatures, above 98.6, are much more rare and are usually consistent with hyperthyroidism, which may actually have similar symptoms. However, hyperthyroidism is also characterized by bulging eyeballs, fast pulse, hyperactivity, inability to gain weight, insomnia, menstrual problems, nervousness, and irritability. In addition to a series of standard allergy treatments for hypothyroid, I recommend a natural thyroid supportive enzyme with minerals (AllerZyme thy).

Other hormonal problems can also play a part in chronic fatigue syndrome. Women and men can be allergic to their own hormones, including adrenaline, epinephrine, norephinephrine, cortisol, insulin, the various thyroid hormones, testosterone, DHEA, and, for women, estrogen, estradiol, estrone, estriol, and progesterone. Many people who are taking DHEA are allergic to it and may be experiencing fatigue or other side effects including loss of hair which I have recently discovered in some patients. Adrenal allergies, which are common in menopausal women, people with exercise-induced asthma, and those who are experiencing a great deal of stress, tend to cause hyperactivity, anxiety, and heat rashes. Treating for hormones can be an important step in healing many of the immune disorders. After treating for female hormones I commonly recommend using progesterone oil or cream, maybe a natural estrogen for women with menopausal symptoms, Pregnenalone, or DHEA. I always use muscle testing to assess whether patients are allergic to the supplements I give them and to determine how many they should take.

Hypoglycemia, another common cause of chronic fatigue and a factor in many other immune disorders, is caused by carbohydrate and sugar intolerance and poor metabolism of sugar. The body naturally strives to maintain an adequate blood sugar supply to the brain. In hypoglycemia, the brain does not get enough sugar, resulting in fatigue, depression, irritability, anxiety, other psychological disturbances, excessive sweating, mental confusion, and in severe cases, bizarre behavior and convulsions. Many studies have shown that depressed individuals tend to suffer from hypoglycemia. The standard method of diagnosing this disorder is with an oral glucose tolerance test. After the subject has fasted for about 12 hours, a baseline blood glucose measurement is made, and the subject is given a very sweet liquid containing glucose. Blood sugar levels are then rechecked at 30 minutes, at one hour, and then hourly up to six hours. If the levels rise above 200 milligrams (mg) per deciliter, it indicates diabetes. If they fall below 15 mg, it indicates hypoglycemia.

Many of the symptoms of hypoglycemia are similar to those of candidiasis which also involves a problem with sugar. Sometimes hypoglycemia can be linked to an allergy to insulin or adrenaline and the symptoms can be cleared by treating for these hormones. Two key allergy treatments in working with hypoglycemia is treating the allergy to sugar and amino acids. Half of our amino acids are converted to sugar and utilized by the body for proper brain function. If a person is allergic to amino acids or not digesting or metabolizing those proteins. they are deficient in sugar and experience hypoglycemia and accompanying sugar cravings. In accessing individuals for hypoglycemia, I usually find a problem with protein, or sugars, or both. This also refers to poor digestion and/or allergies to these nutrients. I will recommend the sugar intolerant diet located in the Resource Guide.

Another cause of chronic fatigue is poor digestion and metabolism. I usually begin my work with new patients by evaluating how well they digest and metabolize foods. No matter how good the diet is, if the person cannot digest properly, he or she will end up with allergies, nutritional deficiencies, chronic health problems, and immune disorders. Most people eat too much sugar and do not digest and absorb it properly. Some people have problems with fats, carbohydrates, or proteins. With CFIDS sufferers, I always recommend one or more digestive enzymes and sometimes other enzymes for the spleen and thymus. Nearly everyone with a chronic immune disorder has poor digestion.

For example, I am currently treating a woman who has one of the worst cases of chronic fatigue syndrome I have ever seen. She could barely make it into my office for our first visit. I immediately put her on an enzyme to help with the digestion of sugar, and within a few days her condition had improved. Her digestion was better, her fatigue had diminished, and she was able to eat a wider variety of foods, which was significant since she was extremely thin.

Another theory suggests that chronic fatigue is caused by a hyperactive immune system. Several studies indicate that CFIDS patients with severe symptoms have a higher number of killer T cells, the white blood cells that fight viruses and other microorganisms. In addition, these people have a reduced number of normal suppressor T cells, the white blood cells responsible for stopping the immune system once it has finished its attack. When this mechanism fails, the symptoms do not shut down and the immune system continues to mount its defensives. This overactivity releases lymphokines, chemicals that may be responsible for symptoms such as fatigue and muscle aches. Further studies are needed to substantiate this theory.

As I mentioned earlier, I treat each case of chronic fatigue syndrome individually, not according to some standard treatment protocol but according to the person's unique allergy evaluation. This approach, which is based on my own research and clinical experience, has been largely successful in clearing up certain allergies and changing the symptoms and quality of life for these people. What I learn on one patient I try out on others with a similar profile; thus I have come to see that there are allergy elimination treatment protocols that seem to correlate with people with chronic fatigue syndrome.

Psychological stress, depression, and anxiety are all factors that can add to the "load" of someone with a weakened immune system. If people digest and absorb their food well, have no allergies, and eat a nutritious diet appropriate for their body type, they will remain physically strong and resilient no matter how much stress they are under. When they have dormant or chronic allergies and are eating foods they cannot tolerate well, however, stress or emotional trauma may cause their immune system to weaken and their body to break down.

There are many symptoms of chronic fatigue syndrome that overlap with those of certain mental disorders.

This can make it difficult to obtain a correct diagnosis. To compound the matter, many physicians attribute CFIDS to emotional rather than physical causes, which in itself can be an added stress for the patient. These and other major stresses, combined with the pressures of everyday life, can contribute to chronic fatigue if the load is overwhelming and may lower the body's resistance to infections.

Depression affects 20 percent of Americans at some point in their lives, and most depressed people feel fatigued. People with CFIDS usually have a symptom of depression that accompanies the fatigue. In contrast to ordinary sadness, depression may last for months or even years. In addition to daily depressed mood, symptoms may include weight loss or gain (plus or minus 10 percent of ideal body weight), insomnia, excessive sleeping, restlessness, lethargy, low energy throughout the day, feelings of worthlessness, suicidal thoughts, and difficulty making decisions and concentrating. The presence of these symptoms in the absence of the physical symptoms of CFIDS—for example, sore throat, fever, achiness and pain—suggests a depressed state and not chronic fatigue syndrome.

Often people start manifesting symptoms after an emotional trauma, such as a death in the family, a divorce, or the loss of a job. In such cases, the depression and the chronic fatigue may be inextricably linked, and it is important to attend both to their emotional state and to their physical condition. Of course, many people simply feel discouraged and depressed as a response to their fatigued state.

Another important cause of chronic fatigue syndrome is candidiasis, or yeast infection, I believe that fungal infections play a major role in every chronic health problem. They are prevalent, insidious, and difficult to get rid of because they can be passed back and forth between people, and they are a leading cause of immune suppression problems. More people than you can imagine have some form of yeast infection, whether it is athlete's foot, eczema, vaginal infections, intestinal bloating, skin rashes, mouth sores, or scalp problems. These infections place a constant burden on the immune system and are usually a primary factor in cases of chronic fatigue syndrome.

A woman in her 80s came to see me with a chronic cough. She lived in a retirement home with its own medical facility, and she worked in the facility as a volunteer. At times her cough got worse, at times it got better, but it was always there. When it became worse, they gave her antibiotics which lessened it somewhat, but never really eliminated it. We cleared bacteria and viruses with NAET which eliminated her depression and fatigue, but the cough remained. I knew it was fungal in origin because she was always fighting a vaginal irritation. Then we treated her with NAET twice for fungus, as described in the resource section of this book, and her cough cleared up and has not returned in two and a half years. In addition, her vaginal irritation has disappeared and she is no longer susceptible to colds and runny noses. In my 20 years of practice, I have never seen anything as effective for fungal infections as NAET in combination with enzyme therapy and dietary recommendations for a ten-day period after treatment with NAET.

The prevalence of yeast infections is due to the widespread use of antibiotics, the use of birth control pills and hormone replacements for women, and the transmission of this mircroorganism through sexual and skin-to-skin contact. Some people are also born with a genetic predisposition to contract it. For example, my young daughter used to experience bloating, and her ears would feel like they were filled up or popping. When I treated her for fungus, her bloating cleared up and her ears stopped clogging. Although she had never been given antibiotics, my husband has always had problems with fungus.

Other contributing causes of chronic fatigue syndrome include both an iron allergy leading to a deficiency of iron, and an excess of iron. Many people are allergic to iron which makes it difficult for them to absorb iron from food. An iron deficiency can cause anemia, low red blood cell count, and fatigue, and clearing people of their allergy to iron can help restore their energy.

The other problem is that iron can be a toxic metal and in excess can cause certain cancers, heart disease, and other illnesses. Dr. Ray Pete, a nutritionist in Eugene, Oregon, cites research suggesting that the regulation of iron is an essential function of the immune system because iron is a basic requirement for survival and growth of cells including bacteria, parasites, and cancer. In a newsletter published in 1996, he writes, "Just like lead, mercury, cadmium, nickel, magnesium and other heavy metals, stored iron produces destructive free radicals. The harmful effects of iron-produced free radicals are practically indistinguishable from those caused by exposure to X rays and gamma rays; both accelerate the accumulation of age pigment and other signs of aging. Excess iron is a crucial element in the transformation of stress into tissue damage by free radicals." Dr. Pete has written extensively about the toxic effects of too much iron and the dangers of taking supplemental iron. Dr. Pete also believes that too much iron can block our absorption of copper, and too little copper can make us store too much iron. He believes copper is a crucial element for skin and hair color and elasticity of the skin and blood vessels, and an important anti-aging element. Copper is also necessary for the normal functioning of nerve cells. The shape and texture of hair can change in a copper deficiency as too much iron can cause a deficiency in copper. When our tissues age, they naturally lose copper as they store excess iron. Treating for iron is actually more important than recommending iron supplementation.

Mineral allergies and deficiencies are another essential cause of chronic fatigue syndrome. Vitamins like C and E get a lot of attention. They are important but an allergy to them could be the cause of chronic fatigue. Allergies to minerals are equally critical in a person's health. Chromium, one of more than a dozen minerals essential for good health, is a trace element that helps the cells break down sugar into energy for the body. An allergy to chromium can cause problems metabolizing sugar, including hypoglycemia or even diabetes. Chromium makes insulin function more effectively, thereby lowering blood sugar and insulin levels. Recent research has shown that high circulating levels of insulin can be destructive to arteries. Insulin resistance is a newly designated risk factor in cardiovascular disease, along with high cholesterol and blood pressure. Interestingly, chromium also tends to normalize abnormally low blood sugar and to lower blood cholesterol, and it may be a factor in building a leaner physique.

The wide use of cortisone and other drugs can also be a cause of chronic fatigue syndrome as well as Candida and other yeast infections. My own research indicates that chronic fatigue syndrome patients tend to have hypofunctioning adrenal glands. These people show decreased levels of the adrenal hormone cortisol and increased levels of the pituitary hormone ACTH which stimulates the adrenal cortex to produce hormones such as cortisol. Cortisol is important for fighting infections because it is an important natural anti inflammatory, helps in the metabolism of fats and carbohydrates, and influences sodium potassium or normal electrolyte levels. It also influences the growth of connective tissue such as bone, cartilage, and tendons, When the adrenal cortex is weak, it cannot adequately produce steroid hormones like cortisol. The pituitary gland continues to secrete ACTH to help the adrenals produce cortisol. If the adrenals cannot keep up with the body's demands, elevated ACTH levels and decreased cortisol levels are the result. This increases the symptoms of adrenal exhaustion, ranging from chronic fatigue to undue water retention and poor sugar metabolism There are certain blood tests and saliva tests to measure cortisol levels. In addition, if the blood pressure decreases from a lying to standing position, it is a sign of adrenal insufficiency. Decreased cortisol levels suggest a possible allergy to the body's own adrenal gland or adrenal gland hormones.

Some of the symptoms of adrenal deficiency, which is related to hypoglycemia, are faintness and lightheadedness caused by diminished cerebral blood flow with hypotension. Other symptoms such as slow pulse, nausea, stomach discomfort, and headaches may also be a result of increased epinephrine and norepinephrine response in the body's compensation for adrenal corticol deficiency. Some of these patients may also be allergic to epinephrine or norepinephrine and to the adrenal cortex or adrenal medulla which can cause.

Adrenal fatigue, or hypoadrenia, refers to adrenal glands that are not functioning to their full and normal potential. This can cause fatigue, depression, dizziness, spaciness, poor memory, muscle weakness, and some of the other symptoms of chronic fatigue syndrome. Treating for the adrenal medulla and adrenal cortex with NAET can cause an immediate improvement. I generally recommend an adrenal enzyme, depending on the person's overall makeup, cortisol levels, and other allergies.

Salt, one of the basic allergens we treat with NAET, is imperative to adrenal gland health and function. People are put on these low-salt diets for many reasons, but the diets can be unnecessary and even deleterious. Sometimes treating for salt, eating foods with natural salt, or taking supplemental electrolytes can improve adrenal gland health. Other nutrients important to the adrenal glands are potassium, zinc, iron, magnesium, calcium, Vitamin C, amino acids, and the B vitamin, especially B[5] and pantothenic acid

Another important gland for chronic fatigue syndrome and for the immune system in general is the thymus which lies below the thyroid gland and above the heart. The health of the thymus determines the health of the immune system because it is responsible for so many immune system functions including the production of T lymphocytes, a type of white blood cell responsible for "cell mediated immunity." (For more information on cell mediate immunity, see the section on the Immune System.) The thymus gland releases several hormones including thymosin, thymopoeitin, and serum thymic factor. Abnormally low levels of these hormones, which occur when the body is allergic to its own thymus or the gland is not functioning adequately, can cause depressed immunity and an increased susceptibility to infection. Most CFIDs patients are allergic to thymus and need to be treated for it. Once they've cleared the allergy, I usually prescribe a freeze-dried live-cell thymus supplement.

With CFIDS patients, I also check the spleen, which is the largest mass of lymphatic tissue in the body, lying in the upper left abdomen behind the lower ribs. The spleen produces white blood cells that can destroy bacteria and other organisms and destroy worn out red blood cells and platelets. The spleen also serves as a blood reservoir, releasing stored blood during hemorrhages and preventing shock, and it secretes many potent immune system compounds that are used in the defense of the body. Treating for an allergy to the spleen, followed by a spleen enzyme, can be helpful for people with chronic fatigue syndrome.

Another major cause of CFIDS is the essential fatty acids (EFAs), or fats in general. The essential fatty acids are essential nutrients for immune system functioning, and poor intake or metabolism of these nutrients can play a role in chronic fatigue syndrome and other immune disorders. There are two essential fatty acids: linoleic acid and alpha linolenic acid. Linoleic acid cannot be made by the body and must be provided by the diet. The conditional EFAs, which are formed in the body from the essential fatty acids, include Gamma Linolenic Acid (GLA), Arachidonic Acid (AA), Eicosapentanenoic Acid (EPA), and Docosahexaenoic Acid (DHA). Essential fatty acids are needed by the body for proper nutrition and health. Essential fatty acids are precursors to the prostaglandins, which are hormones that can control different physiological functions. Essential fatty acids are found in many natural occurring seed oils and in the green leaves of edible plants. Flaxseed, soybean, and canola oils contain alphalinolinic acid and linoleic acid. In fact, more than half the fatty acids in flaxseed oil are alphalinolinic. The essential fatty acid Gamma Linolenic Acid is available in evening primrose oil and black currant oil. Fatty acids provide flexibility and fluidity to all cells, allowing them to change shape and pass through capillaries. The EFAs are also the precursors for the eicosanoids which include the prostaglandins and leukotrienes. The eicosanoids are powerful tools that holds the human body in shape. They are powerful agents that control the body's hormonal function and almost every physiological function. They basically keep us alive and well. They are very important in regulating the immune system as a powerful anti-inflammatory. Like all hormones, eicosanoids operate at a delicate balance for regulators of cellular function. An allergy to EFAs, which is relatively common, can cause a deficiency in these vital nutrients and a resistance to absorbing them from foods. This, in turn, can lead to a deficiency of eicosanoids or prostaglandins and other immune mediators, resulting in immune suppression and chronic fatigue. Clearing the allergy can effect a permanent change in energy level and the body's ability to respond to infection. Supplementation with essential fatty acids has shown benefits in cardiac problems, dislodging plaque from artery walls, decreasing pain and inflammation, increasing oxygen flow and endurance, preventing platelet aggravation, and dilating airways, which makes them especially important for asthmatics.

There are also some major factors that stimulate or inhibit the conversion of the essential fatty acids to prostaglandins which we will discuss later when we talk about the treatment of immune disorders. For example, high carbohydrate diets, obesity, elevated insulin, and certain chemicals and food coloring can inhibit prostaglandin production, whereas a diet rich in fatty acids, along with good protein and fat digestion, can be stimulating. Also, allergies to protein and fat can inhibit the body's conversion of EFAs to prostaglandins.

Another factor that inhibits the production of prostaglandins is the intake of trans fatty acids which are partially hydrogenated vegetable oils found in a wide variety of foods. Among other things, trans fatty acids can lower good cholesterol, increase bad cholesterol, raise total serum cholesterol, lower birth weight in infants, interfere with the storage and metabolism of normal fatty acids, and increase blood insulin levels in response to glucose load, thereby increasing the risk of diabetes. It can directly affect immune response by lowering the efficiency of B cell response. It can also decrease the levels of testosterone in males, precipitate childhood asthma, and escalate potential free radical formation.

Commonly found in foods such as potato chips, salad dressings, breads, and crackers, these oils are not only partially hydrogenated but also include rancid or overheated oils that contain breakdown products such as oxidized fatty acids, oxidized steroids, peroxides, hydrocarbons, and aromatic compounds. They can be extremely toxic to the liver and destructive of cell membranes.

Antioxidant therapy is commonly used and integrated in many approaches to alternative health care. Unfortunately, many people are allergic to the most popular antioxidants which include Vitamins E and C, beta carotene, bioflavonoids, ginseng, gingko biloba, milk thistle, and lipoic acid. All of these nutrients can be important in boosting the immune system, but allergies to them can cause some of the problems that manifest in chronic fatigue. Once people have cleared these allergies, they are able to absorb these antioxidants from the foods they eat, as well as from supplements, if necessary.

Every day in my practice I witness the impact of mercury and dental amalgams on people with chronic health problems, including CFIDS and other immune disorders. For asthmatics, it is almost always necessary to treat for mercury, amalgams, and other toxic metals with NAET. In cases involving chronic fatigue, I check these allergens in the early stages of treatment. There is much debate over whether one needs to have one's mercury removed and replaced, and much research into the impact of this process on the body. I consider it an individual decision, and I will not make a recommendation either way. However, I will refer people to dentists who do this kind of work if they are interested. Whether you have removed the mercury or not, however, an allergy to it will continue to have a strong impact on the body and needs to be treated with NAET.

I read a case history recently about a woman diagnosed with MS whose health improved 90 percent when her fillings and amalgams were removed. Her numbness went away, her tingling disappeared, and her sleep was restored. "I'm a reborn person," she wrote, "enjoying hobbies of woodcraft, knitting, crocheting, passions long ago stolen from me. I am even more thankful for the gift of being able to play vigorously with my grandchildren for the first time. No longer fearing the prospect of a wheelchair, nursing home, or helpless existence is a wonderful weight to have lifted off oneself." I hear similar stories all the time about the benefits of removing and being treated for amalgams and mercury. With chronic fatigue patients in particular, removing the mercury and treating with NAET will often bring about a dramatic restoration of health and energy.

In the literature there has also been some preliminary research indicating that root canals may have a toxic effect on the body and may contribute to chronic fatigue, depression, and other autoimmune problems. Dr. George E. Meinig, a dentist, estimates that 75 percent of patients experience some chronic degenerative illness as the result of root canals. Dr. Boyd Hailey has done research indicating that 45 to 50 percent of root canals show moderate levels of toxicity due to the buildup of bacteria. Because teeth with root canals are essentially dead, they can harbor infections that constantly challenge and compromise the immune system. Dr. Hailey cites the case of his daughter, who, after being diagnosed with chronic fatigue syndrome, had a root canal extracted. Her health improved dramatically. Dr. Meinig explains that many of the toxins are caught in the dentin tubules which make up 90 percent of the tooth structure. It points to the fact that 75 percent of patients whose immune systems have been compromised by illnesses, accidents, and poor nutrition are at a higher risk with root canals because of bacteria coming from root canal teeth.

"To visualize what happens, picture the bacteria trapped in the dentin tubules; see them mutate and become more virulent and their toxins more toxic," writes Dr. Meinig. "In their escape into the blood circulation of the tube socket, these bacteria, like cancer cells, metastasize to other parts of the body. As they migrate they infect the heart, kidneys, joints, nervous system, brain, eyes, can endanger pregnant women and, in fact, may affect any organ, gland, or other tissue."

The spread of these bacteria can further weaken the immune system of people with autoimmune problems. Treating for the bacteria with NAET can help stimulate the immune system to eliminate it from the body. The question of whether these teeth need to be extracted is not within my area of expertise. I do know that NAET treatments can help ameliorate the problem. Many times, I test different teeth with more specific muscle testing to determine which tooth actually harbors the bacteria, what type of bacteria it is, then work with NAET and adjunctive enzyme therapy to treat the specific organism. Bacteria in general can be a contributing cause of chronic fatigue syndrome and other autoimmune problems, and there are many common bacteria I treat with NAET. In combination with the body's own antibodies, bacteria and other major allergens such as foods, environmental allergens, or toxins form these CICs that compromise the immune system. A list of the most common are located in the Resource Guide of this book. Clearing bacteria with NAET not only restores energy but also helps eliminate inflammation. It can, therefore, be successful for those suffering from arthritis, bursitis, or fibromyalgia, and for individuals experiencing sore and painful joints and muscles. In fact, it is one of the most successful treatments we do for people with immune disorders, and some doctors believe that bacteria are among the strongest stressors on the immune system. I would also clear fungus and parasites and viruses for more thorough results with autoimmune problems in general.

Antibiotics, which are commonly prescribed to treat bacterial infections, are overused and are often inappropriate and unnecessary. There are many herbal formulas and enzymes that are more effective than antibiotics in dealing with bacteria, especially in the early stages. Antibiotics often cause allergic reactions and tend to suppress the bacteria rather than eliminate them. These reactions create more CICs that continually compromise the immune system, causing greater susceptibility to other bacteria, viruses, and cancer cells. Antibiotics also destroy natural intestinal flora, leading to an overgrowth of Candida and fungal infections. Except in extreme, acute cases, where antibiotics may be necessary, NAET in combination with natural enzymes and herbs can be an effective alternative.

One patient of mine kept getting sinusitis, and her physician prescribed antibiotics. The infection would go away but two months later it would return. We discovered that it was a fungal rather than a bacterial problem, and we treated her for fungus. Two days later her sinusitis disappeared and she has not had another case in two years.

Hormonal disorders, which are actually caused by allergies, are another cause of chronic fatigue syndrome. As I mentioned before, we can be allergic to any of our own hormones, including melanin, insulin, testosterone, estrogen, and progesterone. A recent article from my local newspaper reports that researchers have found that a hormonal disorder may play a role in the symptoms of chronic fatigue syndrome. They discovered that CFIDS patients tend to have low levels of cortisol, a hormone that controls the immune system and is secreted by the adrenal glands in response to stress. I often find that people with chronic fatigue are allergic to cortisol and need to be treated with NAET. The researchers reported that patients with chronic fatigue also had low levels of adrenocorticotrophic (ACTH), a releasing hormone from the pituitary that plays a role in the production of cortisol. The imbalance can leave patients in a permanent state of fatigue or lethargy. The absence of the proper levels of ACTH-releasing hormone could account for the low levels of cortisol in these patients.

I had a patient with chronic fatigue, although her primary diagnosis was endogenous depression. In her workup, I found that she was extremely allergic both to ACTH and to cortisol. After treating her for these two hormones, and having her take some natural adrenal enzymes she had a major breakthrough and felt better than she had in the past 15 years. Instead of prescribing cortisol, practitioners should consider alternative treatments, particularly NAET.

For women, estrogen and progesterone are important hormones as well as common allergens. Most women over 35 need progesterone supplementation to maintain the thyroid gland and create a sense of well being. In cream form, it can be good for arthritis and joint pain. Estrogen supplementation should be given only when deemed necessary after careful evaluation. Allergy to these hormones can cause fatigue. Allergies to progesterone and estrogen and other female hormones like estradiol, estrone, and estriol can also cause problems. In particular, an allergy to estradiol can produce menopausal symptoms like hot flashes and mood swings, insomnia, and irritability

For men, testosterone and progesterone can be important and may help alleviate chronic arthritis pain. However, an allergy to testosterone can cause hair loss in men, muscle fatigue, weakness, low energy, and diminished libido. Insulin is important in the metabolism of sugar, and an allergy to it can be a precursor to diabetes, especially if the disease runs in the family. Patients who have trouble sleeping may be allergic to their own melatonin. Instead of taking melatonin supplements, which they are unable to utilize in any case, they should be treated for melatonin with NAET.

The liver is the most important center of detoxification and the body's first line of defense against chronic illness. Every day I talk to patients about the importance of maintaining a healthy liver. Unfortunately, the standard liver function test is inadequate in diagnosing some precursors to acute liver problems. Instead, I use muscle testing procedures and several tests described in the resource portion of this book. One of the best treatments for the liver is NAET. In addition to causing chronic fatigue syndrome and other autoimmune disorders, exposure to food additives, solvents, cleaning products, formaldehyde, toluene, pesticides, and other chemicals, as well as heavy metals, such as lead, mercury, arsenic, and aluminum can overburden the liver with toxins and compromise its function.

Besides chronic fatigue, the symptoms of a sluggish liver are headache, digestive problems, and chemical sensitivity. After many years of working with NAET, I have discovered that those individuals who experience many symptoms during the 25-hour clearing, or become even more sensitive to other allergens afterward, tend to be those individuals with liver toxicity. This is an important point for NAET practitioners and patients undergoing NAET treatments. For example, a man in his 50s started to see me for mild asthma, and noticed after I cleared him on the basics, became overly sensitive to pollens, perfumes, and fumes. I immediately performed an abdominal palpation examination and found a positive liver reflex representing liver toxicity. I prescribed a liver enzyme and within 24 hours his sensitivity was diminished. Now, when a person becomes overly sensitive, I automatically presume that the liver needs some support. A liver enzyme (lvr) (see Chapter 20) works successfully for detoxification. NAET treatments not only eliminate allergies but also detoxify the body, so we need to maintain a healthy liver for detoxification to occur adequately.

Conventional Treatments

According to traditional medicine, there is no cure for chronic fatigue syndrome and fibromyalgia. The only treatments prescribed are lifestyle modification and drugs to treat muscle pain and depression, aid in sleeping, and reduce anxiety. The approach is aimed at helping people minimize discomfort while recognizing limitations so they can adjust. Behavior modification is recommended, and patients are instructed to keep an energy diary to identify patterns of energy and fatigue and to aid in planning activities, setting limits, tailoring their behavior to match their energy level, and incorporating rest periods into their day.

Patients are encouraged to adhere to a diet that is low in animal fat and high in fiber, with plenty of fruits and vegetables. In contrast, I will recommend different diets for different individuals, depending on their particular problems with digestion and absorption and their food intolerances. (See specific recommended diets based on abdominal palpation.) For some people the diet will be low in animal fat and high in fruits and vegetables, whereas for others it may be the reverse, depending on what I discover when I evaluate them.

CFIDS patients may respond well to antidepressants, although they generally require smaller doses than those who are being treated for depression alone and cannot tolerate the normally prescribed doses. It can take 3 to 4 weeks before improvement of symptoms is noted. Antidepressants can help alleviate the depression that often accompanies chronic fatigue, and some patients report that their energy level improves as well. Side effects may include restlessness, sedation, dry mouth, fast heart rate, and constipation. The most commonly prescribed antidepressants are the tricyclics like Doxepin and Elavil and the serotonin reuptake inhibitors like fluoxetine (Prozac), sertraline (Zoloft), and paroetine (Paxil). Others include traxodone (Desyrel), venlaxine (Effexor), and bupropion (Wellbutrin).

Hypnotics are often prescribed to CFIDS patients to help reduce anxiety and aid in sleeping. In addition to being potentially addictive, these drugs may cause hallucinations, loss of muscular coordination, dizziness, drowsiness, amnesia, and depression. They include the benzodiazetines clonazetam (Klonopin), traizolan (Halcion), temazepam (Restoril), altrazoam (Xanax), and lorazepam (Ativan). If muscle or joint pain persists, NSAIDs (non-steroidal anti-inflammatory drugs) are typically prescribed or purchased "over the counter." NSAIDS include aspirin, ibuprofen (Motrin), nuprin (Advil), naproxen (Alleve), naprosen (Nanaprox), piroxicam (Feldend), and cyclobenzaprine (Flexeril). Side effects may include gastrointestinal upset and kidney problems. If the joint pain is especially severe and does not respond to NSAIDs, a physician may give a localized injection of a steroid like depomedoral or an anesthetic like lydocaine.

Immune suppressant drugs are currently being used experimentally in the treatment of chronic fatigue syndrome on the assumption that the disease is caused by an overactive immune system. The drugs, which are normally prescribed in kidney transplants to prevent the body from rejecting the foreign kidney, are highly toxic and have serious side effects. Anti-cancer drugs have also been prescribed on an experimental basis.

Patients with chronic fatigue syndrome who are diagnosed with neurally mediated hypertension (MNH) have been treated with calcium channel blockers, which inhibit the contraction of smooth muscle. There is no evidence that NMH causes CFS, and the treatment is considered experimental. Studies show that it is difficult to adjust the dosage of these medications, which are typically used to treat high blood pressure, to minimize adverse side effects like dizziness, low blood pressure, nausea, and headaches. Alternative methods for mediating the NMH in CFIDS patients includes exercising the lower extremities prior to standing, avoiding heavy exercise after meals, support hose to decrease pooling of blood, and increased salt intake to encourage adequate blood flow to the brain.

Some studies have demonstrated a relationship between a tendency to develop allergies and CFIDS. As I've already mentioned, I believe that allergies are the primary cause of chronic fatigue. Unfortunately, many of the drugs used in conventional medicine to treat allergies cause drowsiness, fatigue, headache, dry mouth, impaired coordination, and upset stomach. Non-sedating allergy drugs include terfenadine (Seldane), astemizole (Hismanal), and loratadine (Claratin). Sedating drugs include diphenhydramine (Benadryl) and hydroxyzine (Atarax).

Adenosine monophosphate (AMP) is a naturally occurring metabolite that has been used in the treatment of some herpes viruses and has also been helpful for chronic fatigue syndrome. Because it has adverse side effects like asthma, heart palpitations, and dizziness, however, it is no longer commonly used. Ampligen is an anti-viral that has been used to treat both HIV and CFIDS. Taken either orally or intravenously, it seems to help with fatigue and has few side effects, although it is expensive. Another drug called nephazoline (which is sold over the counter as eye drops with the brand name Clear Eyes) is an ophthalmic drug that stimulates the trigeminal nerve to the brain and helps with chronic fatigue syndrome. A nicotine patch has also been used to stimulate the production of seratonin, which helps with depression and fatigue. Nicotine is a basal dilator and can improve cognitive functions. Unfortunately, many people are allergic to nicotine and need to be treated for it with NAET before they can make use of it.

Alternative Treatments for Chronic Fatigue Syndrome

A long tradition of herbal medicine exists throughout the world, and the value of herbs is unquestioned. In fact, a significant proportion of today's drugs are derived from plants. However, there is little evidence to support the role herbs can play in the treatment of chronic fatigue syndrome. This is due to the inaccessibility of information from the Far East, where herbal medicine is highly developed, and to the lack of studies being done in the West. Like allopathic medicines, herbs can have potent side effects, and the dangers of taking them are increased by the lack of clear standards applied in the dosing. As with any treatment, it is important for the person undertaking it to become knowledgeable about possible side effects or allergies.

"Energy boosting" preparations may contain ephedra or other stimulants, which can have the same problematic side effects as diet pills. Certain products use astralagus, an herb that enhances immunity. *Echinacea purpurer,* the root of the purple cone flower, a member of the daisy family, is used by Native Americans for enhancing the immune system. In laboratory experiments it has been shown to be almost as effective as prescription drugs in inactivating certain viruses. Echinacea can be purchased at most health food stores, and I rarely find people allergic to it. I use it with certain enzymes, as described tin he viral recipe section of this book. Garlic, an edible member of the allium family that includes onions, chives, and shallots, is an important anti-infectant and antiviral.

Ginseng, which is derived from the plant panax ginseng, is usually prepared as a tonic tea. Siberian ginseng (*eleutherococcus senticosus*) is another herb that increases resistance to stress, fatigue, and disease. Ginseng (Siberian or panax) can enhance the ability of humans to withstand many adverse physical conditions, including heat, noise, motion, and exercise, and can increase mental alertness and energy levels under stressful conditions.

I use Siberian ginseng in certain preparations to help improve adrenal function after clearing allergies to vitamins C and B in chronic fatigue syndrome patients. It can also increase feelings of well-being, which can help with depression and insomnia, A possible explanation may lie in its ability to balance the neurotransmitters like seratonin, dopamine, norepinephrine, and epinephrine.

Panax ginseng, as opposed to Siberian ginseng, is especially effective with severely fatigued or debilitated individuals. As with Siberian ginseng, clinical studies have shown it to enhance mental and physical performance, boost energy, and reduce the body's vulnerability to stress in both men and women.

Gingko biloba is an extract from the leaf of a common ornamental tree that can relieve symptoms of cerebral insufficiency related to artherosclerosis and has been used by some people to boost brain power, clarity, and attention. Comfrey is a preparation of the root or leaves of the plant *symphytum officinale* commonly used as a tea; although it contains possible carcinogens, it is effective in helping fractures to heal. Primrose oil is a preparation made from the seeds of the evening primrose (*oenothera biennis*) that helps the immune system and increases the suppleness of muscles and joints. St. John's wart (*hypericum perforatum*) is a shrubby perennial plant native to Europe and the United States that is commonly used to improve mood and alleviate depression. Research indicates that it can inhibit the growth of different viruses, including the enterovirus associated with AIDS and the HIV virus, and can improve the mood in AIDS patients.

Shiitake mushrooms (*lentinus edods*) have been used in Asia for centuries to enhance the immune system and combat cancer. They can be taken as an extract or eaten in the diet. Research from Japan indicates that components from the mushroom have had impressive results in prolonging the lifespan of cancer patients and activating the macrophages and immune mediators in the body.

Magnesium is important for chronic fatigue syndrome because it helps relieve pain, boosts energy production in cells, and aids in digestion. Omega-3 fatty acids and the essential fatty acids are necessary for maintaining normal membrane structure and cell function. Other nutrients, including vitamins B, C, E, beta carotene, and various minerals, are also essential but are deficient in most people because of the deficiency of minerals in the soil. Before prescribing nutritional supplements, I test and clear people for any allergies to them.

In addition to the alternative treatments mentioned thus far, acupuncture, and relaxation techniques can help alleviate pain and increase energy level in CFIDS patients.

9 | FIBROMYALGIA

Bones, bones
Irish bones,
the lickety-click split
of bones
screaming
all the way down
to the marrow.
　　　　　—from "Bones"

Betsy

Betsy, 81, was diagnosed with polymyalgia rheumatica (PMR) eight years before she first came to see me in 1996. PMR is characterized by achiness in the muscles of the neck, shoulders, or hips, especially in the morning. Patients feel stiff all over and have trouble getting out of bed. The disease can strike without warning and can be accompanied by headaches, hearing difficulties, and a persistent cough. Although the cause is uncertain, the standard treatment is cortical steroids.

Betsy experienced severe pain in her shoulder and arms that would wake her up frequently throughout the night. For the past three years she had been taking prednisone, which gave her some relief. But as time went on, she had developed allergies to a number of foods including dairy, grains, and alcohol. Among her symptoms were diarrhea, chronic sinus congestion, and hypoglycemia, and she needed to eat constantly to avoid feeling lethargic or faint. Once a highly energetic woman, she was slowed down by the allergies and the PMR, as well as by the side effects of going off the prednisone.

An abdominal diagnostic exam and a 24-hour urinalysis revealed severe intestinal toxemia, calcium deficiency, low adrenals, and an inability to digest simple sugars and complex carbohydrates. She also evidenced an epigastric reflex, an inflammation in the gastric area that occurs frequently in people who have been on prednisone and whose immune system has been stressed. Prednisone is so damaging to the immune system that the occurrence of food allergies and hypoglycemia is common.

I performed a complete allergy test with the suspicion that Betsy was allergic to calcium. Treatment for calcium often proves helpful in relieving the joint pain associated with rheumatoid arthritis, osteoarthritis, and fibromyalgia, and I was hoping that she might respond to this treatment as well. She proved to be allergic to all of the most common allergens and to most foods. When I perform an allergy test, I am checking for food intolerances as well as allergies. Although they resemble allergies, intolerances generally clear up when we desensitize people to the basic allergens. With real allergies, by contrast, we need to treat for the food to which the person is intolerant as well.

Besty was allergic to most vegetables, fruits, berries, alcohol, grains, seeds, food additives, fungi, bacteria, viruses, and the prednisone she had been taking for three years, which helped explain her difficulty when she went off the drug. After describing the NAET technique to her, I explained the dangers of steroids and the stress they cause a healthy immune system. Then I began treating her for the basic allergies, starting with eggs, chicken, feathers, and tetracycline. Since going off the prednisone, she was again suffering severe shoulder and arm pain, but instead of taking medication, she was seeing an acupuncturist and a physical therapist who provided only temporary relief. When I treated her for calcium, which includes milk products, her shoulder and arm pain completely disappeared for the first time since 1988. She was so happy, she was in tears. Her stamina returned and she was able to sleep all night without interruption. In addition, she could now take calcium supplements which previously made her sick to her stomach. It was one of the most dramatic and exciting improvements I had ever seen in a patient. We still had to treat the rest of her food allergies, however.

We proceeded to treat her for the foods she most enjoyed eating, including grains, nuts, artificial sweeteners, chocolate, and peanut butter, and she began taking the enzymes recommended for her, including a calcium enzyme (para), an enzyme for digestion of sugars (pan) and complex carbohydrates, an enzyme for the strength and nutrition of the adrenal glands (adr), and AllerZyme CFS (or fibromyalgia). After that, I did not see her for some time, although she reported periodically that she was doing fine.

Toward the end of 1996, Betsy came to see me with a severe eye infection. Her doctor had given her eye drops, which did nothing. Testing revealed that she was allergic to a number of bacteria, including *staphylococcus abdominus, staphylococcus aureus,* and *streptococcus viridans.* I generally suspect a fungus or bacteria allergy in conditions such as arthritis, fibromyalgia, and PMR. People being treated for bacteria should avoid contact with anything other than distilled water. This includes not taking a shower, not eating raw food, and wearing plastic gloves when using the toilet. Within 25 hours of her treatment for these bacteria, her eyes cleared up and she has not had a problem since.

This past spring, Betsy returned with a deep cough and severe sinus congestion. I have found that mucus problems like these are generally caused by an allergy to fungi, including molds and yeasts such as Candida. In particular, people who have taken antibiotics or steroids like prednisone for a period of time tend to suffer from severe fungus allergies. Betsy first went to see her doctor, who prescribed two courses of antibiotics. This did nothing for the cough and, in fact, only killed off the healthy flora in her system and allowed yeasts to multiply, affecting not only her intestines but also her lungs. I have also noticed that if mold has not been cleared, a fungus over-growth will often show up during mold season. Betsy turned out to be allergic to quite a few fungi, including *blastomyces dermatoides, epidermophyton floccosum, mucor racemosus, mucorales mutabile, mycosis fungoides, nocardia asteroides, rhizopus nigricans, schimmelpilz II,* and *nos. vaginitis.*

Clearing the fungi was not easy for Betsy because she lived alone and needed to clean her entire house thoroughly, wear a mask and gloves, buy a new toothbrush and hairbrush, and make sure she was drinking and eating with sterile uten-sils. Nevertheless, 25 hours after her treatment, Betsy's cough was almost completely gone. I also prescribed a good aci-dophilus formula that includes an enzyme for combatting fungi (smi). Typically, after patients have cleared a fungus or some other infectant, I have them take certain enzymes de-signed to help the immune system eliminate the fungus from the body (AllerZyme C). Betsy was so pleased by her dramatic improvement that she has become a vocal advocate of NAET.

FIBROMYALGIA

Anyone who has been ill knows how distressing it can be to have a physical ailment. But patients with the ex-tremely painful muscle condition known as fibromyalgia often experience an additional obstacle: the necessity of proving that anything is in fact wrong with them. Though recognized as an illness by the American Medical Associ-ation (AMA) in 1987, fibromyalgia continues to be ques-tioned by doctors who are unfamiliar with the syndrome. In fact, fibromyalgia affects up to 10 million Americans, or 5 percent of the nation's population, making it the most common cause of widespread pain encountered in medical practice.

People with fibromyalgia who present to their physi-cians with complaints of chronic pain all over their bodies originating in the muscles might have their blood tested or X rays taken, only to be sent home with a less than reassuring declaration that the symptoms are a mere creation of their own mind. Since fibromyalgia does not appear in any medical diagnostic test, some in the medical profession have difficulty identifying it or even believing in its existence. However, there is a standardized method of testing for fibromyalgia as described in the 1990 guidelines of the American College of Rheumatology that allows for precise, reliable classification of the disease. A diagnosis of fibromyalgia is based on the patient's report of at least three months of widespread physical pain, as well as tenderness of 11 out of 18 predetermined points on the body when pressure is applied. Fibromyalgia may appear without the presence of any other condition. This condition is sometimes referred to as primary fibromyalgia. However, a patient will frequently have developed accompanying disorders, such as rheumatoid arthritis or systemic lupus erythematosus, in which case the fibromyalgia may be labeled "concomitant." The following syndromes often appear with fibromyalgia or have symptoms similar to fibromyalgia:

1. irritable bowel syndrome—abdominal pain, cramps, audible bowel sounds, loose stools with mucus but no blood

2. inflammatory bowel disease—abdominal pain, weight loss, bloody diarrhea

3. irritable bladder—frequent and urgent urination

4. female urethral syndrome—frequent and painful urination, recurrent bladder infections

5. dysmenorrhea—menstrual cramping

6. restless leg syndrome—uneasy feeling of insects crawling on legs which is worse at night or when lying down

7. headaches—especially muscular tension and migraine

8. Raynaud's phenomenon—reduced blood flow to fingers, toes, and face, especially in cold and stressful situations

9. premenstrual tension syndrome

10. allergies—common allergy symptoms

11. hypertension

12. sleep apnea—snoring, periodic cessation of breathing for several seconds while asleep

13. sicca—dry eyes and dry mouth, reduced production of body fluids, aggravated by antidepressants

14. arthritis—joint pain or failure

15. carpal tunnel syndrome—pain and numbness in the thumb and fingers because of excessive stress or pressure at the wrist

16. systemic lupus erythematosus—an autoimmune disease with symptoms such as skin rash, arthritis, and kidney trouble

17. Sjogren's syndrome—an autoimmune disease characterized by dry eyes and mouth

18. polymyalgia rheumatica—stiffness and pain in shoulders and hips found among the elderly

19. osteoporosis—bone condition characterized by increased risk of fractures and breaks, and chronic pain

20. hypothyroidism—characterized by fatigue, fluid retention, cold intolerance, dry skin, weight problems, depression

21. MS—a disease of neurological dysfunction

Fibromyalgia is not considered an inflammatory autoimmune disease like arthritis. William Wilke, M.D., explains, "Most inflammatory conditions hurt a lot more when you move, while fibromyalgia pain continues and may be worse even when you're not moving." Also, arthritic pain tends to originate in the joints, while the pain of fibromyalgia arises from the muscles. Sometimes people think that fibromyalgia is the same as chronic fatigue syndrome or CFIDS. Although the two conditions overlap significantly—both involve fatigue, sleep disturbance, irritable bowel syndrome, headaches, depression, numbness, and pain all over the body—patients with fibromyalgia always experience pain in at least 11 of the 18 tender points, whereas rheumatolgists do not require pain in 11 points to diagnose CFIDS. According to various estimates, fibromyalgia sufferers are from 65 percent to 95 percent women, and the disease most often surfaces during a patient's 20s or 30s. Childhood is another common time for the onset of fibromyalgia with 28 percent of the cases beginning at that time.

There are two comforting facts about fibromyalgia that long-term studies have revealed. Fibromyalgia is not fatal, and it is not degenerative, progressive, or ultimately crippling. Although the pain is by definition chronic and pervasive[1], the symptoms can wax and wane in intensity, allowing periods of relief and stabilization. Fibromyalgia may follow one of three distinct courses: remitting, in which the symptoms intermittently disappear and reappear; fluctuating, in which they lessen periodically but never disappear entirely; and progressive, in which they become increasingly more severe.

Although a 1995 survey revealed that approximately 100 million Americans have one or more chronic ill-

---

[1]*Persons with Chronic Conditions: Their Prevalence and Costs* 11/13/96, vol. 276, No. 18, p. 1473.

nesses, this country's health care system remains firmly rooted in episodic and acute care according to an article published in the *Journal of the American Medical Association*. In a 1987 study, chronic health conditions accounted for three-quarters of directed medical care costs in the United States, whereas only 46 percent of patients reported suffering from chronic conditions. Fibromyalgia is one of these conditions, needlessly sapping our resources when a more effective, lasting treatment is now available: NAET.

A young woman in her early 40s came to see me about two years ago with symptoms suggesting fibromyalgia. Her symptoms included irritable bladder, dysmenorrhea, constant pain in the muscles at various trigger points, hormonal problems, some hypothyroid symptoms, and severe digestion and bloating problems. I tentatively diagnosed her with fibromyalgia and referred her to a physician for more testing and evaluation. The physician referred her to a rheumatologist who specialized in fibromyalgia and who prescribed antidepressants. However, the patient was reluctant to take them and came back to see me.

Suspecting that food allergies were the problem, I did a full workup and gave her enzymes to help her digest fats. I also put her on the fat-intolerance diet described in the Resource Guide of this book and modified her carbohydrate and sugar intake. She lost weight immediately, and her symptoms improved by about 30 percent. Then we began clearing the 10 basic allergens. After being treated for sugars and calcium, she noticed that her chest pain diminished. A thorough testing of her food allergies revealed that she was allergic to many foods, especially dairy products, meats, and animal and vegetable fats. We desensitized her to these allergens with NAET and her pain was reduced to a minimum. About three and a half months later she came back and was pain free.

The only problem that remained involved early menopausal symptoms connected with allergies to her own hormones. We treated her for her hormones, including estrogen, progesterone, testosterone, estrogen, estriol, and estradiol, alone and in combination with certain emotions, heat, and sugar. We also prescribed a natural hormonal cream derived from yam, soybean, and licorice root. Her symptoms disappeared, including her hot flashes, and she did not have to take any drugs or antidepressants. Subsequently, we also treated her for thyroid, the Epstein-Barr virus, and other emotional allergies. She maintains her diet, continues to take her enzymes, and she remains completely pain free. This case is typical of the results I, and other NAET practitioners, have had with fibromyalgia patients.

There are warning signs and precursors to fibromyalgia. A common one is some previous experience of physical trauma such as an injury, accident, a serious illness, or even a severe and persistent cold or the flu. In traumatic fibromyalgia, the sorest points are generally clustered around the area of injury. Estimates of how many fibromyalgia cases involve a known triggering event range from 20 percent to 50 percent. However, there may be more subtle indicators of future trouble which can be revealed through careful observation and questioning. Sometimes the first sign of fibromyalgia is the recurrence of "growing pains" after they have stopped growing.

Sleep is a crucial factor in the identification and management of fibromyalgia. Insomnia is a common symptom of many of the immune system problems and for people as they age. People with fibromyalgia often feel drowsy much of the time, and some cannot work. In addition, fibromyalgia patients have more "nonrestorative" sleep than average, meaning that they sleep more lightly rather than reaching deep stage four sleep. Sleep disorders are extremely prevalent among fibromyalgia patients.

People usually sleep better after being treated for calcium with NAET. When the body is lacking calcium, which tends to happen with an allergy to calcium, a person is in a constant state of tension and has difficulty sleeping. Other allergens I treat for in cases of insomnia are seratonin, other neurotransmitters, the hypothalamus gland, and the hormone melatonin.

Another common sleep disturbance is called the alpha delta sleep anomaly in which the sufferer does not get enough deep delta-level sleep because he or she is constantly being jolted awake or into a lighter stage of sleep by intruding alpha (waking) waves. Since delta sleep is a time for the restoration of neurotransmitters in the body's self-healing process, an ongoing deficiency of deep sleep can take a toll on one's health and proper functioning. One of the most common sleep disturbances in fibromyalgia patients is periodic limb movement disorder, or nocturnal myoclonus. In the daytime, this manifests as restless leg syndrome in which patients feel numbness or tingling in their legs and seem to be constantly moving their legs for reasons they cannot explain. In my experience, calcium is one of the primary allergy treatments for restless leg syndrome.

Recent research by Robert M. Bennett, M.D., of Oregon Health Sciences University, has found that some fibromyalgia patients have less of a protein called somatomedin-C in their bodies than healthy people. The concentration of somatomedin-C in the blood normally follows the rate of secretion of growth hormones. Research suggests that this protein activates the growth hormone and makes growth possible. Dwarfs, for example, have substantial amounts of growth hormone in their blood, but low levels of somatomedin-C, which explains their small stature. This protein, released during stage four sleep, is also instrumental in the repair of muscle tissue. Some researchers think the lack of somatomedin-C worsens the deterioration of muscle tissue and the tenderness and pain of fibromyalgia. Hence, sleep deprivation contributes to the pain rather than the reverse. I treat for somatomedins all at once by treating for the blood rather than the specific protein.

Sometimes people are genetically predisposed to sleep disturbance, or some accident, illness, or allergy results in the development of unhealthy sleep patterns. Aside from the physical stress, sleep deprivation is known to cause a number of psychological effects including depression, irritability, difficulty in concentrating, and memory problems, all of which are symptoms commonly reported by fibromyalgia patients. Once sleep is normalized, most of the other symptoms clear up.

According to the American Academy of Rheumatology, other factors that may be related to the initial development of fibromyalgia are psychological stress, immune or endocrine abnormalities, and biochemical abnormalities in the central nervous system .

Stephen J. Gislason, M.D., of Environmental Research Incorporated, has a theory that is unusual among medical doctors. "Fibromyalgia," he writes, "is a symptom complex caused by delayed pattern food allergy and is part of a larger illness complex. The general classification is non-specific hypersensitivity disease. Fibromyalgia should be treated for diet revision as the first and most essential form of therapy."

Although I agree with his appraisal, I use NAET to treat the allergies rather than revising the diet. In my experience, people with fibromyalgia and chronic fatigue tend to eat the foods to which they are most allergic. Gialason goes on to describe (with reference to the work of Dr. William Knicker) a "plausible explanation for the immune mechanisms which cause fibromyalgia involving the following steps: the abnormal entry of large food molecules into the bloodstream, the formation of immune complexes, the action of chemical mediators released by activated immune cells, and the activation of cell mediated immunity." In other words, undigested food gets into the bloodstream, forming CICs that then lodge in different parts of the body including the joints, muscles, and head, and provoke autoimmune reactions in which the body eats its own tissue. These mechanisms are responsible for a variety of autoimmune disorders, not just fibromyalgia.

Symptoms of Fibromyalgia

The most notable symptom of fibromyalgia is widespread and enduring pain that patients describe as aching, stabbing, or lacerating. Other common symptoms, accompanied by an estimate provided by the National Fibromyalgia Association of the frequency with which they occur in fibromyalgia patients, are shown in Table 9–1:

Table 9–1

Symptom	Estimate of Occurrence
muscular pain	100%
fatigue and decreased energy	96%
insomnia	86%
joint pain	72%
headaches (tension, migraine, nonmigraine)	60%
restless legs	56%
numbness and tingling (in extremities, limbs, face)	52%
impaired memory	46%
leg cramps	42%
impaired concentration	41%
nervousness	32%
major depression	20%

Other symptoms identified in fibromyalgia patients include cognitive dysfunction, dizziness, parasthesia, cold intolerance, temporary skin color changes, fluid retention, dry or watery eyes, dry mouth, tight skin, abdominal pain (usually related to irritable bowel syndrome), bloating, constipation or diarrhea, urinary urgency or frequency, secondary growth hormone deficiency, inappropriate fluctuations of body temperature, and irregular fingernail growth such as unusual curvature, ridges, or frequent breaking. In addition, sleep deprivation may compromise neurotransmitter function, causing a breakdown in the communication between mind and body resulting in faulty sensory feedback and improper muscle control. For example, because of the inability of the body's musculature to accurately determine its own activity, the fingers may fail to assert enough pressure or the wrist may weaken while attempting to grasp an object .

Fibromyalgia is a sensitivity amplification syndrome which means that certain stimuli such as lights, smells, sounds, and vibrations, are felt more intensely in someone with fibromyalgia than in a healthy person. The body may even interpret these sensations as painful, causing the person discomfort and anxiety. Diagnosed psychiatric disorders, particularly depression, appear in approximately 20 percent to 30 percent of fibromyalgia patients. The association of fibromyalgia with depression has led some to hypothesize that the syndrome has mental origins with the emotional state compromising the immune system. However, this is an unlikely explanation and an attempt to undermine the reality of the disease, since most patients develop feelings of depression after the manifestation of physical pain which is in itself, an emotional and stressful circumstance. Psychological problems, then, are a consequence, not a cause, of fibromyalgia.

Tests and Questionnaires

There is no blood test or X-ray examination to identify fibromyalgia. Laboratory tests are often used to rule out the possibility of other conditions that resemble fibromyalgia such as hypothyroidism, inflammatory muscle or joint disease, arthritis, and polymyalgia rheumatica. The only methods of positively diagnosing fibromyalgia are listening carefully to the patient's history and administering the tender-point test. The established criteria for diagnosis, along with a history of widespread physical pain for a minimum of three months, involve the 18 recognized "tender points" on the patient's body. When a pressure of approximately 4 kilograms (kg) (hard enough to turn the fingertip white) is asserted by the fingers on these 18 specific points, at least 11 must yield an excessively painful response in order to diagnose fibromyalgia as the cause of the patient's suffering.

The location of the 18 "tender points" are as follows (every point occurs twice, once on each side of the body):

1. Occiput—subocciputal muscle insertions into the base of the skull (where the head and neck meet along the spine, on the back side of the body);

2. Low Cervical—at the interior aspects of the inner transverse spaces at C5–7 (approximately halfway between the shoulder and the neck, on the back);

3. Trapezius—at the midpoint of the upper border of the muscle (three fingers widths away from the previous points, on a diagonal, toward the spine);

4. Supraspinatus—at its origins, above the scapular spine near the medial border (four finger lengths down from the previous points, on the neck, but slightly further out);

5. Second rib—pectoralis major lateral to the second costochondral junction (just above the collarbone on the front side of the neck);

6. Lateral epicondyle—extensor origin two centimeters distal to the lateral epicondyles (about three finger widths below the elbow crease on the inner side of the lower arm);

7. Gluteal—upper outer quadrants of buttocks on anterior fold of muscle (above the buttocks, approximately halfway in toward the spine);

8. Greater Trochanter—posterior to trochanteric prominence (below the buttocks, nearly at the outside edge of the thigh);

9. Knee—at the medial fat pad just above the joint line (on the inner side of the knee in front, in the area known as the fat pad).

Physicians have reported that the area between the shoulder blades is the most commonly painful spot among fibromyalgia patients.

Occasionally, a patient will not experience pain at all 11 points, but may still have fibromyalgia and require further testing at a later date since tender points can vary from day to day. In addition to the tender points, researchers are now exploring other psychological ways in which people with fibromyalgia can be recognized. Lawrence Bradley, Ph.D., of the University of Alabama, is leading research into the differences between fibromyalgia patients and people without fibromyalgia. One finding is that the cerebral spinal fluid of those with fibromyalgia has more of a neuropeptide called substance P. Because substance P carries pain signals through the body, people with more P will probably be more aware of their pain. People with fibromyalgia were also observed to have impaired functioning of the part of the brain that determines how many pain signals the brain receives. Both of these factors can result in a fibromyalgia patient's perceiving more physical pain than would be felt by someone with a healthy body.

Treatment for Fibromyalgia

Fibromyalgia is a complicated and delicate condition for which the medical profession has found no universal,

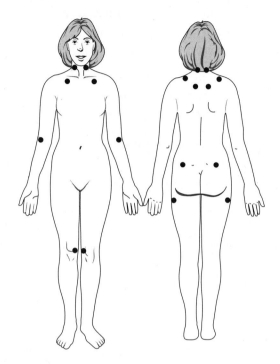

Figure 9–1   Fibromyalgia Syndrome Symptoms

long-term solution. Many different approaches have yielded some improvement in certain individuals, and each fibromyalgia sufferer would be well advised to explore the health care field carefully to find the combination of treatment approaches that best suits his or her needs. As Dr. Robert M. Bennett states, "Effective management of fibromyalgia patients requires a holistic approach demanding skill in such diverse topics as myofascial anatomy, psychiatry, sleep disorders, exercise psychology, physical therapy, and the functional neuroanatomy of chronic pain. . . . Currently, the muscle pain experienced by these patients cannot be completely eliminated. Without being unduly negative, it is important that the patient understand that the total elimination of pain cannot be the goal of treatment. Rather than eliminating pain, the aim is to improve function and restore the patient to a more functional lifestyle."

Fibromyalgia is generally a life-long problem. Without a single proven cure, the treatments prescribed by physicians attempt to control the symptoms and sleep disturbances as effectively as possible. One popular treatment involves trigger-point injections, generally composed of one percent procaine or lydocaine, combined with the technique of stretching the muscle. The painful injection is made directly at the point of tenderness, with only one area treated at a time. The injection brings immediate relief for a few hours and then the return of some pain as the numbing effect wears off. Within two to five days, there is a substantial reduction of the pain (typically between 50 percent and 80 percent improvement) which lasts two to three months. When the pain eventually returns, another injection is required to relieve it again. Some of the problems that result from trigger-point injections are allergic reactions such as dizziness, light-headedness, and very rarely, an anaphylactic reaction.

Many doctors prescribe antidepressants to their fibromyalgia patients, with subsequent improvement in some cases. In particular, amitriptyline (for example, Elavil) and fluoxetine (for example, Prozac) have been shown to reduce pain and other symptoms as well as helping patients to sleep.

One explanation for this effect is that the antidepressants reduce the amount of perceived pain by raising the patient's threshold for pain. The antidepressants are believed to act directly on the central nervous system, changing the brain chemistry to alter pain perception, deepen sleep, and improve moods even when administered at doses far lower than those prescribed for clinical depression. Low-dose tricyclic antidepressants help control sleep disruptions due to their antihistamine content which can induce drowsiness, and to their ability to increase the brain's level of seratonin, an important neuro-transmitter. Side effects of amitriptyline include weight gain and dry mouth. Sometimes, however, these medications produce a stimulating rather than a calming effect on some patients. The drugs may lose effectiveness over time, necessitating increased dosages, and could potentially be prescribed indefinitely.

In my experience, most patients are allergic to these drugs. If they decide to keep taking them while undergoing NAET, I treat for the drug first which minimizes the side effects. Other drugs used to reduce pain for short periods are analgesics such as aspirin and other anti-inflammatories, although they are not always effective. Long-term use of pain killers like Vicodan and Percodan, or sleeping pills like Halcion, Restoril, and Valium can produce serious dependencies and impair sleep quality. Tranquilizers and benzodiazepene sleeping medications actually worsen fibromyalgia symptoms by preventing deep sleep. Alcohol and caffeine may also disrupt sleep and increase discomfort.

A natural coenzyme called NADH has been used to treat fibromyalgia in clinical trials at the Immunology and Nephrology Departments of Georgetown University. NADH has been shown to produce substantial, enduring pain relief, according to participants in the experiment. Another naturally occurring medicine currently being used in alternative health care for fibromyalgia is a combination of malic acid and magnesium that reduces pain and tenderness in some patients. Malic acid, found in some fruits, and magnesium, a mineral, are both involved in the body's processes of energy production. Individuals taking the malic acid-magnesium supplements have reported improvement of symptoms within 48 hours.

One essential component of any fibromyalgia treatment program is exercise. Muscles are thixotrophic, meaning that their function deteriorates when they are not used, causing them to become shorter and stiffer.

Regular aerobic exercise is crucial, not only for short-term health restoration but also as a permanent aspect of a fibromyalgia patient's lifestyle.

Those who become inactive in order to avoid pain are neglecting their responsibility to actively participate in their recovery, and are substantially reducing their chances of improvement.

Of course, if you are in severe pain, you do not want to incur further injury through overexertion. Beginning at a moderate level and gradually increasing the level of exercise can be the best therapy of all. Suggested modes of exercise include walking, stationary or regular bicycling, swimming or other water therapy, and gentle dance programs. Jogging and weight-lifting are generally not encouraged because of the strain they place on the joints. Regardless of which exercise one chooses, effectiveness depends on sustaining an elevated heart rate for several minutes at a time. Twenty to 30 minutes of exercise is an appropriate goal to work up to gradually.

Some experts hypothesize that exercise is beneficial because it increases the supply of several substances that are especially critical to a body grappling with fibromyalgia. Exercise helps to produce endorphins that naturally inhibit pain and improve sleep, as well as seratonin and growth hormone that reduce pain and repair muscle tissue. Exercise also increases blood flow to the muscles to help diminish some of the pain. Some patients for whom exercise has provided major improvement find that they do not need medication to manage their fibromyalgia symptoms.

There are a number of other things individuals can do without a doctor to care for their condition. Learning proper posture can help to avoid back and neck strain. Physical therapy, hot baths, cold treatments, and massage can be valuable in pain reduction. Stress management is another important aspect of fibromyalgia treatment, including such relaxation techniques as yoga, breathing exercises, guided visualizations, and meditations. Patients with fibromyalgia must pay careful attention to their sleeping habits and keep a regular sleep schedule with sufficient hours of sleep each night. And because fibromyalgia can be frustrating and frightening for any patient, emotional support and reassurance must always be available.

10 | CANDIDIASIS

Bands of vandals
roam through my body
looking for trouble . . .
They jump onto their Harleys
burning rubber down my throat,
skid out,
doing wheelies along my spine . . .
                    —from "Hoodlums"

Trudy

Trudy, 35, came to see me for chronic fatigue and excessive weight. For years, she had been plagued with chronic yeast and vaginal infections, bacterial infections, and bloating. Like so many women, she had tried a variety of supplements, alternative treatments, and almost every diet imaginable, with only temporary improvement. The yeast infections made sexual intimacy difficult which put stress on her relationship with her husband and further weakened her system. I have found that NAET and enzyme therapy are excellent interventions for chronic fatigue and chronic yeast infections.

On the abdominal diagnostic enzyme evaluation exam, I found a possible thyroid imbalance and asked Trudy to do a basal temperature test. Most women with chronic yeast infections have low thyroid as well. I also found a problem with absorbing sugars and a positive spleen reflex, indicating a low immune function and an inability to digest sugars. Her diet consisted primarily of sugars and carbohydrates, suggesting

that much of the food she ate was not being digested properly. She also drank a great deal of alcohol.

Her low thyroid helped explained why she had so much
trouble with weight gain and fatigue. In addition, she reported
that her hair was thinning, her menstrual cycle was irregular,
and her libido was low.

The urinalysis revealed severe bowel toxicity which suggests problems with digestion and elimination, backup of the
bowel, and intestinal toxemia. She also had high calcium oxalate in the urine and low calcium phosphate. The high oxalate, the most common constituent of kidney stones, is
usually indicative of an inability to digest fats or possibly an
excessive consumption of fats. The low calcium phosphate, related to problems with carbohydrate and sugar metabolism,
showed that she not only did not digest sugars well but also
had trouble absorbing sugars. We found that her calcium was
very low, her pH was acid, and her uric acid was normal.

I put Trudy on an enzyme to help her digest fats and
sugars (bil) and another to improve spleen function (spl).
Based on her basal temperature test, I prescribed a natural
thyroid supplement and enzyme (AllerZyme thy) and then did
some allergy testing. Our main goals were to help with the
chronic fatigue, strengthen her immune function to combat the
chronic yeast infections, and help her lose weight.

Trudy was allergic to all the basics except Vitamin C. We
had to treat for Vitamins B_2 and B_{12} as well as for fructose,
corn syrup, and cane sugar by themselves. While the basic allergies were clearing and she was taking the natural thyroid
supplements, she lost 20 pounds and noticed an immense improvement in her energy, accompanied by a reduction of the
vaginal irritations caused by the yeast infections. Further testing found her allergic to chocolate, caffeine, nuts, animal and
vegetable fats, turkey, soybeans, fungus, alcohol, wine, some
bacteria, milk products, the adrenal gland, all the hormones,
and shingles, which she had once contracted.

After clearing the basics, I treated her for animal and vegetable fats and then for alcohol. We had to treat her four times

for alcohol, including two separate times for vodka, and she needed to be 40 feet away from anything that had even the slightest alcohol or sugar content (since sugar ferments to alcohol). This was an especially difficult allergy to clear because she had a hard time staying away from alcohol. Both her parents were alcoholics, and she was bordering on alcoholism herself. Once we cleared this allergy, Trudy stopped drinking entirely. In my experience, alcoholism is usually caused by an allergy to alcohol, which causes the person to crave it.

Next, I treated her for yeast. First I did the regular yeast mix, including baker's yeast and brewer's yeast. Then I treated her for fungus and several species of Candida: *Candida albicans, Candida rugosa,* and *Candida tropicalis.* As I always do with this treatment, I emphasized to Trudy that for the first 25 hours she had to adhere to a strict diet free of sugars and yeast and avoid any skin-to-skin or sexual contact. She also had to wear new gloves and a mask and new clothes and personal care products wherever they contacted her skin. Then she had to follow a modified diet for 10 more days. To help the body detoxify itself of the Candida once the treatment had cleared, I also prescribed certain enzymes and a natural antifungal (AllerZyme C) .

Once Trudy had cleared the Candida, we treated her for about 20 different fungi including *Epicococcum, Schimmelpilz 1* and *2, Aflatoxin alterneria,* and *Aspergillis.* This treatment also required that she adhere to the same 25-hour restrictions. When fungus finally cleared, which took three treatments, her energy improved dramatically and her bloating disappeared. It has been several years, and she has not had a single vaginal infection or irritation since then.

After we treated for fungus, I decided to treat Trudy for bacteria because she had frequent bladder infections and was allergic to quite a few bacteria.

Finally, after treating for some leftover foods, we treated Trudy for hormones. Most of the women I see are allergic to one or more of their own hormones including melatonin, insulin, estrogen, progesterone, testosterone, the thyroid hormones, adrenaline, DHEA, and cortisol. With hormones it is important to treat women at specific times of the month. Women should not be treated for progesterone just before, or for estrogen just after, their period, when these hormones predominate. Otherwise, the treatment will fail. Instead, progesterone should be treated postmenstrually and estrogen premenstrually. Women in menopause can be treated at any time, as long as they have not just taken their hormone replacement and have been off the hormone patch for eight hours or more.

By the time we completed our treatment, all of Trudy's symptoms had disappeared. She comes in every six or seven months to reevaluate her enzymes, we do a urinalysis once a year, and we occasionally review her allergies, particularly to fungus.

CANDIDIASIS, FUNGAL INFECTIONS, AND YEAST INFECTIONS

Most people who suffer chronic immune disorders are plagued with fungal infections. Yeast infections, especially Candida, are a growing problem in the population and play an important role in autoimmune problems. Symptoms include fatigue, PMS, depression, insomnia, nervous system problems, poor memory and mental confusion, endocrine problems, bloating, skin problems like eczema and psoriasis, liver problems, endocrine disturbances, irritable bowel syndrome, muscle aches, chemical sensitivities, frequent bladder infections, lack of energy, decreased libido, sexual dysfunction, infertility, bloating, intestinal gas, rectal itching, altered bowel function, menstrual complaints, a craving for carbohydrates, and sensitivities to foods, chemicals, and other allergens.

Candida albicans is probably the most common fungal infection, but it is certainly not the only one. Other species of Candida, molds, and other fungi can pose problems as well. Anyone who has been on repeated doses of antibiotics like ampicillin, tetracycline, and amoxycillin should be suspected of having a Candida infection (candidiasis). Birth control pills, hormone replacements, and steroids can also encourage the growth of Candida. In addition, the yeast is passed back and forth sexually and through skin-to-skin contact.

In my experience, there are people who have high levels of Candida in the system but no symptoms, and people who have very little Candida but many symptoms and feel like they are going crazy because they do not understand what is happening to them. Those people who are allergic to the yeast or fungus are the ones who develop the symptoms, and these symptoms become more and more pronounced as one eats more and more of the foods that feed it. With NAET we can treat the allergy to Candida and other fungus and achieve immediate results.

In his book *Chronic Fatigue Syndrome and the Yeast Connection,* Dr. William Crook reports that most of his patients with chronic yeast-related illnesses also have viral problems. The allergic reaction to the yeast weakens the immune system, and the body is unable to fight off viruses and other infectants, to which they may also become allergic. Also, the yeast may link with viruses or other allergens to form antigen-antibody complexes—for example, yeast and Epstein-Barr virus leading to chronic fatigue, yeast and bacteria leading to sore throats, yeast and calcium leading to arthritis, or yeast and certain foods leading to irritable bowel syndrome.

Together with certain bacteria and other friendly infectants, *Candida albicans* normally lives on the mucous membranes of the digestive tract and the vagina. When the body is not allergic to it, this yeast does not cause any problems. But when the body has been weakened by antibiotics, steroids, or a diet high in sugar, Candida may become overgrown in the system and precipitate a full-blown allergic reaction. In turn, the overgrowth may cause dysbiosis, a poor balance of flora in the digestive system, and leaky gut syndrome, in which undigested food leaks through the intestinal wall into the blood, creating more allergic reactions and bloating.

Many people are unaware that they have candidiasis. To obtain a complete symptomatic picture, I have patients fill out a questionnaire that includes the following questions:

1. Were you breastfed as an infant? If not, explain.

2. Have you ever taken a broad spectrum antibiotic, single or multiple courses?

3. Have you taken antibiotics more than three times in one year?

4. Have you taken cortisone drugs or prednisone?

5. Are you asthmatic?

6. Have you taken birth control pills or hormone replacements?

7. Do you have any fungal infections, for example, athletes foot, fungus under the toenails, jock itch?

8. Do you feel worse on damp days or in musty, moldy places?

9. Do you crave sugar, sweets, alcohol, beer, wine, carbohydrates, or bread?

10. Do you suffer from constipation, diarrhea, bloating, or abdominal pain, especially after eating sugar, bread, or wine?

11. Are you bothered by hormonal disturbances, PMS, menstrual irregularity, sexual dysfunction, sugar craving, or low body temperature?

12. Are you sensitive to tobacco smoke, perfumes, insecticides, or chemical odors?

13. Does your skin itch? Is it unusually dry? Do you have rashes or any kind of psoriasis or scaling?

14. Do some foods disagree with you or trigger symptoms?

15. Do you have any of the following symptoms: constipation, bloating, gas, tiredness, lethargy, depression, poor memory, inability to concentrate, mood swings, burning, tingling, numbness, muscle aches, weakness, pain in joints?

16. Do you experience abdominal pain, spots in front of eyes, fading vision, rashes in groin area, cold hands and feet?

17. Women: do you have vaginal discharge, burning, premenstrual syndrome, severe cramps? Men: do you have prostatitis, impotence, urinary burning?

If one answers yes to eight or more of these questions, it is a sure sign of Candida.

Yeasts, which are single-celled organisms, normally live on the outside of mucous membranes. They need to consume substances like sugars and fats to survive. When the immune system is weakened from an allergy overload, it cannot fight fungi, bacteria, and other infectants. Yeasts will burrow deeper into the system, spread through the blood to different organs, and cause sickness. As Dr. Crook describes in his book, "Candida has been referred to as a Dr. Jekyl and Mr. Hyde sort of critter. Here's why: It can switch from a single-cell yeast form into a branching fungal form. This fungal form can burrow beneath the surfaces of mucous membranes."

When yeasts multiply, they produce toxins, experienced in the body as disturbances like bloating, headache, and fatigue. When the body is fighting a yeast infection, it cannot cope with bacterial or viral infections as effectively. Yeast affects the immune, endocrine, and nervous systems and can create the numerous symptoms listed earlier. If any of these symptoms are present, I test for fungus and, if necessary, treat for it as well.

Most of us have large quantities of yeast in our bodies and pass it back and forth. It is only the people who are allergic to it who have the problems associated with it. Dr. Crook mentions that those who have antibodies to Candida, such as those who are allergic to it, develop more symptoms.

Birth control pills, antibiotics, and the consumption of large quantities of carbohydrates increase the amount of yeast in the body. Until it is eliminated, these substances and foods will continue to pose a problem. Hormonal changes can also encourage yeast colonies to develop.

For practitioners who use NAET, the muscle response test procedure is the most effective diagnostic tool for fungal allergies. Certain laboratories do stool analysis, blood work, vaginal smears, or other tests to determine the amounts of Candida in the system, but the reports are usually accompanied by a note stating that the findings are only meaningful if the symptomatolgy is consistent: in other words, if the patient has the symptoms of candidiasis which I believe are caused by an allergy to the fungus. The implication is that people with high levels of Candida do not necessarily need treatment unless they have symptoms.

If you are allergic to fungus or molds, either one can play a part in affecting or aggravating your symptoms. Like yeasts, molds are members of the vegetable kingdom. Yeasts are oval or elliptical single-celled organisms, whereas molds form colonies in which the cells grow long and intertwine with each other. Sometimes molds can change to yeasts, and yeasts can change back into molds. Molds occur naturally in the soil, air, and water and can be found growing on vegetables and fruits, especially grapes and dried fruits. When appropriate, I have people run tests to determine the amount of mold in their house. Molds will die when exposed to snow, but they can survive in the soil during the winter months. Because they float in the air like pollen, especially where the climate is humid, and are breathed directly into the lungs, they can be a major cause of coughs, bronchial infections, and asthma for those who are allergic to them.

Damp, dark conditions promote mold growth. Hence, damp basements and bathrooms and old, sweaty clothing are primary sources of household mold. The damper it is, the more the mold grows. Once my son started sneezing and coughing, and we wondered what the cause might be. It turned out to be an old sweatshirt that he had worn while exercising several months before and had left it in a corner. Mold can grow in mattresses, carpets, bedding, pillows, rags, sleeping bags, old books, newspapers, flower pots, plants, and soil. Houses in shaded areas near streams tend to accumulate mold, and humidifiers tend to encourage mold growth. Other areas prone to mold are decaying leaves, compost, lawn clippings, hay, refrigerator doors, and the space between a kitchen sink and the wall. Fruits and vegetables stored in a basement can get moldy, especially potatoes.

Patients often respond to moldy environments by becoming spaced out, incapacitated, and depressed. Women on the birth control pill may have particularly severe fungal infections. One of my patients was so irritated by vaginal yeast infections when she started to take the pill that her marriage began to suffer because of the pain during sexual contact. Another woman who had been on the pill for some time for menstrual cramping and bleeding began to be bothered by severe joint swelling, arthritis, migraines, dizziness, swelling, bloating, and teariness. When she drank even small quantities of red wine which is fermented with yeast, she became incapacitated. The yeast problem continued to plague her when she went off the pill, so we treated her for basic allergies and hormones with NAET. Her bleeding ceased and her periods became regular.

Hormone replacement therapy with estrogen or especially progesterone can cause candidiasis or other fungal infections. Treating for the Candida and the woman's hormones can be important in taking care of the problems many women experience. Bad breath, chronic sinusitis, tinnitus (ringing in the ears), irregular menstrual cycles, chronic cramping, and endometriosis are among the many chronic health problems for women that stem from fungal infections. Once the basics have cleared, treatment for fungus can yield dramatic results.

In my experience, fungus puts more stress on the immune system than any other infectant and inhibits one from dealing effectively with life-threatening illnesses like cancer, AIDS, and MS. When I find that fungus is an important part of a person's problem, I recommend the Candida diet (see the Resource Guide) which is high in protein and vegetables and low in carbohydrates, and encourage them to live in a mold-free environment. A dehumidifier in the home can be helpful, but air conditioning, especially in a car, may harbor and spread mold.

There are many foods and other environmental substances and toxins that can be linked with Candida or fungus. When one eats those foods in excess or contacts those toxins, it can aggravate the fungus in the body. Vitamin C and Vitamin C-rich foods can be strongly linked to Candida, as are the B vitamins and sugars, including both simple sugars and the complex carbohydrates found in grains and other foods. One patient with chronic colitis who had tried everything from parasite treatments to strict diets and nutritional supplements came to see me as a last resort. After treating for the basic allergens and certain foods, we treated separately for Candida and mold, including a number of combinations like fungus and grains, fungus and fruit, fungus and nuts, and fungus and spices. When he finally cleared these combinations, his health improved dramatically and he is now able to work long hours at a new job without symptoms.

Other substances that form antigen-antibody complexes in combination with fungus include various naturally occurring minerals, proteins, and toxins such as the lead from gasoline, the mercury in amalgams, the aluminum in cans and cooking utensils, insecticides, pesticides, household chemicals, formaldehyde, soaps, cosmetics, alcohol, solvents, and detergents. Indoor air pollution from smoke, odors, rugs, carpets, carpet pads, perfume, dust, or any of a number of inhalants or contactants may also form combinations with fungus and aggravate the Candida in the body. Any food allergy can be linked with fungus, as can antibiotics, steroids, and hormones.

Medications for Controlling Candidiasis

Three prescription medications are generally prescribed by the medical profession to control Candida and other yeasts and molds: nystatin, nizoral (Ketoconazole), and diflucan (Uconazole). Another antifungal medication called Amphotericin, which is a fungicide by Squibb, has also been used in Europe. The most popular, nystatin, is available in tablets, capsules, liquid, or powder. Dr. William Crook, author of *The Yeast Connection*, recommends using nystatin powder because it is the most effective in eliminating the yeast from the mouth and other areas of the digestive system. The powder is chemically pure, free of additives or food coloring, and is affordable. However, I believe it suppresses the yeast rather than killing it which causes more problems later on. Also, it may be toxic to the liver.

The second drug, nizoral, is a broader-spectrum antifungal and is preferred by some physicians as a slightly more potent alternative for those who have persistent and long-standing Candida and related health problems.

It does have some side effects, and people on this medication need to have their liver function checked every two to four weeks.

The third drug, diflucan, has been used in many foreign countries with favorable results. Its disadvantages are that it can be toxic to the liver, and it is quite expensive and not usually covered by insurance. Dosages range, and a regular liver function test is essential.

Several nonprescription supplements are also effective in inhibiting the growth of Candida. Like the prescription drugs, these preparations can cause yeast "die-off" reactions lasting up to a month in which the metabolic byproducts of the death of the yeast have a toxic effect on the body. Before I prescribe any antifungal supplement, I treat for the allergy to Candida with NAET which minimizes the die-off reaction. An anti-Candida supplement I have used in my practice is tripilic acid, a short-chain saturated fatty acid effective in treating for yeast and available without a prescription. Citrus seed extract under various brand names has also proven to be effective although the die-off reaction can create havoc in the system if the person has not been treated for an allergy to Candida. For example, I remember a severe asthmatic who began taking citrus seed extract and had to be taken to the emergency room with an asthma attack. Many people are also allergic to citrus seed which is cleared in our basic allergy treatments. With Candida, I generally use enzymes containing cellulase, magnesium, and protease.

11 THYROIDITIS

*Bequest of the great aunts   (along with their laughter and
defiance)   the gland that fails   attacks itself
bringing confusion to the rest of the body   regulatory
system gone haywire   Hidden away for a generation
only to resurface.   To be chosen for such an inheritance,
to be remembered in that way.*
                        —from "Meridians of Longing"

Barbara

Barbara, 40, was coughing so badly when she came to see
me that we had to move her from the waiting room into another room. She told me that she had been sick constantly
for the past two years, had taken antibiotics repeatedly, and
had just gotten over a five-week bout with viral pneumonia
and bronchitis. She had also been diagnosed with
Hashimoto's thyroiditis by an endocrinologist who had put
her on thyroid medication for the first time in four years. Although she was extremely fatigued, she was primarily concerned with her weak immune system and her constant
bouts of sickness.

I performed a complete abdominal diagnostic exam on
Barbara and found two things most significant: a reflex or
weakness related to her spleen, an organ important in the manufacturing of lymphocytes and antibodies in a healthy immune
system; and a difficulty digesting fats, common in people with
low thyroid. I prescribed an enzyme to help her digest fats (bil)

and an enzyme to boost the spleen (spl) and help her body fight infection (AllerZyme B). I also showed her how to treat for her own saliva and recommended that she do it daily for a while to prevent any kind of virus from lodging more deeply in her system. Her cough lingered for some time, but she has not had any bronchitis or other respiratory infection since.

Allergy testing revealed that she was allergic to all the basic allergens and many foods, and I began to treat her for the basics. We used an accelerated treatment procedure in which I treated her for two allergens each day, four hours apart, because her health was so poor and she wanted to get better as quickly as possible. We treated her for eggs and chicken, calcium, Vitamin C, all the B vitamins, and sugars. We had to treat her for many different sugars separately, some in combination with others. For example, we did cane sugar in combination with hormones and caffeine. Barbara had always eaten a lot of sugar. For her problems digesting fats, I recommended the fat intolerant diet (described in the Resource Guide of this book), which decreases the amount of fat and increases complex carbohydrates. Then we took a break for three weeks while she self-treated for sugar at home to clear other possible combinations. When we resumed, I treated her for iron, Vitamin A, and salt and then did a thorough retesting of her allergies and reassessed her situation.

With her thyroid problems, Barbara noticed several important symptoms: pressure in the thyroid gland, low energy, and decreased resistance to infections. On synthroid, which she had represcribed after not taking it for a number of years, she noticed that she felt jittery, experienced heart palpitations, and had extreme mood swings. She questioned whether this was the right medication for her and expressed an interest in exploring more natural options. Given her symptoms and her body's resistance to synthroid, I wondered whether her thyroid condition might be viral in origin. Further testing indicated that she was allergic to Vitamin E, amino acids, some neurotransmitters (seratonin, norepinephrine, epinephrine, and dopamine), some phenolics, and especially bacteria and viruses. I also found her to be allergic to beans, meats, shellfish, berries, oils and fats, food additives, hormones, and some vaccines.

Instead of taking her off Synthroid®, I treated her for it, which helped reduce her heart palpitations but did not relieve the pressure in her throat or her low energy. When we completed the sugars, her coughing slowly resolved. As for her resistance to infection, she continued to treat herself every day for saliva and she remained on the enzymes that boosted her immune system. Although she was doing quite well, I wanted her to be even stronger and more resistant to infection, and I wanted to address her hormonal imbalance.

After treating her for amino acids, I prescribed an amino acid supplement which I do only temporarily because I prefer that people get their amino acids from food. I then treated her for the viruses to which she was allergic (influenza, coronovirus, all the coxsackie viruses, Epstein-Barr, echo virus, Herpes I, varicella, and variola). She had more virus allergies than anyone I had ever treated. After three treatments, she finally cleared the viruses and immediately felt a noticeable improvement. She was able to get up early in the morning with no fatigue, she could exercise, she was more attentive, and she could read a book again, which she had been unable to do before because she found it so difficult to concentrate. In addition, most of her congestion and the remaining cough disappeared. It was a dramatic change for her. She looked completely different and people remarked about it.

Clearing the viral allergy also eliminated her sore throat and the pressure in her thyroid, and her temperature rose almost immediately. She asked if I thought she needed to remain on synthroid, and I recommended that she talk it over with her endocrinologist. On her own she decided to discontinue taking it, and I in turn put her on a natural thyroid supplement and enzymes (AllerZyme thy) to ease the transition. As it turned out, my suspicion that a virus might be the cause of her thyroid problem was correct.

I then treated her for bacteria which was not as severe an allergy as the allergy to viruses. People who have been on antibiotics for periods of time generally have bacterial allergies because the antibiotics tend to suppress the bacterial infection rather than eliminate it. Next, I treated for her remaining food and vitamin allergies which had become more noticeable now that she was feeling better. In particular, I find that allergies to oils and fats are closely linked to low thyroid. Barbara recognized that she craved and ate certain nutrients or foods that caused her problems, whether it was congestion in her throat, fatigue, or mood swings. For example, when she took Vitamin E, she would experience excessive heat and severe depression. After I treated her for the vitamin, she became aware of how much she really needed it and how much it worked for her. We ended by treating for some environmental allergens and the thyroid gland itself.

After getting through many of the foods and some other environmental allergens, Barbara is doing extremely well. Now and then she comes in to make sure she is taking the right enzymes but she has not been sick since our first appointment three years ago. She no longer has any thyroid pain, her blood tests are normal, and she feels better than she has ever felt. Over the years, Barbara has referred more than a dozen other patients to me, including her entire family, and she has become an outspoken advocate of enzyme therapy and NAET.

THYROID DISORDERS

Hypothyroidism, or low thyroid function, is one of the most common problems affecting physical and mental health, but it frequently goes unrecognized. A small butterfly-shaped gland located in the neck below the Adam's apple and weighing less than an ounce, the thyroid carries out the vital responsibility of controlling metabolism, the process of converting food into energy through a series of chemical changes. Minute thyroid secretions, less than a spoonful a year, maintain the body's heat production while regulating the circulatory system and blood volume. The secretions are essential for muscle health and heighten nerve sensitivity. Broda O. Barnes, M.D., declares, "Every organ, every tissue, every cell, is affected by the hormone secretions of the gland." The thyroid is one of the group of glands called endocrines which include the pituitary, adrenal, sex, thymus, pancreas, and pineal glands.

The thyroid manages the tempo of the body, from controlling the rate of oxygen use to regulating the speed of food utilization and the function of many organs. The thyroid has been called the thermostat of the body. It secretes hormones that assist the operation of each cell by determining the rate of metabolism; that is, how quickly food is transformed into energy and released. Without a thyroid gland, all metabolic activity, such as heat production, is immediately reduced. When the thyroid underfunctions—hypothyroidism—all metabolic activity is reduced and replacement hormones may be required. Deficient thyroid function also affects human development, possibly stunting growth in children as well as diminishing growth of hair, nails, and skin. Other areas compromised by an improperly functioning thyroid are bone healing, menstruation, mental processes, muscle health, and even sexual development and libido. All of these ailments resulting from thyroid damage have been shown to improve following thyroid treatment.

One of the most common symptoms of thyroid deficiency is fatigue, whether mild or severe. Dr. Barnes explains "It may come on so slowly that a victim, feeling no sudden precipitous decline in energy level, may come to accept fatigability as—for him—a virtually normal state." Although there are over 100 symptoms that characterize low thyroid function, and not every patient suffers from the same ones, the most common are severe headache, repeated infections, skin problems (eczema, psoriasis, acne, and boils), chronic infections, frequent colds tonsillitis, sinusitis, ear infections, menstrual disturbances, memory loss, concentration difficulties, depression, paranoid symptoms (confusion and other psychological conditions), cold intolerance, poor equilibrium, muscle aches and weakness, hearing disturbances, burning and prickling sensations from nervous system changes, decreased frequency of bowel movements, weight gain, relatively slow heart rate, and a firm, bumpy, slightly enlarged thyroid. "Many people with problems labeled 'psychosomatic'—and many who have been classified as being hypochondriacs—are victims of unrecognized hypothyroidism," according to Dr. Barnes.

Unfortunately, many of the standard thyroid diagnostic tests used today do not accurately diagnose hypothyroidism. Researchers have been unable to find a way to gauge the amount of thyroid hormone available inside each of the billions of cells in our bodies. Instead, doctors often use the basal metabolism test which measures the total amount of oxygen consumed by the body every minute while the subject is at rest. This method has a high potential for error, however, since the patient is rarely at complete rest in a doctor's office with all the stimulation and tension involved. Other tests, such as the protein ban iodine and radioactive iodine uptake tests, fail to reliably detect hypothyroidism. Unless the symptoms are severe, patients will be told they are normal even though they are suffering.

These various tests attempt to measure the thyroid activity by determining the amount of hormone stored in the gland and the amount present in the bloodstream. But they fail to do what really counts: measure the amount of thyroid hormone available and used by the body within the cells. Most people who are hypothyroid are actually allergic to their own thyroid gland and hormones. As a result, the body responds to the hormones by creating antigen-antibody complexes which prevent the body from utilizing the hormones and provoke more autoimmune reactions.

Dr. Barnes suggests an alternative method of testing thyroid function that he has found to be successful in determining thyroid problems. Studies have shown that hypothyroid patients generally run below-normal temperatures. The explanation for this finding is that it takes sufficient thyroid hormone to convert food into energy and heat. When the thyroid is deficient, proper oxidation and burning of fuel is compromised, and the body cannot maintain a normal temperature. In the basal body temperature test, an ordinary thermometer is placed in the armpit for 10 minutes on awakening. If the measure of a patient's at-rest, or basal, temperature is significantly lower than the normal range, low thyroid function is indicated. This method has proven successful in diagnosing hypothyroidism as well as determining the progress of the disease during treatment. As the at-rest temperature of a patient rises, the symptoms subside. Women who are still menstruating should take their basal temperature during their period so the temperature does not fluctuate with ovulation. Men can do this test anytime.

Temperature readings below 97.8 strongly suggest low thyroid function. Those above 99.2 suggest some gross pathology, possibly an infection or an overactive thyroid. Dr. Barnes conducted research on the basal temperature test and reported his groundbreaking results to the *Journal of the American Medical Association* in August 1942. One thousand college students were tested using both the basal temperature test and the basal metabolism test, and Dr. Barnes found that an abnormal body temperature was actually a more accurate indicator of hypothyroidism than the conventionally used basal metabolic rate.

In my clinic, I rely on several factors as an indication of poor thyroid function. First, I do an abdominal palpation enzyme evaluation exam to determine inflammation and metabolic imbalances. When I find an indication of abnormal thyroid function, I then recommend a 24-hour urinalysis, a basal temperature test, and several specific muscle tests for thyroid hormones and other related areas.

Hypothyroidism may be related to heart problems and coronary heart disease. The thyroid plays a role in controlling blood cholesterol levels, a common culprit in heart disease. Lung cancer and emphysema may also be associated with hypothyroidism, and a hereditary tendency to thyroid deficiency lowers resistance to infections and disease.

The symptoms of hypothyroidism are difficult to pinpoint because low thyroid function can dramatically impact so many different areas of the body. There are also a multitude of related health problems that emerge from the weakened thyroid condition. One common effect of thyroid deficiency is a weakening of the heartbeat, meaning that less blood is circulated through the body each minute. This can cause both physical and mental fatigue as it reduces the amount of oxygen traveling to tissues that need it.

Skin Problems

When thyroid function is low, which slows down the body's metabolism, blood circulation is also diminished, including the flow of blood to the skin. Bacterial invaders that are normally disposed of through the blood are then given the chance to invade and cause disease. Thyroid deficiency can contribute to skin conditions from boils to acne, exema, excessive dryness, psyrosis, and other serious diseases, including possibly lupus erythematosus.

Infectious Diseases

A weakened immune system and lowered resistance to harmful agents and viruses nearly always accompany thyroid deficiency. This helps to explain why hypothyroid patients are especially vulnerable to such infectious diseases as pneumonia, tuberculosis, rheumatic fever, sinus attack, ear infections, colds, flus, and other respiratory infections.

Menstrual Irregularities

Thyroid function is often related to a menstrual disorders including excessive bleeding, higher frequency of periods, severe cramps, and premature or delayed appearance of first menstruation. Miscarriages, infertility, and complications during pregnancy may also be connected to thyroid deficiencies.

Headaches (Including Migraines)

A low tolerance for stress among hypothyroid patients and the increased likelihood of fatigue can put excessive pressure on the brain and skull, leading to severe headaches.

Hypertension

There is evidence that low thyroid function is one of many factors that may exacerbate high blood pressure. Numerous patients experience a decrease in blood pressure following thyroid therapy.

Heart Disease

Research has indicated that administering thyroid therapy without any other changes in lifestyle or diet can reduce the chances of heart attacks among patients with coronary artery disease. Thyroid deficiency can produce changes in the body that increase the risk of heart attacks, and thyroid therapy can diminish or reverse these changes. For example, hypothyroidism can raise blood pressure and cause blood clotting, but thyroid therapy lowers blood pressure and corrects the ability of the blood to clot. The fatigue that is common in thyroid deficiency plays an important role as well, since overexertion can trigger a heart attack. Also, hypothyroidism causes abnormal levels of compounds called mucopolysaccharides to accumulate in the body tissues, and these substances are known to cause inflammation and atherosclerosis.

Arthritis

Often, a patient will have complaints of arthritic pain in the bones, joints, and muscles that is alleviated after thyroid deficiency is identified and treated. The high levels of mucopolysaccarides mentioned in the previous section can be an important factor in the development of arthritis. The prevalence of thyroid diseases is greater than all the other endocrine diseases combined with the exception of diabetes. Most of the cases of low thyroid are the result of a disease called Hashimoto's thyroiditis.

To understand autoimmune thyroid disease, you need to understand how the body reacts to its own tissue cells. An organism's immune system is designed to protect against foreign agents and infectants. Normally they are eliminated without injury or attack on the organism itself. The ability to distinguish between body's own cells and foreign organisms is an important measure of the strength of the immune system. When this system is compromised, as in autoimmune disease, the body's destructive capabilities are turned against its own tissues.

In essence, what happens is that the body's first line of defense, the macrophages, are not strong enough to destroy the antigen-antibody complexes (CICs) that have been created by the immune system in response to foreign organisms and materials, for example, bacteria or inadequately digested food metabolites. The body then activates B cells and T cells to infiltrate the area and attack the CICs, which by now have lodged in different parts of the body such as the thyroid tissue. In trying to destroy these CICs, the lymphocytes infiltrate the thyroid tissue and destroy the target cells directly. By destroying the target cells, they actually attack their own tissue as well. This process is known as "antibody dependent cellular cytotoxicity" (see The Immune System).

Hashimoto thyroiditis is an autoimmune thyroid disorder in which the body attacks its own thyroid tissue and the thyroid gland ultimately loses its capacity to produce thyroid hormones. The factors that compromise the immune system and inhibit the body's first line of defense include allergies, poor digestion, drugs, and aging. When all of these occur simultaneously, the body's circulating immune complexes grow in size and inhibit the immune system from doing its work effectively such as destroying infectants and keeping us healthy. Autoimmune diseases like Hashimotos is the most common sign of a weakened immune system.

Enzyme therapy and NAET restore immune activity by improving digestion and metabolism, fighting infectants, and eliminating allergies. The NAET treatment for thyroiditis is profound, well researched, and proven to work in every case. Doctors all over the world who practice NAET have used this treatment protocol, and thousands of patients have reaped the benefits. Again, the complete protocol will be discussed in full in the NAET chapter relating to thryoiditis.

Hashimoto's thyroiditis is a chronic inflammatory disorder of the thyroid gland that primarily affects young and middle-aged women. (The woman-to-man ratio of occurrence is 9 to 1.) It is the most common inflammatory thyroid disease, accounting for about 85 percent of thyroiditis cases. Frequently, there is a history of thyroid disease in the patient's family.

Patients with Hashimoto's thyroiditis are at greater risk for developing other autoimmune disorders such as Graves disease and B-cell lymphoma of the thyroid. Also called chronic lymphocytic thyroiditis, this disease can lead to hypothyroidism and possibly result in the complete absence of all thyroid cells. Hashimoto's is referred to as "autoimmune" because it occurs when abnormal blood antibodies, in combination with the white blood cells that normally protect the body against threatening substances, begin instead to attack and destroy thyroid cells. In other words, a person is allergic to his or her own thyroid hormone.

Each of the other immune disorders referred to in this book may have Hashimoto's thyroiditis or hypothyroidism as part of the symptom complex. For example, many CFIDS patients are hypothyroid and may even be taking medication for this problem. The antibodies frequently found in cases of Hashimoto's thyroiditis are known as antimicrosomal and antithyroglobulin antibodies.

Pain is present in only about 10 percent of the cases. The primary symptoms are tiredness, mild pressure in the neck, or enlargement of the thyroid gland. Sometimes patients will have an irregular goiter (growth on the thyroid) which is firm and slightly tender, particularly in the early stages of the disease. Juvenile Hashimoto's is characterized by remissions and recurrences.

One way to diagnosis Hashimoto's is through the identification of high levels of antithyroid antibodies in the patient's blood which attack the thyroid proteins in the body. Blood levels of thyroid stimulating hormone (TSH) are also measured, since irregularities can point to thyroid disorder. In hypothyroidism, TSH is considerably elevated, whereas in hyperthyroidism it is considerably reduced. The reason for the TSH increase in patients with hypothyroidism is that the thyroid destruction causes thyroxin levels to fall, and the body responds with more thyroid stimulating hormones. Doctors can confirm diagnosis with a thyroid biopsy in which a needle is used to remove cells from the thyroid gland and are then examined on a glass side. Blood lymphocytes, a type of white blood cell seen in the smear, provide information about the inflammatory reaction occurring in the thyroid gland.

The standard treatment for Hashimoto's thyroiditis is the immediate introduction of thyroid hormone (thyroxin) replacement. Thyroid hormone therapy is used even if it seems that thyroid function is normal at the time of diagnosis. The proposed benefits of hormone replacement include:

1. Suppressing the pituitary gland's production of TSH, which helps to prevent further enlargement, shrinks the goiter, and reduces the formation of nodules;

2. Anticipating the development of thyroid failure and the resulting low levels of thyroid hormones that may occur if the disease progresses; and

3. Possibly inhibiting the blood lymphocytes that are responsible for the thyroid inflammation.

After treatment begins, the goiter is supposed to shrink over a period of six to 18 months, although in some patients it takes several years to disappear.

Other Treatments for Hashimotos

In a study of Hashimoto's by the Shanghai Research Institute of Acupuncture published in the *Journal of Traditional Chinese Medicine* (March 1993), seventy-one cases of Hashimoto's thyroiditis were treated by moxibustion and their immune and thyroid function were observed. This traditional Chinese technique, which involves burning small quantities of an herb at points near the skin, was found to reduce the thyroid antibodies in the peripheral blood of all of these patients. The results indicate that the treatment of Hashimoto's thyroiditis by moxibustion is probably accomplished by inhibiting the T lymphocytes.

It is also worth noting that synthetic T_4 preparation (or thyroxin), which is the most commonly used thyroid medication, is considered a poor replacement therapy by Dr. Barnes and his coworkers at the Barnes Foundation. They recommend naturally desiccated (freeze-dried) thyroid. Although it may be better for the body, the dosage of natural thyroid is harder to regulate. Therefore, I do not recommend either natural or synthetic hormone, but instead treat the root of the problem so the patient can be weaned from the medication. Until then, muscle testing procedures can be helpful in determining how much hormone the patient needs.

Chapter

12

ULCERATIVE COLITIS, CROHN'S DISEASE, AND IRRITABLE BOWEL SYNDROME (IBS)

> *Too worn down to send the swimmer in,   too discouraged to want to go on.   When the pain hits   in too many places at once. . . .   Abdomen discovering knots even the sailors never thought of*
> —from "Meridians of Longing"

Jeffrey

Jeffrey, 26, came to see me because he was HIV positive and had digestive problems, fatigue, and a variety of allergic symptoms including runny nose, coughing, and teary eyes. He was taking a number of different nutritional supplements that were recommended by other health practitioners or that he had read or heard about from friends— a multivitamin, an antioxidant, some herbs, and some enzymes to help his digestion—even though some of them did not agree with him. He wanted to strengthen his immune system, fight the HIV virus, and clear up any digestive problems and allergies he might have.

When I took his history, Jeffrey complained of bloating and gas, frequent diarrhea, undigested foods in his stools, an inability to tolerate fatty foods, constipation, and tenderness under his right rib cage. Since being diagnosed with HIV, he had also noticed that his energy and his resistance to infections had diminished, and he could be impatient or irritable under stress. He was very muscular and appeared to be in excellent health. As an aerobics instructor, he was especially disturbed by his increased fatigue because he required a lot of physical energy in his work.

On the fasting part of the abdominal palpation exam, we found a positive epigastric reflex reflecting an inflammation of the gastric mucosa that is sometimes representative of an acid condition caused by poor digestion, an inherited tendency, or a bacterial infection. This reflex generally indicates poor digestion and includes bloating soon after eating. I also found a positive liver/gallbladder reflex which denotes toxicity and which seemed to be related to the pain under his right rib cage, near the liver. There was also a positive lower right reflex usually indicative of an inflammation of the ileocecal valve, sometimes related to irritable bowel syndrome or an inability to metabolize protein, and therefore a deficiency in protein and possibly calcium as well.

On the nonfasting part of the palpation, we found a positive epigastric reflex as well as an inability to digest fats and proteins which matched the symptoms he reported in his history. The urinalysis showed digestive incompetence, especially an inability to digest protein and fats. His uric acid was high (.25), usually demonstrative of poor protein digestion, as were the oxalates (.45), representative of poor digestion of fats. His pH was very acidic (5.6) and his calcium was quite low which commonly coorelates with an acid pH. His bowel toxicity was above normal, suggesting a problem with elimination and the possibility of liver toxicity, found on the palpation as well. His specific gravity and chloride were high, reflecting poor digestion of complex carbohydrates. His Vitamin C and kidney concentration were normal, but his calcium and magnesium were deficient.

I immediately prescribed an enzyme to help him digest fats and proteins (bil), an enzyme for liver toxicity (lvr), and an enzyme (SML) as a gentle bowel cleanser that he could use for a short period of time and which would help the liver as well. I also prescribed an antioxidant enzyme (NSL). The epigastric reflex was not as strong on nonfasting, so I was able to give him an enzyme with protease (trauma) which he needed for protein digestion. People with gastritis may find protease irritating and may not be able to use it immediately, even though they may need it. For Jeffrey, however, it seemed to work.

Within four days, his digestion, which had been poor for so long, was almost perfectly normal. This often happens with people with digestive problems once they start taking the right enzyme. After that, we did extensive allergy testing and found that he was allergic to all the basics except salt. He was also allergic to corn, coffee, chocolate, caffeine, animal fat, amino acids, fish, milk, meat, Vitamin E, Vitamin F, and some environmental allergens.

We began by treating him for the basics. Then I treated him for amino acids, generally important allergens for people with hypoglycemia or difficulty digesting protein. Immediately, his energy and stamina improved and stabilized. In fact, this treatment was probably one of the most important for the build-up of his strength and his immune defenses.

Next, I did a thorough retesting to get an idea where we stood. Jeffrey was still allergic to tomatoes, wheat, parasites, food additives, cotton, dust mites, flowers, cat hair, fruits, the HIV virus, some antibiotics, fungus, cold, hydrocarbons, Vitamin F, and grass and tree pollens. With each individual, I evaluate which items to treat first based on his or her symptoms and my experience. For Jeffrey, I wanted to clear some of the infectants, something I generally do with people with chronic health problems. This included parasites, especially intestinal flukes and blood flukes.

Once he cleared the parasites, I prescribed some specific antiparasite enzymes (AllerZyme P) that I include in the Resource Guide in the back of this book. Then I treated him for HIV which we needed to do alone and in combination, in particular with DNA-RNA, certain hormones, and milk which he drank frequently. I then treated him for fungi, including all the different species of Candida, Alternaria, and Aflatoxin, especially important because it can occur in beer, nuts, bread, fruit, and grains. After we cleared the fungi, I prescribed an antifungal diet for 10 days as well as certain antifungal enzymes

(AllerZyme C) to help the body eliminate fungus from the system. There are certain supplements I use just for Candida and others that are specifically used for fungus. Then we treated for bacteria and antibiotics.

Jeffrey was prone to chronic bronchitis that he would treat with antibiotics. One day he came in with a bronchial infection for which he was about to take antibiotics. I urged him to wait 48 hours while we treated for the bacteria. He turned out to be allergic to quite a few bacteria that his body was carrying, including a couple of streps, some staph, yersinia enterocolitica, and klebsiella. When one is allergic to bacteria, the bacteria can link with other allergens and lodge in different parts of the body as CICs, causing autoimmune problems (in which the body tries to attack and destroy these complexes and in so doing attacks the tissue in which the CICs are lodged). This then decreases the body's immune availability, strength, and resistance. I treated him for all the bacteria and had him take large doses of protease and some other anti-infectants including golden seal, garlic, and grapefruit extract (AllerZyme B). Within two days his symptoms cleared up, and in the past four years he has not had a single infection or needed to take any antibiotics. In general, I find that once people clear their allergies, their immune system gets stronger and they no longer get sick or need to use antibiotics.

After we finished with the bacteria, Jeffrey still noticed an occasional runny nose, meaning that we needed to deal with some of the environmental allergies. These can cause as much stress on the body and as much fatigue as any other allergy. I treated him successfully for the pollens of flowers, grasses, and trees. The first year we had to do pollen every two weeks during the spring as new plants bloomed. After clearing the pollens, to which he had been allergic since childhood, his energy improved dramatically.

I then treated him for his remaining food allergies. Even though his digestion had improved, he still noticed some gas and indigestion when eating certain foods. We did tomatoes, wheat, peppers, food additives, corn starch, potato starch, baking soda, baking powder, tofu, gum mix, and some of the thickeners, among others. Then we treated for some miscellaneous allergens and many antibiotics. Even though he had not taken antibiotics for some time, it was possible that his body might have still been experiencing symptoms related to an allergy to antibiotics.

I then treated him for his blood, alone and in combination with HIV, DNA, RNA, and lymph nodes. In his workouts, he noticed that when he overheated, he would develop hives. When we evaluated, we found that he was allergic to adrenaline and testosterone, common allergies for male HIV patients and especially for him because he exercised so often. We treated him for these hormones, as well as for cold and heat, and the hives disappeared completely. We also treated for dental amalgams, mercury, and warts which fell off immediately.

It has been four years since Jeffrey first came in, and he continues to do wonderfully. I see him once every six or seven months just to make sure he is taking the right enzymes, including protease, which is now being recommended by many researchers of AIDS and HIV. He also takes some herbs and antioxidants. His T-cell count is better than ever, and he has sent me many new patients over the years.

Susan

Susan, a 63-year-old teacher, was sent to me by her physical therapist. Seriously underweight at 100 pounds although only five feet seven, she looked extremely unhealthy. She had been suffering from chronic fatigue and daily diarrhea for more than a dozen years. She was susceptible to chronic infections and suffered from dry skin and excessive gas. Although she had undergone extensive tests, the only thing that had helped her with the diarrhea was the drug Immodium, which she had been taking twice a day for many years.

Aware that she was sugar and milk intolerant, she avoided milk. She also noticed an acid stomach, bloating, and gas in

combination with the diarrhea, and she could barely eat anything without developing these symptoms. The approach I had
to offer appealed to her because it gave her hope that a
change might be possible.

Since she had never taken any enzymes, I thought it
would be a good place to start. An abdominal exam revealed
an epigastric reflex, suggesting a possibly preulcerous inflammation of the stomach, duodenum, or esophagus, and helped
explain the gas she experienced right after she ate. I found a
positive liver reflex, suggesting toxicity from the foods she ate
as well as from the Immodium and other drugs she had taken
over the years. There were problems with both the ascending
and descending colon, not uncommon in cases of colitis and
irritable bowel. Adrenal insufficiency and calcium deficiency
were also problem areas for her, and she exhibited serious difficulty absorbing sugar. It was obvious looking at her that she
could not absorb most of the nutrients she ingested.

The urinalysis revealed a trace of sediment in the urine
which echoed the conclusion that her body was virtually unable to absorb any foods at all. Her urine was very acidic and
her kidney was slow in concentrating the urine. On the nonfasting part of the palpation, I found a positive gastric reflex. I
prescribed an upper gastric enzyme devoid of protease which
can be irritating to people with epigastric problems (stm).

Over the next few months, I also prescribed an irritable
bowel enzyme (AllerZyme IB) to help with the diarrhea. Within
two weeks, the frequency of her diarrhea had been cut from six
times daily to twice a day. When we tested her for allergies, she
proved to be intolerant to every food and nutrient, including all
the basics, as well as many viruses, fungi, parasites, and bacteria. Clearly, we had our work cut out for us.

Beginning with the basics, I found that her system was too
weak for us to treat eggs, chicken, and feathers together; we had
to break it down into egg white, egg yolk, chicken, tetracycline,
and feathers which I treated last because it was more important
to get through some of the foods. Then we treated for calcium,
Vitamin C, and all the B vitamins, which had to be cleared sepa-

rately. It was extremely difficult for her to stay away from the targeted foods because she was already so emaciated. Sugar had to be treated several times, as did iron and all the minerals. Just clearing the basics was a major challenge for us both.

By the time we finished the basics, her diarrhea had diminished considerably, her energy had picked up, and she had gained a few pounds. She even had days when she had no diarrhea at all. She was thrilled, and so were her friends. When I retested her, I hoped to find that she had cleared most of her food intolerances, but that was not the case. She was still allergic to quite a few foods including oats, oat bran, rice, wheat, many meats, turkey, fish, virtually all the vegetables, oils, food additives, food colorings, berries, and fruits which she had avoided because of their sugar content. As we cleared each group of foods, they stopped contributing to her diarrhea, and the problem all but disappeared. She continued taking Immodium, however, out of fear that the problem might recur.

Through muscle reflex testing, I discovered that we needed to treat the infectants next. We had to treat for the parasites and bacteria quite a few times before they cleared, but even then she still had an attack of diarrhea every few days. I wanted to eliminate the diarrhea entirely so she could feel safe to discontinue the Immodium.

She kept reminding me that she had chronic sinus congestion and runny nose, but I was so focused on the diarrhea and intestinal problems that I did not suspect a virus. Since then, I have found that many people have viruses they cannot get rid of because they are allergic to them. Symptoms may include not only chronic fatigue and flu symptoms, but also diarrhea, bloating, and other allergy symptoms. Testing for viruses, I found that she was allergic to quite a few of them, including Epstein-Barr, cytomegalovirus (CMV), rhinovirus, cornovirus, and enterovirus. I decided to treat for each one individually because they were so important.

Each time I cleared a virus, her health improved dramatically. She stopped having diarrhea, and her energy increased exponentially. We had to treat for some of the viruses in combination with DNA-RNA and minerals. At some point, I plan to recheck for fungus, minerals, and certain foods. But she has not had any diarrhea for months now, and she no longer takes Immodium. I do not see her as often because she is able to work more and her chronic fatigue is completely gone. She has gained weight, feels younger, and talks about other things besides her health. Quite a miraculous improvement for just eight to nine months of treatment. This case is a reminder not to underestimate the importance of the infectants.

DEFINITION

Ulcerative colitis and Crohn's disease are two disorders known as irritable bowel syndrome (IBS), the most severe digestive afflictions known to medicine. Both result in an irritated, inflamed bowel, and can be difficult to tell apart. The difference lies in the location of the disease in the body. Colitis affects the inner lining of the colon and rectum, whereas Crohn's can occur in any part of the digestive tract including the entire wall of the intestines. Once they are diagnosed, the treatment generally recommended for both these conditions involves the long-term use of potent drugs and possibly serious surgical procedures. Conventional medical authorities agree there is no cure.

Over the past 20 years, I have treated many individuals with colitis using enzyme therapy and NAET, with extraordinary results. Many are now leading normal, pain-free, drug-free lives. My success with this disease is discussed in detail in the NAET chapter for protocol on Crohn's and colitis.

Symptoms

Crohn's and colitis are considered life-long diseases. They may be inactive for extended periods of time, but periodically they become active again, and the symptoms that appear can be worse than, better than, or the same as, previous flare-ups.

The major symptoms of ulcerative colitis are:

- fatigue
- abdominal pain, especially right before bowel movement
- constipation
- frequent passing of blood and mucus with stools
- diarrhea, in some cases, especially late in the disease
- weight loss; loss of appetite
- fever
- possibly painful joints

The major symptoms of Crohn's disease are:

- abdominal pain, often in the lower right area, or bloating and gas
- loss of weight caused by appetite reduction and improper absorption of nutrients
- possible bowel obstruction which may cause vomiting, pain, and distention
- diarrhea, occasionally with blood, and/or constipation
- inflammation or ulceration around the anal area
- fistulas, ulcers tunneling through the bowel walls into adjacent tissues and organs which cause pockets of infection or abscesses that leak pus
- occasional stool passing into urine

- fever

- persistent rectal bleeding, leading to anemia (or low red-blood cell count)

Sometimes other areas of the body are affected by these bowel disorders, particularly the mouth, which may develop sores known as aphthous ulcers. On rare occasions, the skin may form warm, red, tender lumps (erythema nodosum) or ulcerations on the legs. Also, there is the possibility of arthritis-like joint pain and swelling, lower back pain or stiffening, and pain in the spine. Infrequently, the inflammation may spread to the eyes, liver, or bile ducts. Children who are severely affected by the disease may experience a reduction in growth rate and delayed development.

Causes

Medical science has been unable to positively identify a cause for these conditions. One theory is that the immune system reacts inappropriately to bacteria that are normal inhabitants in the body. The aggressive defense against these substances in the bowels leads to the inflammation experienced. Others believe the guilty party is a modern measles virus that somehow fails to fully leave the body once the acute outbreak is over, and which triggers a chronic inflammatory response in the intestinal tissue. The poor diet of contemporary society has also been targeted in the investigation of inflammatory bowel disease with sugars, starches, and processed foods being linked to IBD susceptibility. Studies of numerous chemical substances, from toothpaste ingredients to oral contraceptives, have revealed interesting correlations to the risk of IBD, but no single cause has been confirmed in the literature.

Some possible causes of IBD have been observed, although the causes of particular symptoms are not always clear. These include:

- infections such as colds, flus, or gastroenteritis

- drugs such as aspirin, antibiotics, and anti-arthritis medications

- diet including milk products, cereals, and other foods that may cause a reaction

- stress or emotional disturbances

I have observed that the most common causes of IBD are food allergies, poor digestion of sugars and starches creating CICs and bowel toxicity, bacterial and fungal allergies, and, less frequently, allergies to parasites, drugs, antibiotics, and emotions.

The tendency toward IBD may be hereditary. About 20 percent of people with Crohn's disease have a close blood relative with some form of inflammatory bowel disease.

Associated diseases

Inflammatory bowel disease has been observed to lead to cancer in very rare cases, and only when most or all of the colon has been affected by the disease for many years. Annual colonoscopic examinations by a doctor may be able to detect warning signs of cancer in the bowel before it actually develops. Many patients then decide to remove the colon as a protective measure against the possibility of cancer.

Some systemic complications that can result from Crohn's disease are arthritis, skin problems, kidney and gall stones, liver disease, and inflammation of the eyes or mouth.

Testing

The main procedure doctors use to diagnose Crohn's or colitis is sigmoidoscopy. It involves passing a flexible, lighted instrument through the anus to inspect the inflamed lining of the colon. In a biopsy, a small sample of the lining is extracted to examine under a microscope. Several other tests that may be administered are:

- blood samples (a low red blood cell count means the patient is anemic, possibly from excessive blood loss, and a high white blood cell count could indicate an inflammatory process in the body)

- stool specimens (indicates blood loss or infection by a parasite or bacteria)

- barium enema X rays (running barium liquid, which shows up white on x-ray film, through the anus into the intestines to reveal inflammation or other abnormalities)

- colonoscopy (the passing of an instrument through the anus and colon).

Additional tests used for Crohn's disease of the upper abdomen are an upper gastrointestinal endoscopy (an instrument moves through the mouth to investigate and take samples from the stomach and upper intestine) and a barium X-ray examination of the small intestine.

Treatment

The primary medical treatment for ulcerative colitis is the use of a series of drugs to control the symptoms. In some cases, surgery is performed to remove the colon entirely (proctocolectomy), but this route does not guarantee a permanent cure to colitis and does not prevent further autoimmune activity in other areas of the intestines. The circumstances in which surgery might be considered include severe attacks that do not respond to any treatment, repeated attacks that threaten the patient's overall health, and serious changes in the colon that could precede cancer. If the entire colon is removed, the patient must have an ileostomy, an opening in the abdomen with a disposable bag to collect stool.

The principal drugs prescribed for colitis are Azulfidine® and a form of anti-inflammatory steroid called prednisolone. This steroid may be taken as tablets, suppositories, rectal foams, enemas, or, in severe cases, intravenously. Steroids are used to relieve the inflammation of colitis, but they are sometimes poorly absorbed or inactivated. Side effects may appear immediately and worsen the longer they are taken. Some of the most common and serious side effects include thinning of the bones (osteoporosis), high blood pressure, diabetes, muscle wasting, increased appetite and weight gain, mood changes, depression, rounding of the face, weakened resistance to infections, and cataracts. Because steroids are produced naturally in the body, when additional steroids are introduced to the system, the body usually decreases its own production of them. In addition, most people become allergic to, and dependent on, steroids. Therefore, it is extremely dangerous to stop taking the drugs suddenly, and patients must be gradually taken off the treatment. By desensitizing the system to the drugs, NAET can be a life-saving technique that makes the weaning process quicker, safer, and easier.

For example, a woman with fibromyalgia and colitis came to see me a few months ago. She was in her 70s and had been taking prednisolone for seven years. Due to the brittleness of her bones and her prednisone-induced diabetes, it was recommended that she go off the drug. Reluctantly but steadfastly, she began the weaning. She came to me solely to help her with this process on a referral from her physician. We needed to treat her with NAET for prednisolone three times alone and then in combinations with calcium, nerve tissue, and bacteria. After three treatments over the course of *two* weeks, she stopped taking this medication with no side effects and has been off it for two years now. We have since treated her with enzyme therapy and NAET for the fibromyalgia and colitis, and she is doing extremely well.

Other drugs that are used for colitis are sulphasalazine, mesalazine, olsalazine, and azathioprine. Though there are varying degrees of success with different patients, every one has potential side effects that range from headaches, rashes, nausea, diarrhea, and severe abdominal pain to temporary infertility and blood disorders.

Crohn's disease can also be treated, but not cured, with surgery. The objectives of surgery are usually to remove severely diseased sections of the bowel, to widen a stricture (a narrowing of the bowel), and to drain abscesses. Even after surgery, however, the inflammation can return, often in areas right next to the ones that had been removed. In fact, 85 percent of Crohn's disease patients who have surgery experience a recurrence within the next three years.

Drug treatment is common and depends on the area of inflammation. Some of the drugs used are steroids, antibiotics (metronidazole, ciprofloxacin), azathioprine, mesalazine, sulphasalazine, and olsalazine.

Sometimes going on liquid diets (elemental or polymeric) for two to three weeks can help patients achieve and maintain remission, possibly because they are eliminating the foods to which they are allergic. Patients with Crohn's disease must pay attention to their nutrition, especially children and others who have strictures or difficulty moving their bowels. Conventional literature points out that hard-to-digest foods such as fiber products should be avoided, as well as foods like milk, alcohol, and spicy or fried foods. A study in England found that patients who identified and eliminated foods to which they were intolerant had longer periods of remission than those who ignored the aspect of diet in their treatment. Yeast may be one of those trouble-making foods, as some studies have found a connection between sensitivity to yeast (brewer's and baker's) and these two IBDs.

I was once diagnosed with this disease myself, but I have not had an episode since I began taking enzymes almost 16 years ago. In reviewing the literature and studying this problem for some time, I have seen other effective treatments for IBD such as the dietary recommendations by Elaine Gottschall in her book *Breaking the Vicious Cycle*. Gottschall writes that the fermentation of foods in the intestines, which breeds bacterial and fungal infections, is at the root of IBD, and she describes a diet that eliminates this problem. I would add that intestinal fermentation is at the root of almost all gastrointestinal diseases and that the cause of fermentation is poor digestion and the resultant bacterial and fungal allergies.

Gottschall contends that other causes of fermentation include the use of antibiotics, the lack of breastfeeding as an infant, an over-reliance on antacids, toxic chemicals in food and water, and the use of drugs that inflame the lining of the intestines. She believes that the main dietary culprits are grains, some starchy vegetables, milk (especially the lactose in milk), certain fruits, and cane sugar. She recommends a diet consisting primarily of meat, fish, poultry, eggs, and vegetables, as well as lactose-free milk products and certain beans. However, I have found that once these common food allergens have been cleared with NAET, they can be eaten with enzymes and will cause no recurrent inflammation. Other items I would add to this list of dietary irritants or culprits include oils, alcohol, caffeine, chocolate, and spices. Once the appropriate dietary and lifestyle changes have been made, according to Gottschall, improvement can begin within three weeks, and a complete remission can ultimately be expected.

In a paper on Crohn's and ulcerative colitis, Dr. Ronald Hoffman points out that certain herbs and supplements can be helpful for symptom relief including golden seal, *artemisia sanguinaria, gentian, ginkgo biloba,* garlic, grapefruit seed extract, *quercetin,* and licorice, all of which I have used as antiparasitals, antibacterials, and antifungals.

Aloe vera juice, a potent healing agent, has been used to heal ulceration. The amino acid L-glutamine, fish oil, shark cartilage, and the enzyme bromelain have all been used as anti-inflammatories.

Research has pointed out that antioxidants, as well as the trace mineral selenium and the naturally occurring peptide glutathione, can help reduce the autoimmune reaction of IBD. Acidophilus helps to restore bowel flora and create a more healthy environment for the gut. However, care must be taken to ensure that the person is not allergic to acidophilus; otherwise, it will cause further inflammation, gas, and bloating. Clearing for acidophilus and other probiotic flora with NAET can help to heal and restore balance to the intestinal tract.

The famous psychic and healer Edgar Cayce recommends castor oil packs for IBDs, although I have not seen many patients benefit from this treatment. Dr. Hoffman mentions that a bioengineered EDGF (epithelial-derived growth factor) may eventually be recommended for IBD, and glandular products rich in duodenal extract, similar to EDGF, may have equally beneficial results.

13 HERPES INFECTIONS

I sing the pain that cannot be measured:
the night-time hunter who stalks my bones,
the one-note ringing
no one else can hear,
the squeeze that takes me like a lover
pressing too hard, until sternum meets spine.
　　　　　　—from "Complin"

In addition to HIV, I have had excellent results with the herpes viruses. When I used just enzyme therapy, I could minimize the frequency of outbreaks, especially of herpes simplex I, or cold sores, and of herpes simplex II, genital herpes. Since adding NAET, my success has been even more dramatic.

Research is now suggesting that the active herpes II virus can be a prominent factor in transforming normal cells into cancer cells. Hence, it is important that the virus flare up as infrequently as possible. Herpes is insidious: once it is contracted, it is not expelled from the body but remains dormant and can become active under certain circumstances. Most people who have herpes know what activates it, but they often have no way of avoiding it. For example, exposure to sun may activate the virus. Some sunscreens help, and others do not. NAET treatment and the use of enzymes can help control herpes.

When the body becomes weakened by disease or drugs or everyday stress, and then you eat foods you are allergic to and expose yourself to the sun, the immune system becomes overloaded and cannot maintain control over the virus. In my experience, the more often the virus becomes active, the more serious the problems it can cause.

When these viruses awaken in the body and the defenses are weak, the viruses penetrate healthy cells and reproduce themselves within those cells. Antibodies help delay this reproduction process, but in a weakened and overburdened immune system, they combine with the antigens (viruses) to form circulating immune complexes (CICs) that lodge in different areas of the body, provoking the body 's own aggressive reaction. As I mentioned earlier, these immune complexes can cause various autoimmune problems over time, including inflammation, nerve damage, and pain. For example, the herpes zoster, or shingles, virus can lodge itself in nerve cells and cause permanent pain. With enzymes and allergy elimination, I have had success in treating all the different herpes viruses, especially shingles.

Jim

Jim, 49, came to see me with chronic cold sores, or a herpes I viral infection. He was referred by his wife who had been a patient and had successfully cleared her chronic fatigue. Jim noticed that eating certain foods or, especially, exposing himself to the sun would activate the herpes. No matter what he did, he could not control it, and he believed he would have the problem his whole life.

We found that he was allergic to most of the basic allergens: eggs and chicken, calcium (including all dairy products), Vitamin C mix, Vitamin A, all the B vitamins, all the minerals, all the sugars (which are especially important to herpes), and salt. He was okay with iron

After clearing these, I prescribed enzymes that I use specifically to guard against herpes or minimize herpes activity (AllerZyme H) (see the Resource Guide in the back of this book). These enzymes also contain certain herbs, wheat germ, lecithin, Vitamin C, calcium, and Vitamin E. They are effective for herpes I and II and even for shingles, herpes zoster. There are other enzymes to use for controlling and weakening an outbreak. All the enzymes are high in protease, and the enzymes for an outbreak contain large amounts of amylase which is good for inflammations.

When we retested Jim, we found that he needed to be treated for some heavy metals including mercury, chemicals, dairy products, shellfish, meats and cheeses, and nuts and seeds. Nuts are especially important because they contain lots of arginine which can activate the herpes virus. He was still allergic to strawberries, beer and wine, coffee, yeast, chocolate, coffee, caffeine, vinegar, soy sauce, some herbs and spices, food additives, food coloring, and of course sunlight. We also needed to treat for viruses because whenever he would catch a cold or flu, he would also get a herpes outbreak.

Since I had put him on the enzymes and began to treat the basics, he has not had a single outbreak. We treated him for nuts and seeds, shellfish, beer and wine, vinegar, soy sauce, tofu, soy, and sunlight. Sunlight has to be treated on a rainy or cloudy day when there is no sun at all, and the patient should not be exposed to any other type of radiation including TV, microwaves, or computers. We also treated him for all the herpes viruses themselves in combination with DNA, RNA, and viruses. It has been almost a year now since we began treatment, and Jim still has not had a herpes outbreak.

Aaron

My son, Aaron, who is in college now, used to get frequent herpes outbreaks on his lips when he was young. I knew he was eating foods to which he was allergic, but I did not know what they were or how to treat for them. Because my father also had frequent cold sores, I assumed that it might be genetic, although I do not get them and neither does my husband. When I began working with the enzymes, I gave some to Aaron and he stopped having active outbreaks except when he got too much exposure to the sun, ate too much sugar, or became overly stressed.

After treating for the basics, we treated for certain foods, particularly dairy, which made a big difference for him. We also treated for nuts and some foods related to emotions. Then we treated for the herpes virus with DNA-RNA and several other combinations. It has been about 10 years, and he has not had a single herpes outbreak since then. People do not realize there is an alternative approach to treating herpes, and since the virus may be a precursor to other diseases or problems later in life, it is important to take care of it. Allergy elimination and enzyme therapy can be extremely effective.

Carol

Another patient, Carol, 44, complained of excess weight, bloating, and weekly outbreaks of genital herpes. First, I did an acute symptom examination and a palpation exam, both fasting and nonfasting. On fasting I found upper right quadrant inflammation which usually represents liver toxicity, and a weakness around the spleen, possibly indicating a weakened immune system. I also found inflammation around the lower left quadrant, indicative of irritable bowel syndrome as well as a severe calcium deficiency, and an inflamed lower right quadrant, related to protein deficiency, constipation, or other bowel problems. I also found a positive fungal reflex, suggesting a systemic yeast infection that correlated with her severe bloating and PMS.

The nonfasting palpation, which I performed directly after the fasting palpation, evaluated her digestion of the particular food groups. She demonstrated trouble digesting simple sugars and starches which were the foods she craved and ate the most. In fact, she could not control her consumption of them. I immediately recommended an enzyme to help digest sugars (pan) and starches and gave her some progesterone cream for the PMS. If a person is allergic to progesterone, I generally prescribe a topical cream because taking the hormone internally can sometimes aggravate an existing fungal infection and increase bloating in women.

Since Carol had such frequent herpes outbreaks, I knew there were allergies that overtaxed her immune system and prevented it from keeping the virus in check. I was unable to put her on the herpes enzyme immediately because she was allergic to a few of the ingredients. When I tested her, I found her to be allergic to all the basics: eggs, chicken, and feathers, calcium mix, Vitamin C mix, sugars, B vitamins, iron, Vitamin A, and minerals. The B vitamins were especially difficult for her to clear. She had some strong reactions including bloating, exhaustion, and irritability, and we needed to retreat her for several of the B vitamins separately. With B2 and B12 she needed to be eight feet away from the vitamin and had to wait 40 hours instead of the usual 25. After all the B vitamins had finally cleared, she noticed an immediate decrease in her craving for carbohydrates.

After that I recommended the sugar intolerant diet described in the Resource Guide which helped her lose 20 pounds. When she changed her eating habits, her bloating also diminished. After the basics were done, I retested her and found her allergic to some foods and other allergens, including some neurotransmitters and hormones, especially adrenaline, viruses, many fungi and molds, grains, nuts and seeds, vegetables, berries, oils and fats, herpes II, chocolate, coffee, caffeine, some fruits, food additives, spices, and shellfish.

Other doctors often ask me where to start when someone has so many allergies. The strategies I use are based on a combination of experience and intuition. I find that the more I do, the more easily I can determine the treatment sequence for a particular patient. With Carol, my hunch was to treat her for hormones first, get through some of the foods that seemed to activate the herpes, and then go back to fungus and the herpes virus itself. Once the hormones and viruses had cleared, we treated for grains, including barley, corn, and wheat, nuts and seeds, dairy, coffee, chocolate, caffeine, some fruits, and spices. Then we treated for the herpes II virus which took several sessions plus three weeks of self-treatment with different combinations including DNA-RNA. When herpes finally cleared, her outbreaks stopped for the first time in years.

She did not have an outbreak for months, until her dentist gave her an injection of novocaine. I immediately treated her for all the different local anesthetics such as lydocaine, novocaine, zylocaine, and prilocaine, and the outbreak went away almost completely. If a virus like herpes or Epstein-Barr has been thoroughly cleared, there should not be any more outbreaks.

Again she had no outbreak for several months, until she ate shellfish. I treated for shellfish and had her do some more self-treatments for the herpes virus. I also treated her for all the fungi which cleared up her bloating. Fungus is an important allergen to treat in herpes cases because it can be linked with the virus. After about a year of working together she had had only two outbreaks which pleased her immensely. She even found herself forgetting that she had herpes.

HERPES SIMPLEX

Viruses induce systemic disease by overcoming the body's immune defenses. After they have entered the body, they attach to nearby cells, replicate within them, and spread to other cells. Because viruses are so minute, they can only be seen by a powerful microscope and are hard to diagnose. They can progress slowly or rapidly and can be insidious and hard to eliminate. It has been speculated that cancer may be caused by a virus. Research has suggested that cancer viruses slip into normal cells and change them to cancer cells, thereby turning the body against itself. While trying to defend itself, the body may generate an allergic reaction, sending out antibodies that attack the body's own cells, thereby creating autoimmune reactions and many other symptoms.

One common class of viruses that can transform normal cells into cancer cells is the herpes virus. The effects of this virus differ, depending on the organism it infects. Epidemiologists have calculated that nearly 90 percent of the population of America and Europe have one or more of the various herpes viruses. These viruses can remain in the body permanently and cause skin eruptions and other unpleasant symptoms.

There are three main types of herpes viruses which affect people in different ways: herpes simplex type I (HSVI), herpes simplex type II, and herpes zoster, also known as shingles.There are two other herpes viruses: herpes virus VI has many characteristics of the Epstein-Barr virus and is believed by some researchers to also cause symptoms of chronic fatigue, and the cytomegalovirus (CMV) which can cause a variety of neurological complications and is implicated in some types of learning disability. Similar to Epstein-Barr, herpes virus VI is easy to contract, but differs from it in that it gets inside lymphocytes and is implicated in rashes that occurs in infants because of the body's reaction to the antibodies built against the virus. Herpes virus VI occurs in 25 to 30 percent of patients with chronic fatigue syndrome.

The herpes simplex virus includes the two types most commonly associated with herpes diseases. Although both types can cause sores in the mouth and genital areas, herpes simplex type I, or oral facial herpes, is primarily known for causing recurring cold sores, whereas herpes simplex type II is generally associated with genital herpes. Cases in which the viruses cross-infect are thought to be the result of oral-genital contact.

Herpes is contracted through physical contact with someone carrying the virus. This includes kissing someone with a cold sore in his or her mouth, having oral sex or sexual intercourse, or touching the source of infection on another person's body. Correct use of condoms during sexual activity is crucial if one is sexually active, but even condoms do not guarantee protection from the herpes virus. Since the entire genital area may not be sufficiently covered, herpes can be passed nonsexually through the fingers when the active virus touches a part of the body with thin skin, such as the mouth, genitals, or eye area, or where there is a cut or scratch on the skin's surface. A person with herpes can spread the infection within his or her own system by touching a herpes sore and then touching another area of the body.

For these reasons, direct contact with lesions should be avoided from the appearance of initial warning signs until all scabs have healed and vanished. Use common sense when an infection is active, avoiding not only physical intimacy but also the exchange of articles such as toothbrushes, wash cloths, razors, towels, and cosmetics. Dishes and silverware can be shared as long as they are washed with soap and water which inactivates the fragile virus on inanimate objects. Although herpes can only be transmitted when the virus is active, it can be active even when there are no detectable sores or symptoms on the infected person's body. This type of transmission is known as asymptomatic, or subclinical, shedding, and there is a one-to-four percent chance of contacting the virus through contact on any asymptomatic day.

The first signs of a herpes outbreak are tingling, burning, or itching sensations on the skin. This warning of the onset of the disease is known as the prodrome. Fluid-filled blisters then appear in the area and break, leaving painful sores that scab, heal, and disappear on their own within seven to ten days. During the first outbreak, some herpes patients also experience several weeks of flu-like symptoms such as fever, headaches, and body aches, or whole-body symptoms such as general aches, malaise, and decreased appetite.

In the facial area, herpes simplex affects the lips or nasal region in the form of cold sores, painful sores in the mouth, gums, throat, or lips that can last two weeks or longer if no treatment is received. Most people develop herpes sores on the border of the lip where the lip meets the skin surrounding the mouth. Ulcers or canker sores that recur inside the mouth are usually unrelated to the herpes simplex virus. Oral herpes frequently occurs for the first time in childhood and is not exclusively a sexually transmitted disease.

Common sites of infection for genital herpes include the inner thighs, buttocks, anus, scrotum, the shaft and head of the penis in men, and the vagina, labia, and cervix in women. Patients may also experience enlarged or tender lymph nodes or lumps in the groin area, difficult or painful urination (called dysuria), increased frequency or urgency in urination, painful sexual intercourse, and incontinence. Women may have unusual vaginal discharge. I believe genital herpes is genetic and runs in families.

After contracting herpes, patients can usually expect more than one occurrence of symptoms. Only one third of people with herpes have just one outbreak with no future problems. For the rest, the first outbreak tends to be the most severe. After that, generally milder outbreaks can be triggered by poor diet, illness, stress, fatigue, sexual intercourse, fever, exposure to the sun, menstruation, pregnancy, and allergies to foods and other ingestants and contactants.

The rate of recurrence depends on the type of virus and the individual, with some patients experiencing outbreaks on a monthly basis and others far less often. For the first few years, the average rate of recurrence for genital herpes is every three months. Oral herpes recurs less often, approximately once a year. Genital herpes recurrence is reported in 80 percent of cases, while oral herpes has a 50 percent chance of recurrence. I find that most outbreaks are related to allergies, including allergies to the sun, hormones, and foods. Proper rest, allergy elimination, nutrition, and exercise are the best preventative measures for future outbreaks. The most effective treatment is NAET which can prevent outbreaks altogether.

Herpes simplex recurrences can be explained by the unique activity of the virus once it has entered the body. The herpes virus hides inside nerve ganglia where infection-fighting antibodies cannot reach it. It remains dormant until a sudden stimulus triggers reactivation and the virus moves down the nerve fibers to the area of the body last affected, picking up where it left off.

In extreme cases of herpes without proper treatment, the disease can lead to damage in the eyes and brain. Among women, the herpes virus has been connected to cancer of the cervix, particularly if the patient also has the virus for genial warts, human palpaloma virus. However, a direct cause-and-effect relationship between herpes and cancer is merely speculative and anecdotal, and is not based on reproducible evidence. A pregnant woman can also pass the herpes virus to her baby during childbirth if there are sores around her genital area. People whose immune systems are already compromised—those who have AIDS or are undergoing chemotherapy—have a greater risk of incurring serious infection or organ damage from the spread of the herpes infection.

Most doctors recognize herpes sores by sight and can confirm diagnosis based on the patient's history. Therefore, testing is not always necessary. A swab or viral culture of the sores may be taken to check for the herpes simplex virus and to distinguish between type I and type II. Unfortunately, this method has a 50 percent chance of yielding false-negatives which makes the test relatively inaccurate. Another test, called the EIA test, can diagnose herpes but cannot identify the type. One blood test, the Western Blot, is designed to detect type II herpes through the presence of herpes antibodies, although some experts do not believe that blood tests are useful. The infrequently used Tzanck Test, or lesion smear, involves scraping cells from a herpes lesion and examining them under a microscope. The presence of cells with many nuclei indicates cell damage that may be a result of herpes. This procedure resembles the pap smear that women undergo to test for certain cancers.

Traditional medicine offers no cure for herpes but approaches the disease with the goal of temporary symptom relief. The 10-year-old oral drug acyclovir (brand name Zovirax) has been shown to reduce the pain of sores and the length and frequency of herpes outbreaks. There is also a topical acylovar product which may be effective but must be administered approximately once an hour for the first day of an outbreak. Acyclovar is not entirely dependable, and doctors are now discovering strains of the virus that are resistant to the drug. A number of new antiherpes drugs are awaiting FDA approval. These include Fanciclovir, Valacyclovir, and Foscarnat, but it is difficult to determine the impact they will have on the disease. Sometimes topical and oral antibiotics are prescribed for secondary infections of the skin lesions.

Over-the-counter topical ointments for facial cold sores have proven unreliable for the treatment of herpes viruses, and scientists have not confirmed the effectiveness of any natural home remedies developed over the years. Measures can be taken during an outbreak to help relieve the discomfort such as warm baths and gentle cleansing of the lesions with soap and water. To encourage effective recovery, one should keep the infected area clean and dry, wear cotton underwear and loose fitting clothing, and wash the area after urinating. But once the lesion has healed, the torturous experience of infection can return at any time. The condition is expected to last the patient's lifetime, although it is seldom life-threatening. In my experience, however, NAET, in combination with enzyme therapy, can successfully prevent herpes outbreaks.

At last count, the national incidence of herpes was approximately 20 million people, with 200,000 to 500,000 new cases reported each year. One survey found that genital herpes is epidemic in the United States, and the rate of occurrence continues to rise worldwide. Studies have indicated that 50 percent to 80 percent of American adults have been exposed to HSVI and have produced antibodies in their blood to fight it. The presence of antibodies does not guarantee that the person will experience any symptoms. It does means that a person who has herpes can transmit it.

Shingles, or herpes zoster, is a painful infection of the nerve cells and skin caused by the reactivation of the varicella zoster virus, or chicken pox. The virus settles in the nerve cells and erupts periodically, resulting in chronic pain. It occurs most often in older people and those with compromised immune systems. In the United States, approximately 200,000 to 300,000 cases occur each year, or four out of every 1000 people. The incidence is higher among people over 50. The main symptom is a prolonged, painful, burning rash, frequently located on the face. Other symptoms include numbness and itching in the affected area. Motor paralysis is a rare occurrence but does affect about 5 percent of patients.

Common treatments are topical analgesic preparations and antiviral drugs such as acyclovar. The only studies showing success in resolving pain have been through steroid injections. Some people claim to find relief in megadoses of Vitamins C, E, and B. The best preventative measures are physical exercise, allergy elimination, avoidance of stress, and good nutrition. Enzyme therapy is important in the treatment of all immune disorders, including shingles.

People with shingles have a prior history of chicken pox, and the recurrence of the virus in the latter part of life is often related to immune system suppression. If a patient is on cancer drugs or radiation treatment, has undergone organ transplant, or has AIDS or diabetes, there is a greater likelihood that his or her body will not be able to fight off the varicella zoster virus that causes shingles. Emotional or physical trauma and old age also leave patients vulnerable to the virus. The load phenomena comes into play when the body is exposed to increased amount of allergens combined with emotional and physical stress. The immune system is weakened and the virus resurfaces.

Following an outbreak of herpes zoster, some 10 percent of patients experience a condition called post-herpetic neuralgia in which nerve pain persists for months or even years after the rash has disappeared. There is no proven treatment aside from pain medications which can be addictive and cause side effects. NAET can also be helpful in eliminating the pain. Also, most people are allergic to their medication and need to be treated for it.

Relaxation and breathing exercises can help ease the pain, as can physical therapy, acupuncture, and other alternative therapies for pain elimination. However, I have found the combination of NAET and enzyme therapy to be the most effective approach to shingles and to ending its torturous cycle. Ultimately, I think it is an allergy to this virus that causes it to be reactivated, and once patients have been treated for it, most people will not contract it again.

TROUBLESHOOTING AND PREVENTIVE MEASURES

*I am ready to claim
the space my body takes up in the world
as mine,
ready to take this image of glass
that I am made of
and trade it in for
rock and tree bark and dark solid earth.*
                    —from "Declaration of Intention"

Joseph

Joseph, another HIV-infected individual, was not in good shape when he came to see me. His symptoms included severe gas and digestive problems, constipation, fatigue, forgetfulness, oversensitivity to sugar, chronically swollen lymph nodes and cold sores, and chronic colds, viruses, and bacterial infections. He also had some problems with urination, leg cramps, swollen joints, difficulty falling asleep, and a low T-cell count. He was even considering doing an experimental procedure because of his T-cell count and related problems.

The HIV virus infects the T4 lymphocyte which is one type of white blood cell. When the T4 lymphocyte is infected, other white blood cells of the immune system are activated. After infecting this lymphocyte, HIV can become dormant for a period of time, then reactivate, begin reproducing, and kill the T4 cells. If sufficient numbers of T4 cells are killed, the infected person's ability to activate the immune system may be reduced, and he or she can become more vulnerable to infections. It is not clear why the virus reactivates. It may be that an allergy to HIV and many other allergens compromises the immune system and prevents the body from controlling the spread of the infection. In the same way, harmful microorganisms that normally exist in the body can become life-threatening. For example, such a person may be more susceptible to pneumonia, yeast infections, and viruses such as herpes and Epstein-Barr.

First we did a full evaluation and an abdominal diagnostic exam. The palpation showed a weak spleen meridian, suggesting a possible deficiency in the lymphocytes that the spleen produces. I prescribed the spleen enzymes (spl) I generally recommend to people with HIV and chronic fatigue, and later I treated him for an allergy to the spleen itself. I also found an inability to digest sugars which explained his constant craving for sweets, and palpation points related to fungal infections, a problem for which he was already taking medication. In addition to sugars, he had trouble digesting fats that caused some stress on the immune system by stressing the liver/gallbladder area. Trouble with proteins can cause hypoglycemia, a craving for sugar, and calcium deficiencies, and usually indicates a deficiency of protease, an important enzyme that helps fight antigens and foreign bacteria and viruses. We prescribed an enzyme to digest the fats and sugars (hcl).

His urinalysis evaluation showed severe acidity (5.5 pH). To buffer this excess acidity, his body was using enzymes that should have been available for the digestion of sugars and starches. A high specific gravity and a higher-than-normal volume also suggested the possibility of sucrose in the urine as well as a predisposition to diabetes, problems digesting sugar, hypoglycemia, and a craving for sugar. I therefore prescribed the sugar intolerant diet (see Resource Guide), with an emphasis on lower rather than unlimited fat intake. Next, we did some allergy testing, but Joseph had to stop coming for a while for financial reasons.

When he returned many months later, he reported that his T-cell count was quite a bit higher. He attributed it to the enzymes he had been taking. As a result, he decided not to do the experimental program. We resumed the allergy work because he noticed that yeast was still a problem and he suffered frequent viruses and fatigue.

We treated him for most of the basic allergens, including eggs, chicken, and tetracycline (especially important because he had taken tetracycline for a while as a teenager), Vitamin C, all the B vitamins, sugars, Vitamin A, minerals. and salt. After the initial allergies had cleared, we retested and found quite a few that still needed to be treated, and we came up with a treatment plan based on his particular needs and symptoms.

I decided to treat him first for his food allergies because as a fitness trainer he was very particular about what he ate. We treated him for all the grains, many proteins, fats, beans, coffee, chocolate, caffeine, and some beverages. We got through all the foods to which he was allergic. At this point he reported that he had more energy for his workouts, whereas before he needed to take a two-hour nap every day after he trained, he now felt refreshed after only 15 or 20 minutes. With HIV and AIDS patients, physicians generally cannot do much to help them improve their energy. By contrast, I have had excellent results because I treat patients as people rather than as a particular disease.

Next I treated Joseph for the HIV virus in combination with his blood, DNA, and RNA, which seemed to be sufficient for him. Then we treated for other viruses, including Epstein-Barr, CMV (cytomegalovirus), and herpes simplex (he was constantly bothered by fever blisters and herpes sores). I always treat viruses in combination with DNA and RNA because I find that if I do not, there is a chance they will recur. I have particularly gratifying results with herpes which generally remains dormant once it is treated.

After the viruses, I treated him for many bacteria including pneumonia from which he had suffered three years before. We then treated for all the fungi, one of the most important treatments for most people, and Joseph's energy and digestion improved enormously. Regular blood tests indicated that his viral load was lower and his T-cell count was still good.

Because there had been research suggesting that fluoridated water and vaccinations might exacerbate or even cause HIV symptoms, I treated him for fluoride and for small pox, mumps, measles, rubella, and polio vaccinations. I also treated him for an allergy to antibiotics that can cause immune system problems among people who have taken them for a period of time. I treated him for sleeping pills and an herbal laxative he had once taken, even though he had not used them recently.

Before I treated for organs, I treated him for some chemicals including exhaust fumes, solvents, paint thinner, acetone, and cleaning fluid. Next, I treated him for radiation including the sun, microwave, and television. We also cleared some emotional allergies in combination with certain foods and situations. Then we treated for all the important organs of the immune system including the lymph glands, the lymph nodes, the spleen, the liver, the pancreas, the tonsils, and many of the immune mediators like IgE, IgG, and IgM. I also treated him for DNA and RNA because I find that people can have what are known as antinuclear antibodies, antibodies that are directed against their own DNA, RNA, and other proteins. These can cause serious damage by linking up with other allergens to cause autoimmune problems like Hashimoto's thyroiditis, HIV, and diabetes. Treating DNA, RNA, and the blood can often clear up these chronic health problems. Finally, I treated for other metabolic enzymes and metabolites, some toxic heavy metals, other organs, and muscle and nerve tissue.

Since then, Joseph has come in every few months He has not gotten sick once, his energy is consistently high, and his T-cell count remains stable. Now and then we find something new to treat, but for the most part, we are done. He still works as a fitness trainer, has written a book, made some videotapes, and his life is on the upswing. I taught him how to treat his own saliva for viral infections, and every six to eight months I test for the HIV virus to make sure he has not developed an allergy to it again, either alone or in combination.

Tracy

Chronic gas and bloating and chronic fatigue are the most common complaints that doctors hear every day. I have always had excellent results with gas and bloating with a combination enzyme therapy and allergy elimination. Tracy, however, was an unusual challenge. Nothing seemed to work for her. With the help of both enzymes and NAET, she had excellent results in other areas. She witnessed major changes in her children and her parents, and she sent me many patients who all did well. But we could not seem to eliminate her chronic gas and bloating. We did have one breakthrough when I treated her for chronic appendicitis and she had two weeks of no bloating. But one day she woke up with the same problem again. Her bowel movements were normal, and she ate lots of organic fruits and vegetables.

When I did another abdominal palpation exam, I found that she was extremely intolerant of sugar, true of about 80 percent of the population. The bulk of her diet consisted of fruits and carbohydrates. I kept thinking that perhaps the problem was fungus, but I had already treated her for fungus. However, it was before I realized that patients had to follow a restricted diet, wear gloves and new clothes, and otherwise avoid contact with anything that might contain fungus or mold. Because she was so sugar intolerant, I decided to have her stop eating fruit and I asked her to call me within 48 hours.

When I did not hear from her, I assumed that nothing had changed. As it turned out, when she came in several weeks later, she reported that she had had no bloating since she had eliminated fruit. I prescribed the sugar intolerant diet (see the Resource Guide) with no fruit and minimal grains or other carbohydrates, and she continued to be free of gas and bloating which was a real breakthrough for her. Sugar had been aggravating fungus in her system.

I still needed to treat Tracy again for fungus and mold. The prior clearing had not been successful because she had not taken the necessary precautions. Patients need to disinfect their house for mold, buy new clothes, and wear gloves and a mask. Unless these allergies are properly cleared, they and all the accompanying symptoms will recur. But once they are fully cleared, the changes can be momentous and long-lasting. We treated Tracy twice for about 25 different molds and fungi, and she has been doing well ever since. Because she is sugar intolerant, however, she still needs to keep her fruit consumption to a minimum.

Although the treatment for molds was crucial, the culmination of Tracy's treatment occurred when we treated her for an allergy to oxygen. I had never encountered anyone allergic to oxygen before, but Tracy's digestion problems and occasional bloating improved dramatically after this treatment. We also treated for oxygen in combination with mercury and amalgam.

People with immune disorders tend to have similar symptoms which include:

- joint pain
- irritability
- insomnia
- lethargy
- depression
- poor memory
- headache
- inability to concentrate
- muscle weakness
- bloating
- gas
- constipation
- swelling of joints

They may be fine for a period of time and then within hours, develop symptoms and be unable to move or function normally for days. Patients often tell me that they suspect their problems are related to allergies but they are not sure which ones are the worst. They want to know why their body is reacting the way it is and what they should do to eliminate the most severe allergies causing their problems,

To answer these questions, I do some preliminary detective work beginning with a diagnostic enzyme evaluation which includes an abdominal palpation and a 24-hour urinalysis. Then I test for allergies so they can avoid the substances they are allergic to until they have been cleared using NAET. I also ask them to keep a diary of their symptoms, their daily diet, the supplements they take, and so on. I generally find that the one factor common to all the immune disorders is a yeast or other fungal infection and that eliminating allergies to fungi can be extremely helpful.

If the urinalysis indicates that patients are low in calcium, they are probably allergic to the mineral and should therefore avoid foods high in calcium until they are treated for it. The same is true for imbalances of sugar, sodium chloride, electrolytes, and other minerals. I may also find indications of various allergies that are having a major impact or creating inflammation in the body. When I point these out, patients can note in their diaries whether eating dairy products, for example, increases symptoms such as bloating and other digestive problems, ear plugging, mucus, and sinus congestion. Keeping a diary also helps them determine whether their allergies are mainly to food, environmental toxins, or both. Clearing the basic allergies with NAET often eliminates many other allergies as well, and significantly reduces the symptoms of the immune disorder and the need for medications. At this point, it becomes easier to spot additional allergens that are causing trouble.

For example, one woman who had had chronic fatigue for about 15 years noticed that sometimes she felt fine. Why did this happen? She wanted to know. She knew her problem was allergy related, but which allergies were the cause? As a teacher, she spent her days in the classroom, and wondered whether she was allergic to the students, viruses, the food, the chalk, the furniture, or the mold.

On the abdominal diagnostic exam, I found inflammation around the liver and gall bladder area which usually indicates a toxicity resulting from the burden of too many allergens on the immune system. People who have inflammation in this area tend to be overly sensitive to chemicals, environmental allergens, and perfumes. When the liver is detoxified, these patients improve without the burden of increased sensitivity.

This woman also suffered from sinus infections and congestion, intestinal bloating, constipation, joint pain, insomnia, irritability, and severe depression. I noticed indications of Candida and other fungi, and an inability to digest or absorb sugars. In addition, her adrenal glands, which are intimately involved with inflammation, metabolism of sugars, and the regulation of energy, were not functioning properly. The urinalysis showed that she was sugar intolerant and her consumption of large amounts of sugar was compromising her immune system by fueling the growth of Candida and fungus. I recommended a diet with far fewer carbohydrates and prescribed enzymes to digest sugars and relieve nasal congestion, support the liver, decrease toxicity, and fight fungus. If a person is allergic to these enzymes, I treat them immediately and then go on to treat for the other allergens.

Her most severe allergens were to foods such as wheat, dairy, cheeses, spices, and corn; neurotransmitters including seratonin, dopamine, and gaba; some phenolics; and Candida and other fungi. Her urinalysis showed a sluggish kidney which usually indicates a congested lymph system resulting from liver toxicity and an overwhelmed immune system. There was also a reduced sediment index of carbohydrates in the 24-hour urinalysis, confirming that her absorption and digestion of sugars was poor, one cause of hypoglycemia.

After embarking on a low sugar diet, she kept a diary to record what she ate, what she was feeling, and what allergic symptoms she experienced. As a result, she became more aware of her sensitivities. We treated for the basic allergies and then the food allergies that were not eliminated when the basic allergies cleared. After this initial clearing, her symptoms were reduced by about 90 percent. Her depression lifted, she lost weight, her bowels began functioning normally, and her fatigue improved somewhat. She then began noticing that phenolics in foods and certain environmental factors were causing her fatigue, and we targeted these in our treatments. Ultimately, we succeeded in clearing her essential allergies, and today she is doing extremely well and has no sign of chronic fatigue.

Both the patient and I must act as detectives so we can create an individual treatment program. Through testing, I can usually determine which allergies are the most serious for particular patients. They, in turn, must become more aware of what they are bombarded with each day and which substances provoke reactions. I also need to know what they are digesting and not digesting, absorbing and not absorbing, and what they are deficient in so I can make adjustments. Most patients, even children, become excellent detectives. They know that it was a food additive that triggered their mucus production or chocolate or perfume that caused their headache. They get to know their own bodies, and I listen to what they tell me.

Because most people with immune disorders are infected with fungus and Candida, I usually recommend a reduction in their intake of sugars and other carbohydrates, including junk foods, sweet potatoes, grains, and fruits, and yeast-containing foods and beverages until we treat for Candida and fungus. Most of these people are allergic to yeast and can have some severe reactions, especially when the yeast is linked with certain foods. Avoiding milk products (especially cheese), pesticides, and hormones is also important.

LIVER TOXICITY

To a large extent, our health, vitality, stamina, and energy is determined by the health of the liver. It is one of the most important organs in the human body, and it is irreplaceable. Therefore, we must take care of it.

Liver toxicity can result in psychological and neurological symptoms, depression, headache, mental confusion, mental illness, tingling in the extremities, abnormal nerve reflexes, and other signs of impaired nervous system function. Some liver detoxification can be achieved with liver enzymes that support the function of the liver by facilitating the conversion of glycogen into glucose, increasing protein metabolism, and inhibiting cholesterol secretion in the bile. These enzymes can also help stimulate regeneration of damaged liver cells.

The liver deals with a constant onslaught of toxic chemicals and heavy metals from both outside and inside the system. These toxins are everywhere: in our water, soil, air, food, and even our mouth. For example, lead and other heavy metals in the body come primarily from industrial sources and leaded gasoline. More than 600,000 tons of lead are dumped into the atmosphere and are inhaled through our air and eventually ingested through our water. I always check and, if necessary, treat children for lead.

Other common sources of metals that can cause liver toxicity include tin cans, pesticides, cooking utensils, cadmium and lead batteries, DDT found in tobacco, mercury in dental amalgams and fish, cosmetics, and solvents. Aluminum ingested in foods contained or cooked in aluminum foil, cans, or utensils can be a major toxin for the immune system. Insecticides leach into the water supply, and DDT, even though it is not used in this country anymore, reenters the country in imported produce and can still be found in our bodies from previous exposures. Other chemicals in the soil and water make their way into the body and cause health problems, and chemical sensitivities to soaps, cosmetics, detergents, formaldehyde, and petrochemicals can overload our immune system and increase our susceptibility to problems. Even human breast milk can contain these toxins and pollutants. When appropriate, I treat for these substances with NAET.

I also treat for the liver itself, and other organs related to it such as the gall bladder, spleen, intestine, and stomach, in combination with other allergens, if necessary. This approach has been dramatically successful in restoring strength and vitality to the organ and to the body as a whole. For example, a woman who came to see me for multiple chemical sensitivities had been doing extremely well. After clearing many allergens, including chemicals, mold, animals, perfumes, and formaldehyde, she felt like a new woman and could attend a party with perfumes and cigarettes and eat anything that was served. One day, she was very distraught because it seemed that many of her allergies had returned. When I retested her, I found that all her treatments were holding quite well. In my experience, this indicates a liver problem. NAET treatment, especially for fungus, heavy metals, and toxic chemicals, can cause a rapid detoxification of the body. If the liver is overloaded and not functioning optimally, one can experience signs of liver congestion and toxicity that can mimic the symptoms of multiple chemical sensitivities. Generally, I prescribe a liver enzyme and/or a liver cleanse and test for a liver allergy. This woman turned out to be allergic to her own liver which explained the return of her old symptoms. I treated her for liver, alone and in combination with various emotions, and within 24 hours, she was once again symptom-free and has been so ever since.

In my initial examination of a patient, particularly on their fasting palpation, I can usually detect any liver dysfunction and recommend an enzyme that will support the liver in the detoxification process. Because this woman was sent by another physician who started her on NAET, however, I just took over her treatment and did not do an abdominal palpation, as I ordinarily would have done.

CANDIDIASIS AND FUNGAL INFECTIONS

Yeast infections, especially candidiasis, are a growing problem in the population, and play an important role in causing autoimmune problems. For more information on the causes, symptoms, and treatment of yeast infections, see the section entitled Candidiasis, Yeast, and Fungal Infections.

Until one is cleared of yeast infections, there are precautions that can help in the reduction of symptoms. Fortunately, however, yeast infections can be successfully cleared by treating for an allergy to yeast with NAET.

I recommend that patients, especially those with yeast infections, eat organically grown vegetables and grains and organically raised, hormone-free meats as much as possible. Pesticides, nitrates, food additives, and hormones can often be found in red meat, chicken, and other poultry and should be avoided whenever possible. Patients also need to learn the foods to which they are sensitive and avoid them or treat for them with NAET. After the basic allergies have cleared, we always do some testing to determine which foods are still causing problems. The revolutionary aspect of this work is that such foods need not be avoided indefinitely, but can be cleared using NAET.

One patient from out of town had improved so much over a year of treatments that she could lead a normal life. She came to get some retesting and a repalpation to determine where her digestion had improved. While she was here, she ate at a restaurant and had a severe reaction which included dizziness, insomnia, heart palpitations, and nausea We finally discovered that the cause of her symptoms was a food additive that had not been treated. Everyone, whether they have symptoms or not, should know what they are eating, where it comes from, what it contains, and how it is cooked. You have to be extremely clear in stating what you can and cannot have. If you do not know, cook your food yourself until you are cleared.

I encourage people with Candida to use fresh vegetables instead of canned ones and to avoid bottled, frozen, and canned juices. In general, juices are filled with sugar and tend to exacerbate yeast infections. Water is the best beverage. Most children with chronic ear or sinus infections are filled with yeast because they have been overdosed with antibiotics. Taking them off sugar helps until they can be treated with NAET. Peanuts and peanut butter should be avoided because they contain mold, and most commercial breads, cakes, and crackers contain yeast. My daughter grew up with yeast-free breads and developed a taste for them. It is also important to use cold-pressed vegetable oils that are not rancid and to make your own salad dressings. I recommend flaxseed oil because it has all the essential fatty acids. Vinegar is best avoided because it is fermented with yeast.

For the same reason, people with Candida and fungus should stay away from alcoholic beverages, especially beer and wine, because they are made with yeast and large quantities of readily available carbohydrates that feed the yeast. Even one sip can cause bloating, dizziness, fatigue, and all the other symptoms of an immune disorder. Once you clear the yeast, then you can clear the wine and drink it without problems. By that point, however, you usually do not crave it anymore. NAET treatments tend to eliminate food cravings and addictions and restore balance to the body, so food choices are based on what the body needs rather than what it craves.

If you have Candida or fungal allergies, coffee and tea, including most herb teas, should be avoided because they are subject to mold contamination. Green tea is a suitable alternative as well as pau d'arco tea which some people use to boost the immune system, and seem to be helpful for yeast infections. Diet drinks, which contain caffeine, phosphates, saccharin, food coloring, and food additives, have no nutritional value, can be addictive, and do as much damage to the body as beverages with sugar. Sometimes it takes a few treatments to clear people of diet soft drinks. Instead, use bottled water or put a filter in your house. Avoid leftovers because they are a breeding ground for molds. Spices and condiments, too, are loaded with mold and should be avoided.

Cereal grains including wheat, oats, barley, and rice, tend to contain a great deal of mold and I generally encourage people to eat only a minimal amount of grain. Dry, processed cereals often contain yeast-derived B vitamins and large quantities of sugar. Children who eat them every day end up coughing and sneezing in school. Most people, especially children, are sick more often between Halloween and Christmas because of the high consumption of candy. Their body is weakened and cannot prevent the many viruses and molds which add stress to the immune system.

Nuts are loaded with protein and other nutrients and can be a good food alternative, especially for children on a Candida diet. I recommend roasted nuts, which are free of mold, but not peanuts which tend to accumulate mold.

Keeping indoor humidity below 50 percent can reduce dust mites and molds. Central air conditioning is the most effective way of controlling humidity, although some people react to the cooler air. Car air conditioning especially provides a prime location for the buildup of molds, but this problem can be prevented by asking the car dealer to install an antimold vent or ingredient. Swamp coolers may increase humidity, and window fans may draw mold into the house.

Air cleaning devices that filter the air in the home to remove airborne allergens are invaluable for anyone who has a problem with molds. Several filtering devices are available and some can be used in conjunction with forced air cooling and heating systems. One type of filter uses standard disposable fiberglass filters that are changed monthly. Permanent air filters should be cleaned periodically. An electric filter that uses an electrostatic precipitator requires frequent cleaning and produces irritating ozone if not well maintained. The most effective filter is a high-efficiency particulate air (HEPA) filter. HEPA filtration systems require no maintenance and their efficacy only increases with use. An air cleaner that uses a true HEPA filter is the most efficient and reliable method of cleaning the air of odors, chemicals, and mold.

When choosing an air filter, consider the amount of air the unit can circulate and clean. There are various advantages and disadvantages to the mechanical and electrical methods of air filtering. A mechanical filtration system becomes more efficient with use and does not produce ozone, an irritant to the lungs. They require frequent cleaning, may become coated with tars from tobacco smoke, and may lose static charge capability. Ion generators are effective air purifiers that do not require filter replacement but they do produce ozone which can be serious for asthmatics, and they create an ion imbalance in room air and cause cleaning problems when air particles stick to walls and furniture. Although few air cleaners are listed by the FDA as medical devices because the agency has not established performance standards, one kind of purifier, the HEPA filter, is used in operating rooms where human life, health, and safety are most at risk.

Electric and hot water radiant heaters are the best heating alternatives. Forced air can disperse mold, and, even if there is a central filter, ducts can accumulate large amounts of mold. If forced air is used, the ducts should be cleaned once a year and bedroom air vents should be closed to keep out allergens from other parts of the home. Fireplaces and wood-burning stoves are not recommended sources of heat because they emit toxic particles and gasses. Kerosene heaters produce sulfur dioxide and carbon monoxide in the home, both of which can be hard on the immune system.

To prevent mold, humidity should be kept as low as possible. It may be useful to use a gauge to measure the humidity. Keeping the windows closed and using an air conditioner or dehumidifier may also be helpful. A dehumidifier must be emptied regularly or attached to a drain, and the air intake on air conditioners should be sprayed with a nonallergenic fungicidal spray if the air conditioner develops a musty odor. Special air conditioning filters can be added to trap airborne allergens, and air purifiers can be used to help clear mold spores from the air. Walls should also be cleaned and a mold inhibitor added to any paints before they are applied if the occupant is not allergic to the product. Mold flourishes in dark, damp spaces that are poorly ventilated and in areas where water pools. Moisture and warmth accelerates the growth of dormant mold spores on most surfaces.

Once areas of molds are identified, they should be washed with a mold-inhibiting solution, and ventilation and draining should be improved. Some humidifiers prevent mold growth by a special heating process. Central humidifiers should be checked and cleaned frequently. Window condensation can lead to mold growth on the window frames. Books, leather products, wood paneling, and wallpaper paste all support mold growth and should be avoided or treated with the appropriate mold-inhibiting solutions. Indoor plants are not a major source of mold but may have mold in the soil with spores that become airborne when the plant is watered or repotted. Since wood bark harbors mold, fireplace wood should not be stored inside. Keep cupboards and garbage pails clean and dry. Dry shoes and boots thoroughly before storing, and wash and dry clothing that is damp with perspiration immediately after use.

In the kitchen, exhaust fans can be used to remove water vapor during cooking. Mold grows in refrigerators, particularly around door gaskets, in water pans, and on spoiled foods. Mold also grows on garbage, so containers should be emptied and cleaned frequently. In the bathroom, excess water should be removed from shower doors, tiles, and tubs with a squeegee or sponge. Shower curtains, tiles, shower stalls, tubs, and toilet tanks should be washed with mold-preventive solution. Do not carpet the bathroom. Vent the dryer outside and dry clothing immediately after washing. In a basement, do not lay carpet on a concrete floor; use vinyl flooring instead. Dirt floors should be covered with a vapor barrier. Keep the basement free of dust and remove stored items likely to harbor mold. Allergic individuals should not have their bedroom on the basement level. Avoid cutting grass or raking leaves, or use a tight-fitting mask while doing so. Avoid exposure to soil, compost, sand boxes, hay, and fertilizers. Correct drainage problems near the house to get rid of any pooled water. Avoid camping or walking in the woods where mold grows around moss or other vegetation. Remove rotted logs from around the house and yard.

Antique shops tend to harbor mold, as do sleeping bags, greenhouses, summer cottages, hotel rooms, and automobile air conditioners. Farmers, gardeners, bakers, upholsterers, paper hangers, mill workers, florists, food preparers, plumbers, librarians, and other people working around moldy materials all have occupational exposure to mold.

DIETARY SUPPLEMENTATION AND ENZYMES

For dietary supplementation, I recommend enzymes, vitamins, minerals, and the enzyme recipes in this book. Before I prescribe a supplement, I make sure the patient is not allergic to it or the fillers it contains. I also have people bring in the supplements and drugs they are currently taking and check them for each one. After I clear any allergies to vitamins and minerals, I supplement with these nutrients in combination with enzymes that enhance their absorption in order to make up for deficiencies that may have resulted from the allergies. For example, an allergy to calcium usually indicates a deficiency of calcium revealed in the urinalysis and abdominal palpation. After treating for the allergy, I recommend a calcium supplement with enzymes to help the body absorb calcium from foods. Before patients take it, I test to see how much they need and if they are allergic to any particular brand.

Recently, when I appeared on a radio show in New York, a man called in to say that he had read in my first book that people can be allergic to vitamins. His wife had chronic fatigue and was taking about $200 worth of high-quality supplements each week. He suggested that she stop taking them for a while, and she improved so dramatically that they immediately made an appointment with an NAET practitioner.

TREATMENT FOR DRUGS WITH NAET

In treating individuals with chronic immune disorders, it is extremely important to test and treat for their medications because these can be the cause of many symptoms. For example, a patient with endometriosis used birth control to regulate her bleeding. Once we cleared the basic allergies, we treated for the birth control pills, and for the first time in years, her symptoms of depression, insomnia, and irritability disappeared. She is now considering going off the birth control pills altogether.

Whenever possible, I work with the physicians of patients taking allergy medications to help them decide how much, if any, medication is needed. I do not take people off medications or prescribe them myself. I do provide enzymes, nutritional supplements, and cleanses and help people manage their allergies.

Allergy Management Plan

An allergy management plan defines the goals for getting patients' symptoms under control. Although the ultimate goal is to function normally, free from symptoms, different patients have different individual goals such as working or exercising again, eating a normal diet, eating out, having a social life, living independently and not with their parents. In addition to their goals, their plan should incorporate a list of their allergens, medications, and supplements and should be kept in a place where it can be referred to often. Management plans may evolve as symptoms clear, allergies are eliminated or controlled, or the environment changes. The NAET practitioner may want to formulate and adapt this plan in conjunction with a physician who specializes in immune disorders.

All patients should be able to answer the following questions:

1. Do you have an allergy management plan?

2. Is it written down?

3. Do you understand it?

4. Do you know how to recognize and respond to something that is bothering you?

5. Do you understand what is causing the sensitivity?

6. Do you need help?

7. Were you instructed in muscle testing or the O-ring test so you can assess yourself?

8. Do you know what to do when recovering from an allergic reaction?

9. Do you understand what enzymes to take and how to self-treat for viruses?

10. Do you know how to treat yourself in an emergency?

11. Do you understand the diet?

12. Should you continue taking medications when you feel better (this should be discussed with your physician)?

13. Do you know how to keep symptoms from recurring?

Many people suffer side effects from medications and they should be aware of what each medication and supplement is doing. Ask yourself the following questions:

1. What is the name of the medication?

2. Why are you taking it?

3. What is it supposed to do?

4. How long after starting the medication will it have an effect?

5. When and how often should you take it?

6. For how long ?

7. What happens if it doesn't work?

8. Are there any foods or other medications you should avoid while taking this medication?

9. Are there any side effects? If so, what should you do if they occur?

10. Is there any other information you should have about your medications?

11. Where can you go if you need more information?

As much as possible, patients should manage their condition with alternative therapy and a nonallergic environment to avoid stressing their immune system further with drugs. Until being successfully treated with NAET, they should also avoid foods to which they are allergic, use air purifiers, and eat a nutritious, yeast-free diet. As they undergo NAET treatment, there will be fewer symptoms and less need for medication, and they should consult with their physician to adjust medications as needs change.

Many adolescents have symptoms resembling immune system problems, particularly chronic fatigue, that are caused by allergies and a poor diet. They may be difficult to communicate with and reluctant to take responsibility for their health, but it is essential that they realize what their problem is and what they can do to prevent it from getting worse. Most adolescents feel a need to assert their independence from their parents and are sensitive to the influence of their peers. They may resist or ignore the suggestions of their parents or physicians. Nevertheless, they should participant in their own health care and be educated about their condition, including how to treat it, how to prevent symptoms from occurring, what foods to eat, and what supplements to take to stay healthy. My son, who is now in college, has been brought up to understand good nutrition. Even though most of his peers live on foods high in simple sugars, he has no desire for these foods and tries to eat a balanced diet at school which, needless to say, can be very difficult. NAET can be especially helpful for adolescents because it reduces the number of allergens to be avoided, reduces the cravings, and makes the management of their condition relatively carefree instead of overwhelming.

Like other stages of life, adolescence has its stresses, peer pressures, competition, and temptations in the form of drugs, alcohol, tobacco, and eating disorders. Teen smoking has increased in recent years, and teenagers need to understand how damaging smoking, or just being around smoking, can be for them. Secondhand smoke is actually more dangerous because one is not filtering the smoke through the cigarette but inhaling pure chemicals into the lungs. More than 90 percent of new tobacco smokers are children, and each day an estimated 3,000 from 10 to 15 begin to smoke for the first time. Studies have shown that three-quarters of those who use cigarettes continue to do so because they find it hard to quit. President Clinton signed a bill in August of 1996 designed to prevent the sale of tobacco to underage users. The tobacco and chemicals in cigarettes such as tar, nicotine, carbon monoxide, formaldehyde, aluminum, sulfur, and lead have all been shown to cause health problems, irritate the body, and inflame the airways. Exposure to these toxins, either by smoking or by exposure to secondhand smoke, can be devastating to the immune system.

Animals can create a problem because mold clings to fur and may come off when touched. Wash animals weekly for three weeks and then at two- or three-week intervals. Wear a face mask while brushing a dog or cat or cleaning the cage of a rodent, and wash hands and change clothes afterward. Because vacuuming may blow animal dander and molds around, use a vacuum with a high-quality filter. Parasites can also be picked up while touching an animal. NAET has been quite successful in treating for pet allergies, and it is important to avoid contact with the allergens for 25 hours after treatment. The patient may have to wear gloves and a mask or stay away from the home to avoid contact.

When people with immune disorders are exposed to flu, cold viruses, or other infectants, there is a high risk of developing symptoms. To prevent the spread of viruses, cover your mouth when sneezing or coughing, wash your hands frequently, dispose of used tissues, and keep your hands away from your face. Viruses spread from person to person through the air from coughs and sneezes, through hand contact with an infected person, or by touching surfaces that have been contaminated and then rubbing the eyes, mouth, or nose. Although flu vaccines are supposed to reduce the incidence of flu in healthy adults, I recommend that my patients, particularly those with immune disorders, be tested for an allergen sensitivity to the vaccine before taking it. Otherwise, it may result in flu symptoms that can lead to further problems. I usually manage to get a sample of the vaccine each year and test people for reactions. NAET treatment for flus and virus can be a strong preventative measure for both children and adults.

Healthy individuals who have been treated with NAET have strong immune systems and are able to resist infection. Their bodies are not laden with bacteria that keep resurfacing. When we pollute our bodies with environmental toxins, a poor diet, or medications, including antibiotics and birth control pills, we put undue stress on the immune system. As a result, the liver cannot detoxify the body properly and microorganisms invade the body with little resistance.

Once people with chronic immune disorders are cleared of their long-standing allergies to certain bacteria and viruses using NAET and their bodies encounter a new virus, the section on emergency treatment in this book can be an invaluable resource (see Chapter 5).

The goal of the approach described in this book is to clear the system of all allergens, strengthen the immune system through good digestion and proper absorption of nutrients, and prevent an overload of toxicity in the body by way of a healthy liver and other critical organs of detoxification. Food allergies are the most serious problem for people with immune disorders, especially chronic fatigue. The best way to master them is to treat with NAET.

The benefit of allergy treatment for pregnant women is that the allergy is not then passed on to the child. There are additional ways to prevent the development of food allergies in children. Babies should be breast-fed for at least one year, and it is preferable to wait six to eight months before starting a baby on solid food. If the mother does not breast-feed, the child should be put on a milk-free formula. We test infants for various allergies, including breast milk, and treat them with NAET when necessary.

A mother should not eat large amounts of common or known allergens while breast-feeding because the allergies can be passed on to the child. Children should not be introduced to foods such as dairy products, wheat, nuts, and other foods discussed in the food allergy section until they are at least one year old. When children start eating solid food, they should be introduced to them one at a time to see if they are allergic. Muscle testing help to determine these allergies.

A mother of a young boy who knew that her husband had a serious peanut allergy asked me to check her son for the allergy. In the test, both the child and his father showed an allergy to peanuts. The child was treated and never did develop a reaction to peanuts. After being treated, the father stopped having reactions which had consisted of airway constriction and difficulty breathing.

Massage and chiropractic care are preventative measures that have been proven to be effective with immune disorders. Research indicates that weekly upper body massage may help relieve fatigue, muscle tightness, and stress which play a major role in any immune disorder. Chiropractic care also contributes to strengthening the immune system by reducing structural misalignments, restoring nervous system integrity, and enhancing musculoskeletal flexibility.

Under psychological stress, people with immune disorders generally experience an immediate exacerbation of their symptoms. However, a body that is free of allergens, in a state of homeostasis, with good digestion and absorption, should be strong enough to deal with any emotional situation without experiencing physical symptoms.

Other alternative therapies that can be helpful include qi-gong, acupuncture, yoga, meditation, and psychotherapy which can help provide an understanding of the emotions behind the disease. Herbs such as ginseng can be beneficial in boosting energy and combatting fatigue. Exercise is essential, not only for the muscles and bones, but also for the lungs, heart, brain, other internal organs, and for a sense of well-being. Any enjoyable exercise is suitable. Love, support, and acceptance are also invaluable because without love and affection, one cannot thrive. Those who suffer immune disorders need this more than anyone else.

Plenty of fresh air is also extremely important for people with immune system problems as long as they are not allergic to oxygen. It may sound strange, but I have occasionally treated patients for this unusual allergy. For example, a woman struggling with fungus allergies received NAET treatment, and her symptoms diminished completely for several months. Then they started coming back, especially during waking hours. She would wake up feeling well and then notice, as she moved about and prior to eating anything, she would experience bloating. This puzzled me for some time until I realized I had seen these symptoms in other individuals. Careful investigation indicated that she was allergic to fungus in combination with oxygen. After she was treated for this combination, her symptoms disappeared and never returned. Never underestimate an allergen and the problems it can cause.

III NAMBUDRIPAD ALLERGY ELIMINATION TECHNIQUE (NAET)

15 | DEFINING THE NAMBUDRIPAD ALLERGY ELIMINATION TECHNIQUE (NAET)

There's a big/strong/spirited hunk
inside this disappearing frame
and I'm ready to come out swinging.
　　　　　　—from "Declaration of Intention"

STEVE'S STORY

Steve came to see me with severe food allergies. His diet was very limited and he was frequently distressed physically. He could not tolerate, digest, or assimilate most foods. I decided to introduce the NAET chapter with his testimonial, not because he is an asthmatic, but because his life was so dramatically changed with NAET. He is now able to eat all foods without any problems and can live a more enjoyable, relaxed, and normal lifestyle. The dramatic changes Steve has experienced epitomize the power of this technique. NAET should have far-reaching effects on the way we view and treat chronic diseases and ailments such as asthma, chronic fatigue, migraines, and so forth.

I am writing to thank you for helping me to get my health back. When I came to see you in January 1994, I had such severe digestive problems that I had to curtail many of the activities I had enjoyed much of my life. These problems were also intruding on my business life, and I was becoming seriously depressed and withdrawn. All of that has improved significantly since our work together.

As children growing up in the fifties, my sister and I felt fortunate that we could eat everything we wanted without the hives and other problems my allergic mother experienced when she was not careful about what she ate. As a teenager I was obese, and when I was 21 I went on an all-protein diet over the summer that reduced my weight from 235 to 165 lbs. (I'm 6'1"). Nobody recognized me that autumn until they heard my voice. I was thrilled by the weight loss, but I felt weak and experienced some unpleasant side effects for a while, such as double vision. Around this time I also noticed that I would get diarrhea after eating dairy products, so I began to avoid them. My weight stabilized at about 180 to 185 pounds, and for many years my health was fine except that I couldn't eat any dairy.

When I was around 40 (I'm 47 now), my weight increased to 210, and I began to notice symptoms such as gas, diarrhea and bloating after some meals, even when I avoided dairy products. Fortunately, a doctor was willing to try a relatively new technology at the time, IgA allergy testing using blood samples. The doctor found that I was allergic to 35 of the 70 foods he tested. He said that mine were among the worst results he had ever encountered, and he urged me to avoid the foods to which I was allergic. He also offered me a reducing diet.

His advice was very helpful in eliminating the symptoms and losing the extra weight. To the extent that I avoided the allergenic foods, I had no gas, diarrhea, or bloating and my weight fell again to about 185 pounds.

As helpful as this was, however, it was actually a way of coping with a serious disability. Each time I went to a restaurant (once a source of pleasure), I had to interrogate the waiter about the ingredients in every dish. I read menus with fear because I could not eat wheat, rye, corn, barley, oats, most spices, most oils, or any of the other 35 foods to which I was allergic. Often, waiters would assure me that all of my food requirements would be met, and then my dinner would appear, covered with black pepper or some other item I could not eat.

Whenever I ate one of the forbidden foods, the symptoms came swiftly. If there was dairy in any form, I would experience cramping, gas, diarrhea and bloating within five minutes, and this would become much worse about two hours later. Other foods had similar though less dramatic effects that were just as predictable.

For me this was more than a minor inconvenience. My work as an attorney required me to travel extensively and to take clients and witnesses to meals. I learned how central the sharing of food is to our social and business life, and I began to feel excluded. When friends would invite me to a dinner party, I would arrive with take-out sushi (which I knew contained none of the forbidden foods). After a time, I noticed fewer dinner invitations, and in a way I was relieved because I would no longer have to explain my restrictions to my hosts.

Travel for work or pleasure became something to avoid. Imagine carrying an extra suitcase full of food to Europe just to feel secure about finding something to eat. In each city, after I checked into a hotel, I would locate a food market to buy canned goods, which I would then eat in my hotel room rather than braving the restaurants. Explaining to a Parisian client that I could only have lunch with him if there was no sauce on my salmon was a task that I would not want to repeat.

When I discussed all of this with my sister, I was not entirely surprised to learn that she had had similar experiences. After eating at a McDonald's once, for example, she had been hospitalized for internal bleeding. Later she discovered that they soak their french fries in milk before cooking them, and the milk had caused her to bleed. We spent many hours on the phone sharing information about which foods caused which symptoms and what foods to avoid.

Around this time, when I was 44, an attorney friend told me of her success in treating allergies with you. Thinking that

I had nothing to lose, I came to see you. When you assured me that I would be eating dairy again within a few weeks, I was incredulous. By this time, I considered my body to be as reliable as a laboratory: give me something that had even the smallest amount of dairy in it, and within five minutes the symptoms would begin.

You performed some diagnostic exams, prescribed a number of food enzymes to eat with meals, and did some allergy testing. It was the beginning of a year of treatment that led to my recovery. Today, with a few minor exceptions, I eat whatever foods I choose, in any location, have no symptoms, and again weigh 185 pounds.

The path from being a disabled person who had to refrain from many important activities to being an ordinary person with normal health and a regular diet was a fascinating and surprising one for me and sometimes required faith and patience. Although I am open minded about alternative approaches in any discipline, I am also schooled in Western science. For example, I know that acupuncture and other methods have been used in the East for centuries with success, but I also know that we do not understand how or why they succeed. Still, everything else had failed, and my friend's allergies had improved dramatically, so I decided to give NAET a try, whether I understood it or not.

The first set-back came immediately. The initial treatment for an allergy to chicken and eggs did not work, and I had to be treated a second time. Fortunately the next several treatments went well, and I was soon eating foods I had not eaten in years—without any symptoms. I felt like a child eating certain foods for the first time. It had been so long since I had eaten a strawberry or Wheaties®, for example, that tasting them was an indescribable new experience. At times some symptoms would return, especially after eating at restaurants, where I was experimenting with a broader selection. The reactions were far less severe than before, however, and we would work to identify what foods were causing the reaction and then treat for them.

For me the real test came a couple of months into the treatments, when you told me that I was ready to eat dairy. Given the painful and serious symptoms that I had experienced over the past 20 years, it was no wonder that I felt fear when I faced my bowl of chocolate ice cream. Waiting until the house was empty, I ate the ice cream expecting the worst. After 5 minutes, when the cramping and bloating would ordinarily begin, nothing happened, much to my surprise and relief. The next test, I knew, would be in two hours, when the diarrhea and gas used to become far worse. Again, nothing happened. I have been eating dairy products now for over a year without incident. Though there are many dairy products I don't like and seldom eat or drink (like milk), I am not afraid of dairy and eat some every day.

It has been several months now since we ended the treatments, and I continue to enjoy a wide variety of foods. On rare occasions, I will have minor symptoms after a meal, but probably no more often than most people in their late 40's. For the most part, I eat what I want without any difficulty. I continue to take food enzymes because I find them helpful for maintaining my health. I have far more energy than I used to, and my friends have told me how much better and healthier I look. I am no longer a disabled person and can again participate fully in life. To me, the treatments were a miracle.

THE STORY BEHIND THE DISCOVERY OF NAET

Dr. Nambudripad originally discovered this technique by accident while caring for her own extensive health problems. When she was an infant, she suffered from eczema, and when she was eight her parents started feeding her white rice with special herbs to treat a chronic skin disease. In 1976 she moved to Los Angeles where she became more health conscious and changed her eating habits. Nevertheless, she continued to suffer from bronchitis, pneumonia, arthritis, insomnia, depression, sinusitis, and migraine headaches. She was tired all the time but unable to sleep. Although she experimented with a wide variety of techniques, medicines, and herbs she only became sicker. As she puts it, "Every inch of my body ached. I lived on aspirin, taking almost thirty a day to keep me going."

At the time she was a student at the Los Angeles College of Chiropractic and her nutritional teacher advised her to go on a juice diet. In two days she had bronchitis, laryngitis, and a fever of 104 degrees. To care for herself, she cooked some soft white rice which she had learned to do as a child when she was sick. We now understand that white rice is probably the least allergic food although it has few nutrients.

After hearing an acupuncturist speak at the chiropractic college, Nambudripad was so impressed that she decided to study acupuncture as well. One of her acupuncture teachers noticed her raspy voice and told her he thought she had food allergies. Tests showed that she was allergic to almost all foods except white rice and broccoli. This acupuncturist suggested that Nambudripad try eating white rice and broccoli for a few days. Within a week her bronchitis had cleared, her headaches had become infrequent, her joints had stopped aching, her insomnia had disappeared, and her concentration and thinking had become clearer and more focused.

When she began eating other foods again, her complaints slowly reappeared. She decided to return to rice and broccoli and ended up remaining on that diet for three and a half years. Once in a while she would try something else, but her symptoms, particularly the arthritis, would come back. She could not eat any salads, fruits, or vegetables other than broccoli. She was allergic to all grains, sugars, fish, eggs, and spices. She was also allergic to environmental factors such as fabrics and radiation. She assumed she would live on white rice and broccoli for the rest of her life.

One day she absent-mindedly ate a few pieces of carrot while waiting for the rice to cook. In a few minutes she felt tired, as if she were about to pass out. Recognizing that she was experiencing an allergic reaction to carrots, she called her husband, who was also an acupuncturist, and asked him to get some acupuncture needles and treat her. While she waited for him, she massaged certain acupuncture points to keep from fainting. He inserted the needles and she slept for forty-five minutes. When she woke up she felt strangely different. She was not feeling sick or tired; in fact, her energy level was high. As she got up from the bed she noticed that some pieces of carrot were still stuck to her hand. In a panic, she dropped them immediately. She wondered if there was a connection between accidentally holding the carrots and waking up feeling so good. Her study of electromagnetic fields and acupuncture meridians suggested a possible connection.

Using the muscle testing technique, she found she was no longer allergic to carrots. She ate them the next day and had no reaction. When she treated herself for other foods, those allergies disappeared as well. She began using the technique on herself and over time developed the system she calls the Nambudripad Allergy Elimination Technique. NAET is now used by more than 600 practitioners throughout the world, all of whom are having excellent results desensitizing people to allergens. To locate a practitioner in your area refer to internet site http://www.allergy2000.com.

MY FIRST ENCOUNTER WITH NAET

I first came across the Nambudripad Allergy Elimination Technique through another practitioner. After doing well on enzymes for many years, I noticed that I still had trouble eating certain foods such as grains (wheat and rice) and dairy products. My digestion was not affected but I noticed that I felt fatigue and depression after eating the grains. As a result I was on the lookout for other techniques or products that would help my allergies and those of my patients.

An acupuncturist began working in my clinic who had been treating people with an allergy technique that used vials of different materials to diagnose and treat allergies. I observed her work and talked to her about her success rate. Impressed, I began to refer patients to her who had severe mold, dust, and environmental allergies that I had been unable to treat successfully with enzymes. She had some extraordinary results. Allergies just completely disappeared. I began to send her more and more of my patients.

One patient I referred was a long-time chiropractic patient of mine named Judy who consistently complained of severe nasal congestion, chronic wheezing, and shortness of breath. I suggested that Judy consult with this acupuncturist about diagnosing her specific allergies and then clearing them so she could be symptom free. Judy followed my suggestion and the acupuncturist found her to be allergic to dust, mold, pollen, cats, Vitamin C, some fruits, some vegetables, and all the B vitamins. After several NAET treatments for these allergens, she was completely free of symptoms—no more runny nose, coughing, wheezing, or chronic congestion.

After watching her success with amazement, I went for treatment myself. I was treated first for the basics including egg white, calcium, and sugars. I clearly remember my sugar treatment. Whenever I ate sugar, I would immediately get a reddened cold, runny nose, cold hands, headaches, and depression. After the sugar treatment I stopped craving sugar, then found that I had no reaction when I ate it. I also felt energized after the basic treatments.

Then I was treated for grains—including rice, which I could never eat without feeling fatigued, and wheat, dairy products, fruits, and hormones. After the treatment for hormones, I no longer experienced any premenstrual tension or irritability during my period. These NAET treatments opened many doors in overcoming my allergies and I became increasingly curious.

Eventually, the acupuncturist told me she was moving to Hawaii and suggested that I take the training to learn the technique myself. I followed her advice and signed up for a seminar. I ended up taking five because I could not believe that such a simple technique could have such success. I also continued to get treatments from another doctor and had more extraordinary results. I was no longer allergic to alcohol, sun radiation, dust, or any food. With NAET treatments and enzymes, I no longer had to limit my food intake in any way.

In light of this success, I added NAET to my enzyme and nutritional techniques and have been using it ever since. Over ninety-five percent of my practice is now NAET and enzyme work. Besides the successes with immune disorders that have been significant, I have had tremendous results with headaches, arthritis, hay fever, sinus problems, asthma, obesity, female problems, and symptoms ranging from warts to nail biting. I have also treated many people with depression and various kinds of skin and glandular problems. I have devoted this book to immune disorders. Many immune disorders can be prevented. I feel confident that after a period of treatment, a person's symptoms can be reduced by 80 percent.

WHAT IS NAET?

NAET is a breakthrough treatment that uses chiropractic, kinesiology, and acupuncture to permanently desensitize people to all kinds of allergies. The technique can be practiced by any health practitioner including doctors, nurses, acupuncturists, chiropractors, dentists and, to some extent, allergy sufferers themselves. Clinical studies with NAET have demonstrated that it is by far the most successful and succinct treatment for the elimination of allergies. The theory of NAET is based on viewing the body as made up of pathways for the flow of electromagnetic energy. It is easier to understand how and why NAET works if one understands the theories that underlie it.

The whole concept of the body as an energy field was not new to me when I learned NAET. As a chiropractic student, I was introduced to a philosophy that regards the body as more than just matter, muscles, and tissues coming together without any real intelligence. Chiropractic acknowledges that the body is a holistic complex and that the universal or innate intelligence or organizing force that pervades the vast galaxies also pervades the simplest cells of the body. The founder of chiropractic, Dr. D. D. Palmer, talked about the concept of electromagnetic energy fields. He said that mind does not control the functions of the body. Instead, there is an innate intelligence that controls the mind and its functions as well as the functions of the body. This innate intelligence has the power to conceive, judge, and reason about matters pertaining to the internal welfare of the body. The healing art of chiropractic has been around for over one hundred years and has been successful at treating the body and appreciating it as more than just matter.

In the chiropractic view, when a bone is out of alignment or the spine is distorted or misaligned, the energy force in the body is cut off. This, in turn, causes serious disease. When the misalignments or imbalances are corrected, the energy can flow again through the nervous system to the brain and homeostasis is restored.

The work of Dr. Devi Nambudripad is similarly based on the idea that the body is a flow of electromagnetic currents. According to her theory, when an allergen enters or contacts the body, there is a clash between the energy field of the allergen and the energy field of the allergy sufferer.

The brain identifies the allergen and alerts the immune system which locates the allergen and responds with antibodies and delayed reactive T and B cells. This type of immune reaction causes the release of toxic substances from the T cells. The fighter cells, called macrophages, then invade the area, intent on digesting the antigens. Immune mediators such as histamine are released. These reactions cause blockage in the electromagnetic pathways as well as abnormal tissue response, delayed tissue destruction, and possible autoimmune reaction. These responses can produce any number of symptoms such as constriction of the sinuses, throat, or breathing passageways to keep the invader from entering the body, or vomiting, diarrhea, tearing, and sinus discharge to remove it from the body. The brain makes an all-out effort to protect the body from any substance that it perceives as harmful.

Any time there are energy blockages in the body, health problems result. Some areas of the body are weaker for **genetic** reasons and they will react the most, weakening other areas of the body. Some of the common symptoms that can be produced by such blockages are aches and pains in the body, sore throats, fevers, chills, painful lymph nodes, weakness, extreme fatigue, headaches, sleep disturbances, irritability, confusion, depression, forgetfulness, a burning sensation in the body, frequent urination, crying spells, suicidal behavior, sores in the mouth, indigestion, bloating, and water retention. Virtually any symptom can be the result of a blockage caused by contact with an allergen. After working with NAET for some time, my experience has been that most health problems are ultimately caused by allergens.

If blockages continue or the body is constantly exposed to an allergen, the blockages spread throughout the system and more serious problems occur. When the immune system becomes overloaded and compromised, autoimmune problems develop. Over time, as it is bombarded with allergens, the body becomes more susceptible to chronic health problems, decreased energy levels, migraines, tumors, and mental problems.

Blockages of different meridians produce different symptoms. If there is a blockage of the lung and large intestine meridians, a person suffers severe respiratory distress, asthma, cold, sinus problems, constipation, or diarrhea. If the blockage is in the kidney meridian, the person suffers water retention or frequent urination. A gallbladder blockage produces pain and swelling in the breast, pain in intercostal muscles, abdominal cramps, heavy menstrual bleeding, severe mood swings, aggressive behavior, or anger. Blockages in the heart and small intestine meridians cause heart palpitations, cardiac arrhythmia, insomnia, dry mouth, heavy sensations in the chest, night sweats, fatigue, and insecurity. Blockages in other areas cause a whole array of symptoms. When allergens repeatedly cause blockages of the lung meridian, the person may develop asthma.

HOW DOES NAET WORK?

NAET uses chiropractic techniques to stimulate the areas of the body that are connected to the blockages in the energy system. If a blockage affects a certain organ, the practitioner stimulates areas of the nervous system connected to that organ by autonomic nerve impulses. For example, a wheat allergy might affect the spleen and liver or cause a blockage in the spleen or liver channels, causing chronic low energy, fatigue, and muscle pain and spasms. To treat for the wheat allergy, the practitioner stimulates areas of the nervous system related to the spleen and liver. By stimulating those areas located along the spine while a person is holding the allergen, the electromagnetic repulsion to that allergen is eliminated and a chemical or enzymatic change occurs neutralizing the immune mediators and interrupting the allergen or antigen-antibody complex reaction. This clears the energy blockage for the area involved and sends a message to the brain stating that wheat has been desensitized. The body no longer identifies wheat as an allergen and energy blockages in response to wheat no longer occur.

The **desensitization** process is not instantaneous, however. It takes two hours for energy to pass through each of the body's twelve energy pathways or meridians. To circulate through all twelve meridians takes twenty-four hours. As a result, a patient should avoid contact with an allergen for twenty-five hours after the treatment to ensure complete desensitization. Otherwise, the effect of the treatment may be lost when the brain identifies the substance as an allergen again.

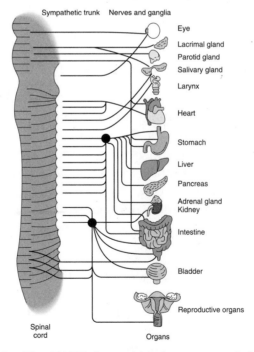

Figure 9–1 The NAET desensitization process is based on the relationship among the spine, organs, and tissues by way of the autonomic nervous system.

During the twenty-five-hour treatment period, patients are told not to expose themselves to the substance or food for which they are being treated. They must not come within four feet of the substance or eat the food or foods. If they do, they can lose the treatment immediately or in the future, and their symptoms might reappear. People who expose themselves to allergens during the treatment period can experience severe allergic reactions (refer to the NAET Treatment Rules in Part VI).

I remember treating a patient named Karen for a severe sugar allergy. On her way home from my office she accidentally ate a hard sugar candy, immediately passed out, and woke up with an excruciating headache. She learned the hard way how potent these treatments can be. After the twenty-five hour waiting period, however, patients can generally eat foods they have been treated for with no reaction.

ELECTROMAGNETIC PATHWAYS (MERIDIANS)

The concept of twelve primary channels, or meridians, and two governing vessels is important in understanding how NAET works. The treatment with NAET diagnoses and treats blockages in the meridians in relationship to specific allergens. Throughout this chapter the words electromagnetic or energy pathways, channels, and meridians are used interchangeably. They all refer to the same concept. There are fourteen channels in the body, and I will discuss each one separately.

The first channel is the *lung meridian*. It regulates the body's entire energy system and oversees the intake of oxygen. Disharmony in this channel is evidenced as coughing, asthma, allergies, skin problems, bronchitis, and fatigue.

The second channel is the *large intestine meridian* that regulates the body's waste removal activities. Disharmony here results in a distended abdomen, constipation, and diarrhea.

The third channel is the *stomach meridian.* It regulates the body's ability to take in food and fluids. Disharmony here leads to mouth sores, nausea, and vomiting.

The fourth channel is the *spleen meridian.* It regulates the transformation of food into energy and maintains the blood supply. Disharmony results in poor appetite, anemia, menstrual problems, chronic hepatitis, and fatigue.

The fifth channel is the *heart meridian.* This channel rules the head, houses the spirit, and regulates the blood vessels. Disharmony or unbalanced flow here leads to heart palpitations or insomnia.

The sixth channel is the *small intestines meridian* that regulates the organ that draws out energy from food and leaves the remains as waste. Disharmony results in vomiting or abdominal pain.

The seventh channel is the *bladder.* The bladder regulates the receiving and excreting of urine (fluid) waste. Disharmony results in burning sensations when urinating or in incontinence.

The eighth channel is the *kidney meridian* that stores reproductive energy and oversees maintenance of bones. Disharmony results in backaches, chronic ear problems, and chronic asthma.

The ninth channel is the *pericardium meridian.* This protects and oversees the heart channel. Disharmony results in stress, sensations of chest tightening, and a variety of breathing problems.

The tenth channel is the *triple burner* that oversees the body's water processing, retaining what is needed and excreting the rest. Disharmony is experienced as edema, a stiff neck, or water retention.

The eleventh channel is the *gallbladder.* The gallbladder regulates the storage and secretion of bile, a fluid that helps transforms food into energy. Disharmony is experienced as a bitter taste in one's mouth, nausea, jaundice, and gallstones.

The twelfth channel is the *liver meridian* that regulates the entire energy system and oversees the maintenance of blood supplies. Disharmony leads to high blood pressure, dizziness, PMS, muscle spasms, and eye problems.

The thirteenth channel is the *governing vessel* and the fourteenth is the *conception vessel.* They circulate energy through the other twelve channels.

INNER ENERGY

In *The Energy Within: The Science Behind Every Oriental Therapy From Acupuncture to Yoga,* Richard M. Chin, M.D., O.M.D., writes that every person has an inner energy flowing through his or her mind and body that is a reflection of universal energies. When these energies are out of balance or stop flowing, we experience illness or disease. Keeping our energy moving and in balance prevents illness and creates a maximum state of health. He refers to the body as "a matrix of interacting multidimensional energy fields."

This energy, known as *qi* (sometimes spelled *C'hi*) in Chinese, is thought to be the source and the destination of all creation. Qi must keep moving in order to sustain life. In order for energy to move it must have an inherent polarity relationship: it must have somewhere to go.

Eastern practitioners who look at the body from a holistic perspective that considers the energy imbalances of the entire system instead of simply the disease of a particular organ or body part, have discovered a highly organized system of energy channels or pathways. It is another circulatory system, similar to the cardiovascular and nervous systems. Chin describes three types of energy:

Genetic or prenatal energy The energy level to which people are genetically disposed. It is programmed in the genes like the color of their eyes and hair, their height, and so on.

Core energy A combination of the energy people are born with and the energy that forms their bodies. It is a combination of two prenatal energies.

Acquired energy The energy people acquire during their lifetime by their lifestyles and practices. This is within their control.

Pain or illness results when the flow of energy becomes blocked or unbalanced in some way, because this disharmony then upsets the balance of the body's entire energy system. . . . Although some energetic healing techniques engage the entire system, many only need to work with the body's twelve primary channels and two governing vessels (channels that oversee all others) to create complete balance and health. One method of balancing the body's energy system is acupuncture in which tiny needles are used to stimulate specific points along the twelve primary energy channels and two governing vessels.

Each of the twelve primary energy channels corresponds to one of the twelve primary organs listed above.

ELECTROMAGNETIC FIELDS

The whole universe, from the tiniest atom to the largest galaxy, is controlled by electromagnetic forces. These forces are responsible for the shape of all things and govern their movement, interrelationships, replication, and functions. The electromagnetic forces in the bodies of animals and humans can be seen as lines of force that run near the surface of the body and then pass into deeper structures (the organs).

Acupuncture practitioners employ a variety of techniques to eliminate imbalances or blockages in the natural flow of energy in the body. NAET uses techniques drawn from acupuncture, chiropractic, and kinesiology to locate and remove blockages in electromagnetic pathways that are related to allergens.

Galvanic Skin Response

Several other areas of scientific study give indications of how these energy systems in the body operate and are detected. Studies of **galvanic skin response (GSR)**, for example—the bodily response measured by "lie-detectors"—have provided interesting data. One study found the presence of an organized system of highly electroconductive points on the skin, similar to the system of points used for centuries in traditional Chinese medicine. These points are related to the human autonomic nerve reflexes. Irregularities in the points correlate with clinical medical diagnoses. With a new technique, scientists are now able to use photography to locate and identify those points.

Neurophysicists have known for a long time that when they measure the GSR at different points on the skin, it varies in direct relation to the amount of energy being discharged from the autonomic nervous system. The decreased electrical resistance at certain points on the skin is influenced by autonomic sweat gland activity on the skin's surface, by the concentrations of nerve fibers beneath the skin, and by muscle motor points. This means that any physical disorder that intensifies autonomic activity decreases electrical resistance on those areas of the skin related to the autonomic nervous system.

Ryodoraku: Electrodiagnosis

Skin resistance has been measured in the laboratory by having a person hold one electrode and passing the other over the skin. As early as 1950, one researcher, Y. Nakatani, proposed a system of electrodiagnosis and electrotreatment that was based on correlations he found between differences in skin resistance at certain points and physical illness. His system, called Ryodoraku, is based on the fact that one of the ways internal disease manifests itself is by causing a disturbance in the autonomic nervous system. The disturbance is manifested systematically by increased nerve response at certain points.

Nakatani found that internal disturbances could be detected before they manifested clinically by measuring skin resistance. Nakatani also noticed that anatomical locations of electroconductive points in unhealthy subjects varied with the disease. Subjects with the same disease had most of their points in the same location. All of these electroconductive points were remarkably close in location and about equal to the number of points found in Asian acupuncture charts of the human body. Nakatani used electrical stimulation to normalize highly conductive points.

Kirlian Photography

Another approach to the study of this phenomenon was developed in 1961 by B. K. Kirlian. He devised a method of photographing the electromagnetic discharges emanating from various objects. This Kirlian phenomena and its possible relationship to electroconductive body points triggered much new research on the topic. Researchers wondered if the Kirlian effect was a result of discharges coming from galvanically detectable electroconductive skin points.

Kirlian photography is a good illustration of electromagnetic forces in the body. Perhaps visual and photographic analysis of these points can assist in the detection of diagnosis of diseases that have not yet manifested clinically.

Electromagnetic Points

The interesting thing about traditional Chinese medicine, studies of galvanic skin response, and Kirlian photography is that they all produce evidence of a pattern of electromagnetic points on the skin and all the patterns look more or less the same. We know that these points are related to underlying autonomic nerve activity and that they respond to stimulation by electricity, needles, heat, and pressure.

Researchers who have tested traditional acupuncture meridians to see if they are direct current paths have found that these meridians conduct electricity toward the spinal cord. The researchers concluded that the meridians carry messages to the brain which responds by sending back the electrical current needed to stimulate healing. This concept also helps explain how NAET works. NAET practitioners stimulate the nervous system to send new messages to the brain.

In addition to the acupuncture meridians, many systems identify seven energy centers, called chakras, located in the body along the spine. There are two contradictory views that attempt to explain the body's electromagnetic structure and the chakras. The first is that the biological structures produce the electromagnetic field in the body. In this view, electrochemical activity within nerve plexi is thought to create the energy vortices called chakras. The body is thought to produce an electrical current that is transformed and processed by boosters—the acupuncture points—and carried by power circuits—the acupuncture meridians—throughout the body.

The opposite view is that the electromagnetic energy produces the physical body. In this view, order begins to emerge from random activity in the quantum realm, replicates itself, and becomes a pattern. More precise patterns develop until a physical form emerges from information and energy carried on an electromagnetic wave. The energy pattern of the body, before it becomes physical, is the aura, or what Sheldrake calls the morphogenic field. The role of the chakras—according to this theory—is to process information carried on particular frequencies.

DESCRIPTION OF NAET TREATMENT

When an allergy is suspected, patients are muscle tested while holding a sample of the suspected allergen. When patients are allergic to the substance, a strong muscle weakens in response to a message from the brain. Once the allergy has been identified, patients continue to hold the offending substance while the practitioner checks to see what parts of the body are being blocked in response to the allergy. The practitioner can determine what areas are blocked by palpating or touching reflex areas on the abdomen and chest. A strong indicator muscle weakens in different areas, corresponding to areas of blockage in the body. When the blockages have been identified, patients turn over, still holding the allergen, and the practitioner uses a tool to stimulate areas along the spine that correlate with the areas of blockage.

Stimulation of those areas balances the electromagnetic fields of the body in relation to the allergen and reprograms the nervous system to stop identifying this substance as an allergen. Patients are then retested. If the muscle responses with the allergen(s) are now strong, patients receive acupressure or acupuncture treatments while continuing to hold the former allergen. They are then told to avoid contact with the former allergen for twenty-five hours. At the end of that time they are tested again. If they do not expose themselves to the allergen during the twenty-five-hour period, they usually become desensitized. If they do come in contact with it, their allergy reaction may return over time.

For the first twenty-five hours following a treatment, I recommend that patients do not overstimulate their autonomic nervous systems by taking hot showers, running, watching scary movies, or doing anything that excites the body, either positively or negatively. The first six hours are especially critical because such activities compete with the allergy treatment's stimulation of the autonomic nervous system.

SELF-TREATMENT FOR VIRUSES

The NAET treatment can be self-administered. I teach my patients and their families how to do muscle testing on each other so they can test for certain foods and for saliva when an infection is suspected. Treating for saliva within the first few hours of the symptoms of an infection stops the progression of viruses and bacteria. By using specific acupressure points, the symptoms can be eliminated almost immediately. For example, if a child has a runny nose, coughing, or sore throat, he or she can spit into a thin glass and use it as a sample for muscle testing. If the muscle is weak, it shows that there is something in the saliva that is causing a reaction in the body, usually a virus. Stimulation of the acupressure points while the subject holds the saliva sample for 15 minutes stops the allergic reaction, fights the virus so it does not progress, and allows the immune system to effectively get rid of the pathogen.

Treatment for Emergencies

Any substance can be treated for in an emergency. For example, if one eats a cookie that causes abdominal pain or wheezing and coughing, he or she can hold the cookie in the hand and treat for it using the acupressure points, preferably every half hour to two hours until symptoms subside. If something in the cookie requires a complete NAET treatment, this might prove to be only a temporary solution. It certainly helps in an emergency, however. For more details on Emergency Treatment, refer to Chapter 3. For more information on Self-Treatment, refer to Figure 5-1 in Chapter 5 and to Part VI.

16 | NAET TREATMENT PROTOCOL

I've had enough of being invisible/
breakable/vulnerable.
I want flesh
I want padding
I want to be the fat goddess
who feeds all the earth from her milky breasts.
I want pillows of meat
to pad the soles of my feet
the curve of my hips
the wand of my back.
                    —from "Declaration of Intention"

Jonathan

Jonathan, 45, came to see me complaining of severe fatigue, chronic bloating, hemorrhoids, dry skin, painful joints, sore throat, poor digestion, and poor appetite. He had been diagnosed with Candida and parasites by another practitioner, and he knew he had allergies to cats, dust, pollens, and certain foods. He was depressed and discouraged and was having difficulty in his relationship with his partner because of his symptoms. He needed help quickly.

The fatigue was the most debilitating symptom for him, and he had to make an effort most days just to smile or do any exercise. He was at the end of his tether and was hoping this approach might work for him. When I explained enzyme therapy and allergy work to him, he responded that he was willing to give it a try.

On the abdominal diagnostic exam with fasting, we found a positive kidney reflex, suggesting sluggishness in the kidney meridian causing some water retention and increased toxicity. He had poor absorption of sugars and simple carbohydrates, a positive reflex related to yeast infections which explained his bloating, and very low adrenals.

On the nonfasting after a complete meal, I determined that he had trouble digesting sugars and proteins. People who have a problem digesting proteins tend to have hypoglycemia and difficulty with calcium absorption. Calcium absorption requires good protein digestion, and poor calcium absorption can lead to achiness in the joints, fatigue, and lower right quadrant bloating and pain. People who cannot digest sugars tend to have a tendency toward asthma, which he had as a child, as well as bloating, digestive problems, and a weakened immune system. He tended to crave foods, become full quickly, and then his appetite would disappear completely.

First, I prescribed a sugar-digesting enzymes (pan) and a kidney enzyme (kdy) to help increase kidney function and reduce water retention. I also prescribed a preliminary antifungal enzyme (AllerZyme C) to help with some of his symptoms. Over the next few weeks, he noticed less bloating, better appetite, a decreased craving for certain foods, and slightly less gas. He still felt fatigued, and as a result he continued to feel frustrated and depressed. I also recommended the sugar intolerant diet with a modified amount of protein because of his difficulty with protein.

He turned out to be allergic to all the basics except salt. When we treated for minerals, we needed to do some individual ones separately including magnesium and potassium. After we cleared sugar, he noticed a slight improvement in his energy. He felt stronger and less depressed. When I did a complete allergy test, I found that he was allergic to fungus, including *Candida albicans* and *Candida parapsilosis*, animal dander, cat and dog hair, dust, weeds and shrubs, miscellaneous pollens and flowers, wheat, soy, pork, turkey, apples, white wine, beer, yeast mix, and chocolate.

I treated him first for the yeast mix, including food yeast, baker's yeast, and brewers yeast, and instructed him to follow the diet in the Resource Guide of this book which includes no grains, vinegar, or milk products. Then I treated for all the bacteria. Despite his doctor's diagnosis, I did not find an allergy to parasites. When we cleared the bacteria allergy, his joint pain disappeared. In my experience, bacteria allergies tend to cause autoimmune problems that localize in the joints. I then treated him for turkey, pork, and soy to prepare for the 10-day antifungal diet, which would require that he eat more meat and vegetable protein.

Although his energy increased, Jonathan was frustrated by his lack of improvement. I suspected that the treatment for fungus would be pivotal for him, since people with Candida or yeast infections tend to become more symptomatic around mold, and he lived in a damp area of Marin County. As well as Candida, we found that he was allergic to *Schimmelpilz I* and *Schimmelpilz II*, *Sporothrix schenckii*, some penicillins, and a few other molds.

In addition to buying new clothes, wearing a mask, and following the antifungal protocol, Jonathan decided to stay in another place that was completely mold-free. We thought it would take about 30 hours to clear.

When he returned the next day to be retested, he felt a little better. We had to do two more treatments with mold and fungus. I prescribed two antifungal enzymes along with the other enzymes he was already taking, and I told him to stay on the diet for 14 days and then come in to be retested. I always retest for Candida and yeast until I am sure the treatment has held and the allergies will not return.

Two weeks later he was a completely different person. He felt happy, he looked healthier, he had more energy, he was no longer bloated, and his relationships had improved.

He had even started taking dance classes with his girlfriend. It was amazing to watch Jonathan turn around.

We cleared a few more allergies, and then he had to take some time off for financial reasons. When he returned recently, he said that he continues to do quite well. He occasionally has some bloating, but the enzymes help. Most important, his chronic fatigue and Candida symptoms are a thing of the past, and he is deeply grateful for what this work can offer.

BASIC ALLERGIES

In my clinic we have a set treatment procedure for allergies, no matter what symptoms or complaints the patient presents. We always test and treat for the basic allergies in the prescribed sequence developed by Dr. Nambudripad after years of research, testing, and experimentation. After years of working with this sequence myself, I recognize how important it is. The complete clearing of each basic allergen in the proper order is crucial for successful results in treating all individuals with immune disorders.

For example, I remember treating one of my first NAET patients, a young man in his thirties with severe candidiasis and chronic fatigue. Not knowing how critical it was to clear the basic allergies in sequence, I immediately treated him for Candida. When the treatment was completed, he was so fatigued he could not get up off the table. When I called Dr. Nambudripad for help, she explained that we do the basics first to strengthen the immune response. She said he was not ready to treat Candida because his immune system was weak and could not clear such a severe allergen. I treated him again that day for eggs and he was fine. Three months later, after a series of NAET treatments including Candida, he could not remember what it was like to have chronic fatigue.

The basics are vitamins, minerals, and foods that are among the most allergenic and the main ingredients in many foods. When the allergies to these basic allergens are cleared, many other foods are cleared at the same time. These basic nutrients provide support for the immune system and are important coenzymes and cofactors of metabolism. Once they are utilized by the body, health improves dramatically. Before undergoing an NAET treatment, I recommend my patients review ahead of time the list of NAET restrictions so they are prepared to avoid the allergen physically when they leave the clinic. For a list of restrictions, refer to Part VI.

Chickens, Eggs, Feathers, and Tetracycline

The first basic is eggs and chickens. Sometimes it is necessary to treat separately for egg white and egg yolk and for white or dark meat in chickens. Included in this treatment are feathers and tetracycline, an antibiotic commonly given to chickens. When this treatment is done, a patient must stay away from eggs, chicken, feathers, and tetracycline for twenty-five hours.

I always treat for eggs and chickens first, even if people say they never eat them because they are ingredients in many foods and products such as shampoos and conditioners. Twenty-five hours after the treatment I retest patients to ensure they are cleared for each part of the allergen.

Sometimes treatments need to be done in combination. For example, eggs may need to be cleared in combination with another food, an organ, or an environmental condition such as heat or cold. This is important because treating eggs alone may not clear a serious allergy to a combination of eggs and some other substance or condition. On the other hand, clearing eggs may clear other allergies at the same time. Each individual is different. For example, one female with fibromyalgia was tested for the ten basic allergies. When we treated her for eggs and chickens, most of the other allergies went away without being treated. After one treatment, her muscle pain decreased by 75 percent.

Calcium and Dairy Products

The next basic allergy we look at is calcium, an important mineral for the body. Milk, dairy products, and root and green vegetables are high in calcium as are sesame seeds, oats, navy beans, dry beans, almonds, walnuts, peanuts, sunflower seeds, sardines, and salmon. When people, especially women, are allergic to calcium, they are likely to be calcium deficient that causes joint pain, aching, crepitation in joints, osteoporosis, menstrual cramps, tetany, and headache. It also causes leg cramps, hyperactivity, restlessness, and an inability to relax because calcium is important in relaxation and sleep. Many patients with fibromyalgia and CFIDS with chronic muscle pain respond well to treatment for calcium as well as people with abdominal pain, insomnia, skin problems, nervousness, canker sores, herpes, hyperactivity, obesity, and arthritis. Calcium is an important nutrient for everyone, particularly for individuals with immune disorders. To make up for deficiencies it may be necessary to take a calcium supplement after the allergy has been cleared.

One three-year-old boy came to me who had trouble sleeping. His mother thought it was because of his pollen allergies. After we treated him for calcium, he never had trouble sleeping again.

Vitamin C, Fresh Fruits, and Vegetables

The next allergy we treat for is Vitamin C. People wonder how anyone could be allergic to such an essential vitamin, but plenty of people are. In fact, the body can be allergic to virtually anything. Vitamin C is found in fresh fruits and vegetables, rose hips, citrus fruits, black currants, apples, strawberries, guavas, cherries, potatoes, cabbage, broccoli, tomatoes, turnip greens, green bell peppers, green and leafy vegetables, cauliflower, and sweet potatoes. Foods are the best source of Vitamin C, not the high-dosage supplements that many people take. When a Vitamin C allergy is cleared, allergies to many fruits and vegetables are automatically cleared.

Scurvy is caused by a lack of Vitamin C. One of the main symptoms of scurvy is fatigue. One of the main symptoms of Vitamin C allergy is also fatigue. People who have chronic sore throats often start taking Vitamin C immediately when symptoms begin. This is helpful for most people, but if they are allergic to Vitamin C, it may be the allergy itself causing the problem. Sometimes I find that Vitamin C allergies are linked with infectants such as bacteria or viruses. When a person who is allergic takes Vitamin C, it triggers the infectant and starts an infection.

This allergy is particularly important to CFIDS patients because a Vitamin C allergy also causes fatigue, respiratory infections, and canker sores. I always check for and clear this allergy. People who get frequent colds and the flu usually have an allergy to Vitamin C and are therefore deficient in the Vitamin C they need to prevent these problems. If the twenty-four hour urine report shows a deficiency, I put people on a Vitamin C enzyme (opt).

Vitamin C, especially ascorbic acid, has been shown to be helpful for asthma, but only if the patient is not allergic to it. One woman asthmatic I saw came from another health practitioner who had put her on high doses of ascorbic acid for severe wheezing and restricted breathing. The patient noticed not only that the Vitamin C failed to help, but also that she started experiencing fatigue, joint pain, kidney pain, headaches, and indigestion after taking it.

When I tested her I found her to be allergic to, and deficient in, Vitamin C. I treated her for the Vitamin C allergy and put her on high doses of a Vitamin C enzyme (opt) instead of ascorbic acid. I prefer not to use the ascorbic acid which is perceived as sugar by the body. I use the whole Vitamin C instead.

After the treatment for Vitamin C allergy, the patient needs to avoid all foods that contain it for twenty-five hours. If they don't, their allergy symptoms will return over time. This is crucial for individuals who suffer from a chronic and potentially fatal condition and need to clear the allergy to Vitamin C.

B Vitamins

The next, and perhaps most important, allergy we treat is an allergy to the B vitamins. This allergy is vitally important because the B vitamins are found in virtually every food. The only foods I have found that do not contain them are tapioca, Jell-O®, and Cool Whip®, something other than a healthy diet. I am working with others to create a nutritional powder without the B vitamins that will give patients something more substantial to eat during the post-treatment waiting period.

There are eleven different B vitamins, but I include B_{13}, B_{15}, and B_{17} as well in my treatment. The B vitamins were described in detail in Chapter 6. I treat all the B vitamins together, then test them separately to make sure each one has been cleared. Since they are so common in foods, allergies to any of the B vitamins cause serious problems for individuals with immune disorders. Most allergies to the B vitamins clear in one session, but some patients take two, three, or even four treatments to clear. Occasionally a patient needs to be cleared on several of the B vitamins separately.

B vitamins are essential for the emotional, physical, and psychological well-being of the body. They contribute to maintaining a healthy nervous system and aid in the digestion of fats and proteins. People allergic to B vitamins suffer severe depression, cloudy thinking, exhaustion, mood swings, and nervousness and can react to virtually any food.

B vitamins are used for the treatment of skin disorders and respiratory problems and help prevent colds and improve memory. Inositol, biotin, and choline prevent hair loss and are essential for healthy hair. Folic acid is needed for the formation of red blood cells and the prevention of anemia. Allergies to the B vitamins must be cleared if good health is to be maintained. Because Vitamin C and the B vitamins are so essential for individuals with immune disorders, I usually put the patient on supplements after I have checked and cleared for those allergies. I often include adrenal support as well (adr enzyme).

One woman with CFIDS came to see me because her condition had worsened. She was taking large doses of medications, and had become noticeably weaker. We started treating for the basic allergies. After we had desensitized her to Vitamin C and the B vitamins, I put her on an adrenal enzyme that included those vitamins. Overnight her condition improved dramatically.

Most people who suffer from a chronic health problem have a Vitamin B allergy that needs to be cleared. Clearing it may also clear other allergens such as wheat, carbohydrates, many grains, some vegetables, potatoes, brewer's yeast, meat, and other foods high in B vitamins. Whole grain allergies seem to be the most commonly affected. People who crave carbohydrates usually have a strong B vitamin allergy.

Sugars

The next basic allergy to clear is to sugars. All the B vitamins must be cleared first, however, because they are important cofactors in the metabolism of sugars. Sugars are implicated in many different health problems, especially chronic fatigue, candidiasis, and colitis. If people are allergic to sugars and intolerant of them as well, eating sugars can cause chronic immune system problems, accumulation of mucus, malabsorption, indigestion, mood swings, weight problems, and a weakened immune response. The sugars we treat are maltose, glucose, dextrose, lactose, fructose, brown sugar, honey, corn sugar, raw sugar, cane sugar, molasses, high-fructose corn syrup, grape sugar, and maple sugar.

Frequently we treat all the sugars at once, although some people are only allergic to one or two of them and should be treated for those separately. During the next twenty-five hours sugars must be avoided. This rules out all foods except meat, fish, or poultry.

Treating for sugar allergies is extremely rewarding. People who have craved sugars all their lives stop craving them. Children who have chronic ear infections, sore throats, or sinus congestion get better. Asthmatics with chronic coughs stop coughing overnight. In fact, sugar allergies seem to be involved in most chronic illness.

Iron and Meats

The next basic allergen to treat is iron. People with an iron allergy do not absorb the mineral from their food and become deficient, causing anemia. Their physicians then prescribe iron supplements for long periods of time which doesn't help because they can't absorb iron. Allergic reactions include backaches, headaches, dizziness, menstrual problems, and fatigue. Iron is an essential nutrient that aids in growth, promotes resistance to disease, and prevents fatigue.

Clearing this allergy clears allergies to many foods that contain iron including apricots, peaches, bananas, prunes, raisins, black molasses, brewer's yeast, whole grains, cereals, turnip greens, spinach, beet tops, alfalfa, beets, asparagus, kelp, sunflower seeds, walnuts, sesame seeds, beans, egg yolk, liver, red meat, oysters, and clams. After an iron allergy is cleared, the patient must avoid all contact with iron for twenty-five hours. This involves wearing plastic gloves because iron is used in cars, cooking pots, and metal alloys.

Vitamin A, Betacarotene, Fish, and Shellfish

The next basic allergy treated is to Vitamin A. Vitamin A and betacarotene are important immunostimulants and protective agents crucial for healthy mucus membranes and the prevention of respiratory infections. Many physicians recommend Vitamin A supplements for asthmatics and skin problems. This is fine as long as they are not allergic to it. A Vitamin A deficiency disturbs white blood cell production in the body and lowers immune function. It is necessary to maintain good vision and prevent night blindness, skin disorders, acne, colds, influenza, and other infections. It helps heal ulcers and wounds and is necessary for the growth of bones and teeth. Vitamin A is an antioxidant and helps protect the cells against free radicals. Betacarotene, found in vegetables and converts to Vitamin A in the liver, is good for the prevention of chronic health problems and is a powerful antioxidant.

When people are allergic to Vitamin A, they do not absorb it properly and become deficient. A deficiency causes skin tags, warts, blemishes, acne, rashes, hair loss, and premature aging, bronchial, lung, and respiratory problems, lowered immunity, infertility, joint pain, vomiting, and GI problems. Vitamin A works in conjunction with other vitamins such as the B complex, Vitamins D and E, calcium, and zinc that are required to mobilize it from the liver where it is stored. Large doses of Vitamin A should only be taken under proper supervision or it can accumulate to toxic levels in the body. Similarly, people who are allergic to Vitamin A and take large amounts are unable to absorb it and accumulate toxic levels in the liver. After clearing the allergy, supplementation may be helpful for a period of time.

Clearing a Vitamin A allergy clears allergies to such foods as papayas, peaches, yellow fruit, asparagus, beets, broccoli, carrots, Swiss chard, kale, turnip greens, watercress, parsley, red peppers, sweet potatoes, squash, yellow squash and other yellow vegetables, pumpkin, corn, spirulina, milk, butter, other dairy products, egg yokes, fish, and fish liver oil.

I saw a four-year-old boy who suffered from chronic eczema and ear infections. He had been on and off antibiotics for over a year. We tried high doses of Vitamins A and C and took him off dairy products but he continued to get the infections. We noticed that he always had problems after taking Vitamin A and realized it was probably a major allergen for him. When we started the basic allergy treatments, we had to do the Vitamin A treatment three times because his mother forgot and kept giving him the Vitamin A supplement. After the allergy was successfully cleared he was symptom-free for nine months and continues to do well.

Minerals

The next basic allergy we clear is to minerals. Some of the minerals individuals with immune disorders are most often allergic to are calcium, chromium, cobalt, copper, selenium, potassium, phosphorus, sodium, sulfur, vanadium, zinc, and magnesium. There has been considerable study of the use of magnesium for those with sleeping disorders and constipation but I have found it necessary to treat them for the allergy before they take the supplement. Once the allergy is cleared, magnesium can be helpful in reducing these symptoms.

After treating for minerals, the patient needs to avoid contact with metals and should use distilled water for washing and drinking. Calcium is usually cleared in a separate session and sometimes other minerals need to be treated separately as well. I test all people with immune disorders for allergies to each mineral mentioned.

Table Salt and Sodium Chloride

Another treatment is for salt allergies. I use a combination of table salt and sodium chloride when treating this allergy. Salt is hard to avoid because it is in so many foods including most canned foods and restaurant dishes.

Clearing a salt allergy clears allergies to other foods such as pineapples, watermelon, celery, lettuce, carrots, beets, artichokes, avocados, Swiss chard, cabbage, cucumbers, tomatoes, asparagus, shellfish, and processed foods.

These are the basic allergies I treat in all my patients. For immune disorders there are a few other allergies that are also basic.

Phenolics

The first is to phenolics, naturally occurring compounds that color, flavor, and preserve food. They help in the germination of seeds and protect plants against other invaders. There are certain phenolics that are often problems for immune disorders. When allergies to these phenolics are cleared, many other food allergies clear at the same time. Phenolics also cause problems in combination with other allergens such as chemicals. I have had a lot of success with CFIDS and other immune disorders by treating for this allergy.

The problematic phenolics are acetaldehyde, alanine, androsterone, apiol, beta alanine, butyric acid, caffeic acid, carnitine, coumarin, ferrous fumerate, glutamine, 5-hydroxytryptopan, hypericin, lactic acid, malvin, menadione, nicotine, oxalic acid, phytic acid, peperine, proline, threonine, uric acid, indole, and skatol. Although these are the most common allergies, I check for all the phenolics because any of them can be a potential allergen.

Amino Acids

If an individual with immune disorders has symptoms suggesting hypoglycemia or severe sugar problems, I treat for allergies to amino acids immediately. When people are allergic to amino acids, they do not absorb the protein they need from food. Protein, an essential building block in the body, is important for healing, healthy tissue, stamina, and prevention of fatigue.

The most remarkable aspect of NAET is the sequence developed by Dr. Nambudripad for the treatment of basic allergies. In her genius and her profound understanding of the body and acupuncture, Dr. Nambudripad realized that adherence to this sequence is crucial for success. If it is followed correctly, the results surpass any other treatment method available for allergies. After treating the basics, I go back and test each basic again (using muscle testing) to make sure they are all cleared. I test all the B vitamins, sugars, and minerals separately. If these basic allergies are cleared, a foundation has been laid for a healthy immune system and it is easier to clear other allergies.

I continually research to discover other allergens that should be added to the basic allergy treatment. Every day I have worked on this book, I have learned something new from my patients. They are truly my teachers and have educated me more than anyone else. Not a day goes by that I do not learn something about the mystery of the human body. The complications of the individual with immune disorders and allergic condition and the number and combinations of possible allergens boggle my mind, whereas the incredible accomplishments of this allergy work amaze me. I deeply thank Dr. Devi Nambudripad for her contribution to the field of health and alternative healing and for her genius in discovering and developing this work.

This work has been an incredible gift to my family, my extended family, my patients, and myself. I cannot imagine living without NAET or raising my children without teaching them about NAET. It is an inextricable part of our lives. I believe no one should get sick. With the help of NAET and enzyme therapy, we can live completely free of sickness and physical disorders.

There are conditions other than immune disorders and asthma that I have treated and researched. I will talk about them more fully in later books. These include migraines, menopause, PMS, female problems in general, eczema, infertility, multiple chemical sensitivities (environmental illness), and children's disorders including ADD, autism, and learning difficulties.

Chapter

17

NAET TREATMENTS OF ALL IMMUNE DISORDERS AND INDIVIDUAL IMMUNE DISORDERS

The doctors have given up on us   And since they have no fix   no answers   they just want us to go away.   If only we had the grace   to be terminal.
— from "Meridians of Longing"

Leonard

Leonard, 57, knew that he was allergic to eggs and chicken, rice, and some dairy, and he wanted to be able to eat those foods again. His chief symptoms were fatigue in the morning and evening and difficulty with the assimilation of food. He complained of feeling "edgy and eternally agitated, bloated, and constipated." He also had mid-back pain, insomnia, and disturbing dreams, which added to his feelings of irritability and agitation. He had a history of hepatitis, prostatitis, hearing loss, and tinnitus (ringing in the ears).

When he first came to see me, I was running behind in my appointments, and my receptionist came to my office three times to tell me that this man was pacing back and forth in the waiting room, asking how long it would be. When we finally met, he told me that he was like that all the time—any little thing would make him edgy and irritable. In addition, he was chronically tired and depressed, and he felt like he was constantly at war with himself. He sensed that some of his food allergies were contributing to these problems, and he hoped that he could clear them so he could feel more peaceful and relaxed.

The abdominal diagnostic palpation exam indicated that he had trouble absorbing and assimilating sugars and was very low in calcium as I had suspected. He was currently taking some vitamins, enzymes, and other supplements that another chiropractor had given him. Because he was about to leave town for an extended period of time, we needed to do something immediately.

I prescribed a complete enzyme to help him digest sugars and fats (hcl) and explained how important proper digestion was for his overall health. Once he had cleared calcium, I planned to prescribe a calcium enzyme (para) that I find helpful for anxiety and irritability. I also recommended the sugar intolerant diet in the Resource Guide.

Testing revealed that Leonard was allergic to all the basic allergens including Vitamin A, B vitamins, minerals, calcium, magnesium, salt, and sugars. After clearing the basics, we retested and found that he was allergic to cheeses, soybeans, stringbeans, lentils, tofu, nuts and seeds, vegetables, coffee, malt, tea, chocolate, soy sauce, herbs and spices, food additives, food coloring, and bacteria which explained the prostatitis. I prescribed a calcium enzyme (para) and another enzyme made up of protease and calcium especially designed for anxiety (trauma), and then we began to treat for the food allergies. Within the first few treatments, while also supplementing with the calcium enzyme and the digestive enzymes, his irritability diminished 50 percent. He was able to sleep more soundly, and he was not as anxious or as fatigued. His energy seemed more balanced, largely because he was not wasting as much of it by being irritable. He was pleased and hopeful.

After we finished clearing him on the bacteria and most of the foods, his energy was fine, his agitation was gone, and his health was completely restored. I think most of the change

could be attributed to treating for the basic allergens, especially calcium. In fact, over the years I've seen more remarkable results with NAET for calcium and the B vitamins than for
any other allergen.

For example, at three years of age my daughter had trouble sleeping and would get up throughout the night. The day I
treated her for calcium she slept through the night for the first
time in months, and she continued to do so from then on
without any problem. As soon as a mother reports that her
child has difficulty sleeping, I look for a calcium allergy because it means they are not getting the calcium they need
from the milk they drink. Calcium allergy may also be an important factor in rheumatoid arthritis, osteoarthritis, or any
other joint problem.

After the basic allergens have been treated, I have specific protocols for each immune disorder. In preparing
this chapter, I noticed that there are several treatments
that all these disorders have in common. Therefore, this
section will present the allergens I generally treat for with
the immune disorders in general. Then I will discuss
each disorder and its NAET protocol or treatment program separately.

Food allergies are central to all the immune disorders. We naturally eat the foods we are most allergic to,
and these in turn cause us to be ill, lethargic, and depressed and prolong our chronic health problems. After
we have cleared the basic allergies, the phenolics, and
the amino acids, most food allergies disappear automatically. In fact, most people do not have many food allergies; they have food intolerances. To the body, these two
terms are interchangeable because they both cause disturbances in the system. But the difference lies in the fact
that when one clears the basics, the phenolics, and the
amino acids, the food intolerances clear up immediately.
Because we are allergic to some basic food groups,
whether that is Vitamin A, Vitamin B, or tyramine (phe-

nolic naturally occurring in beans), we are intolerant to many foods. Once these basics are cleared, our intolerance disappears.

This explains why standard allergy tests don't uncover many of the food allergies people complain of, and why many mainstream practitioners fail to detect any problem when their patients are clearly reacting unfavorably to certain foods. These tolerances can be eliminated through NAET.

After the basics, phenolics, and amino acids are treated, I retest individuals to see if there are any food allergies still remaining. These are the true allergies that require separate treatment. Some of the most common ones are allergies to milk, nuts, corn, soy and soy products, wheat, fatty acids, yeast, artificial sweeteners, alcohol, and spices. However, any individual can present with any number of different allergies. Both acid and alkaline foods can cause allergies. Common acid foods are sugars and starches, tomatoes, onions, peppers, and potatoes. Mold-containing foods, such as dried fruit, nuts, and cheese, can also cause problems, and clearing for mold will usually eliminate the problem. Gluten can be an allergy for many individuals, but not everyone who does not tolerate wheat is gluten intolerant. In fact, I do not find gluten to be as common an allergen as some proclaim. But when it does occur, clearing an allergy to gluten can clear wheat, rye, oats, malt, and barley. The most common cause of a grain allergy is actually maltose. Most people who have immune disorders are extremely allergic to maltose and consume large amounts of grains. Clearing maltose is essential and can enable one to make great progress in their healing. Since it is a sugar, maltose gets cleared among the basic allergens.

Corn is another common food allergen that should be mentioned as an important irritant for those with immune disorders. One reason it is so important is that we consume it in large quantities in its various forms because it is found in many packaged and precooked meals. Some commercial adhesives, talcum powder, and starched clothes can all provoke reactions in corn-sensitive patients. Even licking a stamp can cause a reaction in an individual allergic to corn.

Sulfites prevent the discoloration of foods at room temperature and are used to preserve wine, raw potatoes, and fresh vegetables. Ingestion of these chemicals by those who are sensitive to them can cause bloating, dizziness, ringing in the ears, or headaches. By desensitizing people to sulfites, we can sometimes clear other foods that contain sulfites naturally such as avocados, baked products, beet sugar, dried fruits, fresh shrimp, fruit drinks, cider, gelatin, wine, beer, potatoes, starches, vegetables, and cellophane. Sulfites are commonly used in the manufacture of many drugs.

Food additives such as BHA, BHT, sodium benzoate, sodium nitrate, sodium sulfate, tartrazine, and food dyes should also be checked. By clearing these, we can clear allergies to foods that contain them. Likewise, treating for oxalic acid (a naturally occurring phenolic) can clear foods high in oxalates including chocolate, caffeine, coffee, tomatoes, citrus fruits, spinach, some beans, and mushrooms. (Refer to Chapter 20 for a more complete list.)

Also important are the fatty acids. The absolutely essential fatty acids, linoleic and linolinic, are needed by everyone for proper nutrition and health but cannot be manufactured by the body and must be consumed in foods. The conditionally essential fatty acids—gamma-linolenic acid (GLA), arachidonic acid (AA), eicosapentanoic acid (EPA), and docasahexanoic acid (DHA)—can be made by cells in the body, but people are allergic to them. These allergies can cause illnesses and immune dysfunction and are important to treat.

Trans fatty acids, created by the partial hydrogenation of vegetable oils, have proliferated in the processed foods we consume, and recent research points to them as a possible cause of immune problems, heart disease, and even low birth weight and obesity. Dr. Mary Enig, Director of the Nutritional Sciences Division at Enig Associates, Inc., states that many people in the United States consume 20 percent of the total fat in their diet as trans fatty acids. She writes, "In the U.S. typical french fried potatoes have about 40% trans fatty acids, and many popular cookies and crackers range from 30 to 50% trans fatty acids. Doughnuts have about 35–40% trans fatty acids. . . . Several years ago we documented nearly 60 grams of trans fatty acids in one typical daily diet. More recently the diet of a young student was found to contain nearly 100 grams of trans fatty acids every day because the foods being consumed included a pound of snack chips made with partially hydrogenated vegetable oil." Trans fatty acids are chemically unstable and cause adverse effects, such as poor immune response, by lowering the efficiency of B cell response and causing alterations in membrane transport and fluidity.

Unlike healthful fats and oils, which do not oxidize easily, trans fatty acids oxidize readily and contain toxic compounds such as peroxides, hydrocarbons, and toxic aromatic compounds. They are not safe and can be a danger to those with immune disorders. It has been reported that free radicals, derived from these trans fatty acids, are destructive to the membranes and tissues of the body.

Fats and oils are important components of our daily diet. Unfortunately, many people with immune disorders are allergic to them and equally allergic to the fatty acids of which they are composed. When these people are cleared of any allergy to the fatty acids, they can consume unprocessed or minimally processed fats and oils without any problem. Supplementation with omega-3, omega-6, and other essential fatty acids may also be used, when appropriate.

Other foods that regularly cause allergies among people with immune disorders are artificial sweeteners, yeast, and food coloring. I often recommend that each patient keep a diet diary for a week or two so we can test the foods she or he eats most often and treat with NAET, as necessary. This approach is helpful, especially with children, in targeting the foods that cause the most symptoms. I also frequently test for food combinations and mixtures of foods together. People can be allergic to the combinations of foods even though they are not allergic to the individual foods. I will have them blend up a whole day's meal and bring it with them to test for food combining. Treating for this mixture has proven to be effective, especially for those with chronic diarrhea, constipation, and bloating.

The minerals are also important, and even though they are included among the basic allergens, I always retest for magnesium, potassium, selenium, zinc, chromium, and manganese because these allergens tend to be invaluable in the treatment of immune disorders.

Finally, I test all the digestive enzymes for allergic response, treat as necessary, and then recommend a set of enzymes based on the abdominal diagnostic examination and 24-hour urinalysis. The most important enzymes are amylase, protease, lactase, maltase, pepsin, hydrochloric acid, cellulase, and lipase.

I would say that 50 percent of patients with immune disorders, and especially CFIDS sufferers, feel more vitality, less depression, increased motivation for living, and greater clarity of mind after clearing their foods allergies. If a NAET practitioner did nothing else but food desensitization, the results would be very satisfying.

INFECTANTS: VIRUSES, BACTERIA, PARASITES, AND FUNGUS

Infections caused by viruses, bacteria, parasites, or fungi can be an underlying cause of chronic immune disorders.

Frequently, allergens are linked to infectants, creating and causing chronic infections that cannot be eliminated until the underlying allergies are cleared. By treating for the infectants, we can stop the cycle of chronic infections and chronic antibiotic use. With the infections gone, the body's immune system strengthens.

Candida

Infections of the yeast Candida in all its many forms are a chronic problem among people with immune disorders. After being treated for Candida and other fungus, individuals suffering from chronic fatigue, bloating, fibromyalgia, eczema, infertility, and vaginal infections can show dramatic improvement. Yeast organisms convert sugars to a chemical called pyruvate, which is then converted to acetaldehyde and carbon dioxide. Carbon dioxide is the main culprit in bloating and gas.

When I treat for yeast infections, I also treat for alcohol. Some scientific studies have shown that Candida albicans in the body can produce enough ethanol to make the infected individual drunk. Ethanol, one of the phenolics, is sometimes cleared by treating for phenolics.

People who have been treated for a sensitivity to Candida must remain on a special diet for ten to fourteen days and curtail their sexual activity (or use a latex barrier) to ensure that the yeast is not passed back and forth sexually. Candida can also be spread through toothbrushes, dentures, fabrics, and skin-to-skin contact. For this reason, there is a strict protocol that must be followed for 25 hours after treatment for Candida and fungus. It includes wearing gloves and a mask, avoiding skin-to-skin contact, and following a completely yeast-free diet. Once the Candida allergy has been successfully treated, the body will be able to eliminate excess yeast from the system and the symptoms will not recur, even if the person is reinfected by another.

The other primary infectants, parasites, bacteria, and viruses, can cause symptoms such as insomnia, fatigue, bloating, constipation, gas, frequent bouts of infections, chronic sore throats, flu-like symptoms, sinusitis, headaches, depression, and muscle and joint pain. (Refer to the Resource Guide for a list of the most common infectants in immune disorders.) Some I check for routinely are giardia, blastocystis hominis, enteroviruses, EBV, CMV, coronovirus, influenza, mononucleosis, streptococcus, staphylococcus, and pseudomonas. These infectant allergies are extremely important to treat and clear because they can be the cause of a suppressed immune response, the build up of CICs and autoimmune activity, and resultant fatigue and ill health.

When treating for the infectants, especially viruses, in immune disorders, I insist that we treat for the person's blood, and when necessary, other tissue fluids such as urine, saliva, and feces (helpful when treating parasites). Blood treatments have yielded especially dramatic results. I treated a woman who was just days away from being put on prednisone and possibly given an emergency splenectomy for a very low platelet count. Nothing her physician had tried worked. I decided to treat her for her blood. In one week, her platelets had doubled, and they have continued to rise ever since. I always treat for the blood every six months with HIV patients and those with athlete's foot and other fungal infections. Urine can be used for treating bladder and prostate infections, even though fungus is also a significant factor in both these conditions.

Environmental Allergies

After clearing infectants, I move on to environmental allergies and begin treating for pollens, molds, and other outdoor allergens, animal dander, dust, fabrics, wood, chemical irritants, gas, and other indoor irritants. There is a process called "outgassing" in which certain products give off VOCs (volatile organic compounds), chemicals that can be picked up by contact or inhaled into the body and enter the bloodstream. Perfume, new carpets, new furniture, new car interiors, heated plastic, even flowers on a table all outgas. Many of these can be smelled, although chemicals without smell can also be toxic. Chemicals such as formaldehyde, toluene, zylene, hexanes, nitrous oxide, ozone, carbon monoxide, carbon dioxide, alkanes, and other petrochemicals and hydrocarbons can all be health threats to people with immune disorders. Photocopy paper outgasses tricholoroethylene (TCE), a solvent used in dry cleaning fluids, carpet shampoos, floor polishes, and furniture glues. Paint fumes can also be a problem, along with cleaning solvents, aerosol sprays, and tobacco and wood smoke.

Multiple chemical sensitivity syndrome (MCS), also known as environmental illness (EI), may develop as the result of a single massive toxic exposure, many repeated exposures, or long-term exposure. Once the sensitivity occurs, it takes less and less of an exposure to elicit a reaction. Many people with immune disorders, especially CFIDS, are environmentally sensitive.

Gulf War Syndrome is the name given to the illness developed by veterans of the Persian Gulf War who now experience multiple chemical sensitivity and chronic fatigue symptoms. Many of these veterans have been disabled, and recently I have seen quite a few in my practice. Among the possible causes are exposure to jet and diesel fuels, exhaust fumes, pesticides, immunizations, chemical warfare agents, heavy metal exposure, paint with cyanide decontamination solution petrochemicals, medications, and very poor sanitation. Many of these people feel their health has been severely damaged and no one is really listening. I had a chance to talk with a veteran of the Gulf War who is now severely asthmatic and has nearly died twice as a result of it. He is extremely sensitive to his environment since returning from the Gulf War.

When patients are not aware of which chemical in a room is causing their problem, I have them put out a small jar of water and leave it open for twenty-four hours. They then close the jar and bring it with them on their next visit, and I treat them for a sensitivity to the water, which by now has trapped whatever chemicals are outgassing into the room. I do the same with outdoor allergens: I have the patient put a bowl of water outside the house to collect pollen for forty-eight hours and then treat them for the water. Sometimes I still need to treat for individual allergens such as specific molds and mildews in a patient's bathroom. When I am treating for an inhalant such as tobacco smoke or perfume, I have the patient inhale the substance while being treated rather than just touching it.

Sick building syndrome may be caused by exposure to any of hundreds of common chemicals and substances including industrial cleaning solutions, outgassing office products, furniture, and carpets, and mold and mildew in air-conditioning vents. Many of these chemicals pass into the blood and the brain when inhaled or touched and may cause or exacerbate immune disorders. NAET can successfully treat for these chemicals, but it is imperative that the patient be prepared for the clearing. Their basics need to be treated and retested, their liver needs to be healthy (which may require a liver cleanse and the use of a liver enzyme), and they need to be cleared of Candida and fungus. When these requirements are met, I have seen people breeze through this treatment. When they are not prepared, however, they may not clear, and their symptoms worsen. This applies to chemicals, perfumes, smoke, and other environmental toxins.

Perfumes, Cosmetics, and Toiletries

Perfumes and cosmetics can definitely contribute to the problems suffered by people with immune disorders and they should be tested and treated. Some of the common ingredients that cause trouble are alcohol, aluminum, acetone (found in nail polish remover), ammonium compounds, chloride (a preservative used in some cosmetics to prevent the growth of bacteria), BHA (a synthetic antioxidant), mercury, and dyes and color additives that contain coal tar substances. These chemicals can also cause hyperactivity in children. Other potentially allergenic substances in these products are detergents, soaps, petroleum derivatives, fluorinated hydrocarbons (used in aerosols), mineral oils, crude oil, and liquid hydrocarbons found in hair sprays, a potential problem for both hairdressers and clients. In all, cosmetics and toiletries contain about 8,000 chemicals and chemical compounds, many of which have not been tested by the FDA.

Perfumes and cosmetics derived from petroleum or coal tar can be as harmful as cigarette smoke. Even many essential flower oils are chemically extracted with petroleum ether. Unfortunately, it is becoming impossible to walk into a store, wash clothes, or flush a toilet without being assailed by scents and chemicals. Perfumes can linger in the air, on clothing, on furniture, and in busses, theaters, restaurants, and workplaces long after the people wearing them have gone. An effective air purifier can be helpful in reducing exposure to tolerable levels, at least in the home or workplace. Fragrances are among the few chemicals in products for human use that are not regulated, although they pose an extreme danger to many people. They should be clearly labeled, with precise information about ingredients and restrictions on chemicals used.

Clearing patients for cosmetics and perfumes is often difficult because they must avoid these ubiquitous products for 25 hours after the treatment. During this period, they must wear a mask and gloves unless they are in a room that is perfume-free. When I do a treatment, I wear a shower cap and gown over my clothes because I spray a little perfume for the patient to inhale. I do the same when treating for smoke allergies.

Chemicals

Another major chemical we treat for is formaldehyde, synthesized from methyl alcohol and found in insulation, particle board, plywood, resin, glue, concrete, polyurethane foam, detergents, carpets and carpet padding, new clothes and other textiles, newsprint, household and industrial cleaners, paints, propellants, and dyes. It is also found in name tags, correction fluid, leather goods, decaffeinated coffee, and embalming fluid. Formaldehyde is so prevalent in our environment that patients must wear masks and gloves after the treatment to keep from being exposed. Fingertips are sensitive and should not be exposed within four feet of an allergen unless covered with gloves during the 25-hour period.

Occupational Allergens

In treating all immune disorders, I also treat for occupational allergens to which people are frequently exposed in the workplace. If a person works in a gas station, I treat for gas fumes, chemicals, gas, and diesel exhaust. If a patient is a painter, I treat for paints, chemicals, and other work materials. A person who works in a hair salon is treated for hair dyes, and a photographer for photographic chemicals. People in detergent factories are exposed to chemicals that remove stains, artists to adhesives and epoxy resins, and bakers to dyes, flour, and cornstarch. Cannery workers are exposed to bleaches, chrome, fish parts, foods, and oils. Carpenters are exposed to adhesives, wood, plastics, fiberglass, and varnishes, and chemists to antibiotics, formalins, acids, and ammonia. Electricians deal with electricity and isocyanates, florists with mold, and gardeners with dried pots, pollens, fertilizers, and mulch. Garment workers are in contact with cotton, nylon, acrylic, polyester, feathers, formalines, and solvents while metal workers come in contact with platinum, chromates, and metal dusts and printers with cobalt, glue, solvents, zinc, chromates, gum arabic, and pine resin. All of these are potential allergens that can be irritating and symptom provoking for individuals with immune disorders.

One man I treated sold bread and suffered severe sinus allergies and candidiasis. When we cleared his wheat allergy, he no longer had problems being around bread. Treatment of occupational allergies such as these keep people from leaving work or going on disability.

Medications

Every individual who comes to my clinic is asked to bring their medications to test for allergies. Most people are allergic to the drugs they take, and I will begin NAET treatments with many acutely ill individuals by treating them for their medications. Some of these people are dependent on and addicted to their medications. NAET can be helpful in relaxing the addictions and decreasing the many side effects. For example, I usually find that women who are on hormone replacement medicines suffer many symptoms, from weight gain to depression and bloating. After I treat for the hormones, the symptoms generally disappear within 24 hours, and they may lose 10 to 20 pounds within a couple of days. I treated one woman for the prednisone she was taking and her need for all other medication disappeared. Doctors who treat their hospitalized patients for their medications with NAET witness quicker improvement and happier patients. It would be a major breakthrough if all physicians understood and utilized this approach.

Among the many medications I have treated for in individuals with immune disorders are the tricyclics

(Elavil® and Sinequan®), serotonin reuptake inhibitors (Prozac® and Zoloft®), sleeping medications (Klonopin® and Restoril®), analgesics (aspirin and Motrin®), and anti-histamines (Seldane® and Claratin®).

Unfortunately, my experience over time demonstrates that most medications are not permanently desensitized. Perhaps the reason is that many manufacturers change the composition of their formulas and fillers over time. Therefore, I recommend testing and treating for medications every 6 months. In the process of NAET treatments and enzyme therapy, the need for these drugs usually diminishes.

Vaccines

I also check for reactions to vaccines that people have received, either as children or as adults such as tetanus, DPT, polio, measles, mumps, rubella, and any vaccine taken for travel abroad. I test and treat each vaccine individually. I find that these vaccines can suppress the immune system for years unless allergies to them are cleared. Polio, tetanus, and flu vaccines are especially important in immune disorders; I have found them to be implicated in fibromyalgia and chronic fatigue as well as shingles and depression.

Dental Amalgams

Mercury can severely compromise the immune system and be a major contributor to ill health. Therefore, I always treat for dental amalgams when indicated. Mercury is a poison that can penetrate and destroy bodily tissues, notably the liver, kidneys, nervous system, blood, skin, and mucous membranes. It can cause inflammation and degenerative changes, as well as pain in the bones, edema, headaches, bad breath, tooth pain, an unpleasant metallic or salty taste in the mouth, excessive fatigue, and an inclination to sleep. Aside from physical symptoms, mercury can cause psychological symptoms such as fear, agitation, and memory loss.

Many other materials can be used to restore a cavity in a tooth, from plastics to gold and porcelain, although all of those materials should be checked for allergic reactions before they are used. Some dentists do this kind of testing, or people can be checked and desensitized by a NAET practitioner.

There is quite a bit of controversy about the advisability of removing mercury fillings. At some point, it is probably best to remove all mercury from the mouth, but there should be careful preparation. I recommend that people who suffer severe symptoms consider it sooner rather than later, as mercury may play an important part in their symptoms. People should be treated for, and desensitized to, mercury and other parts of the amalgam fillings before the old fillings are removed. During removal, these substances are released into the bloodstream and can cause a strong allergic response that could last a lifetime. It is also good to take antioxidants when preparing for mercury removal.

Pesticides

I always treat for pesticides when necessary, including insecticides, fungicides, herbicides, fumigants, and rodenticides, There are several families of insecticides: organophosphates, chlorinated hydrocarbons, botanicals, and chemical sterilants.

Any individual suffering from candidiasis or colitis needs to be treated for these chemicals, as they can be a constant irritant in these disorders. Given the well-publicized link between pesticides and breast cancer, we can imagine the impact they can have on our immune system.

Although DDT was banned as toxic many years ago, it lingers in the soil and air and is reintroduced through the import of foreign produce. Some of the so-called inert ingredients in commercial pesticides are among the most harmful. Carbon tetrachloride and chloroform, for example, are powerful liver and central nervous system toxins. Even natural repellents such as vinegar and garlic can be toxic to someone who is allergic to them.

Authorities are reluctant to issue warnings about pesticide exposure levels because exact toxic levels are not known. Measuring pesticide levels in one food does not accurately determine whether it is a health hazard, however, because chemical combinations can have a synergistic effect. Since pesticides can also leak into water supplies, I always check people for the water they drink, whether it is bottled, filtered, or tap.

Just because people are desensitized to pesticides, however, does not mean the chemicals are no longer harmful. Ingesting them can cause cancer, liver damage, stomach problems, and other symptoms. Washing fruits and vegetables is generally not an effective way to get rid of them. Certain natural products such as grapefruit extract and borax can be used to remove pesticides, but people should make sure they are not allergic to those products before using them. By far the best way to avoid pesticides is to eat organically grown food.

Fabrics

I always test for fabrics, including cotton, rayon, nylon, dacron, polyester, and acrylic. Usually, I have patients wear cotton while I treat first for all the other fabrics, and then we treat for cotton, if necessary. Treatment for fabrics is especially important for those with candidiasis and herpes because fabrics can aggravate or mimic these conditions when one is allergic. For example, some women who suffer vaginal irritation think they have an ongoing Candida infection, whereas they are in fact allergic to the fabric they are wearing. Of course, a fabric allergy may simply exacerbate an existing case of candidiasis. This can also happen with a sanitary napkin or tampax.

Miscellaneous Allergens

Miscellaneous allergens include freon from air-conditioning, radon, plants and ferns, all the various gums, kapok
from mattresses, poison oak and poison ivy, rubber adhesive tape, cement, chalk, all the pesticides, hydrocarbons,
paper mix, newsprint, photocopy paper, plastics, radiation, benzene, labels, nail chemicals, and hair chemicals.

Hormones

I also check for sensitivities to the body's own hormones
such as adrenalin, estrogen, testosterone, progesterone,
cortisol, melatonin, gastrin, insulin, glucagon, DHEA, and
the thyroid hormones. Candida and fungal infections can
be aggravated by an allergy to progesterone or estrogen,
whereas thyroid hormones are an integral part of the
treatment protocol for thyroiditis. Women with immune
disorders who experience more symptoms during the
premenstrual cycle are usually allergic to progesterone. If
their symptoms increase after the menstrual cycle, they
are probably allergic to estrogen. These sensitivities respond well to treatment with NAET.

Melatonin is an important hormone that has received
media attention in recent years as a promoter of human
health and longevity. Production of melatonin is stimulated
by the waning of the light at the end of the day. Twilight
signals neural processes that stimulate the pineal gland to
begin releasing melatonin, which in turn prepares the
body for sleep. Blood levels of the hormone slowly rise
over the next six hours until they peak and then slowly return to daytime levels. Melatonin production can be
caused by jet lag, stress, depression, or an allergy to the
hormone. Treating for melatonin has been successful for
those with sleep disorders, common among CFIDS and fibromyalgia patients. Other problems that have responded
well to treatment for this hormone are migraines related to
the menstrual cycle and seasonal affective disorder.

Organs, Glands, and Cells

With patients suffering from immune disorders, the next group of allergens I test and treat for includes organs, glands, and parts of the nervous system. The specific organs and glands will be discussed in the sections on the individual immune disorders. However, I always check the liver, spleen, kidney, and large intestine, as they are important organs for the elimination of toxins. If a person becomes more sensitive to allergens after beginning treatment, I test for a weak liver and treat with NAET. I also determine the body's different organ dysfunctions when I do my initial abdominal enzyme palpation examination and 24-hour urinalysis. Aside from the liver, the organs that are generally most in need of NAET treatment and enzyme supplementation are the spleen and kidneys.

The Immune System

The immune system should be thoroughly checked and treated, if necessary. There are three major parts of the immune system: the thymus gland, the lymph nodes (or glands), and the bone marrow. Frequently, it will be necessary to treat all three to boost the immune system. These organs produce two major types of blood cells: B cells and T cells, which are the main warriors that defend the body against invaders such as bacteria, viruses, cancer, and other diseases. To protect the body against microorganisms or other substances seen as a threat, the B cells produce antibodies and immunoglobulin, and the T cells secrete chemicals called cytokines. For example, when someone is exposed to an antigen, the B cells produce antibodies and the T cells produce cytokines designed specifically to fight that antigen. The next time the person encounters this antigen, the antibodies block it and the cytokines neutralize the toxin. During a lifetime, the body makes many different antibodies, most of which protect it from diseases.

The body produces IgE antibodies to protect itself against parasites, pollens, and dust. Unfortunately, these antibodies can also be harmful because they can trigger allergic reactions by attaching themselves to mast cells in the skin, nose, intestines, and bronchial tubes. The other antibodies such as IgA, IgE, IgD, IgG, and IgM are produced when confronted with other infectants such as viruses, bacteria, and fungi. If people are allergic to these antibodies, their body either does not produce the proper antibodies or produces too many. Either situation can be dangerous.

Researchers at the National Institutes of Health have suggested a correlation between CFIDS and an overactive immune system. When the body is fighting infection, cytokine hormones such as lymphokines and interleukins are produced by lymphocytes to stimulate the immune response, particularly the production of macrophages. Although the production of these substances is part of a healthy immune response, they can actually cause some of the characteristic symptoms of CFIDS, including severe fatigue, muscle aches, and memory problems. The discomfort associated with these cytokines is a signal that the body is fighting infection. In the body of a healthy individual, when the infection is gone, cytokine production ceases and the symptoms disappear. But in CFIDS patients, the NIH researchers speculate, the production of cytokines continues, and symptoms persist. One possible explanation is that an allergy to the infectant being attacked stimulates the ongoing production of cytokines which in turn leads to chronic symptoms. And an accompanying allergy to the cytokines might cause an overreaction to its production and continual symptoms. This explanation is supported by the success I have had in reducing symptoms by treating for the cytokines and infectants.

Other allergens in this group include immune mediators like histamine, prostaglandin, and leukotreienes. These mediators can cause increased mucus, swelling, and edema and cause smooth muscles to contract. If one is allergic to these immune mediators, symptoms can become more severe.

When allergens are introduced into the body, certain cells such as eosinophils, lymphocytes, T cells, macrophages, epithelial cells, and neutrophils in the bloodstream, form the first line of defense. If the body is allergic to any of those cells, an autoimmune reaction can occur that causes the breakdown of the body's immune defenses, leading to greater inflammation and more serious degenerative and chronic health problems.

SYMPATHETIC AND PARASYMPATHETIC NERVOUS SYSTEM

The nervous system controls all our bodily functions. The brain and spinal cord constantly send and transport nerve impulses throughout the body. There are specific parts that should be checked in individuals with immune disorders.

The nervous system is made up of the sympathetic and parasympathetic systems. The sympathetic nervous system slows down certain functions, whereas the parasympathetic nervous system stimulates organs and tissues. These two systems should act in harmony with each other. But if a person is allergic to one particular system, the body can overreact and cause symptoms. An allergy to the sympathetic nervous system can cause constipation, irritability, slowed reflexes, clouded sensorium, and an inability to fall asleep at night. The parasympathetic nervous system can cause a history of bone disorders, nocturnal leg cramps, restlessness, hyperirritability, low blood pressure, hypoglycemia, and depression. An allergy to one or both parts of the nervous system can lead to an imbalance in which one part is dominant. With NAET and enzyme therapy, we can treat for these allergies and eliminate the imbalances.

Neurotransmitters

Our brain makes certain chemicals called neurotransmitters directly from amino acids in the food we eat. Dopamine and norepinephrine are alertness chemicals, whereas serotonin is inhibitory and calming. Dopamine and norepinephrine are made from tyrosine; serotonin is made from tryptophan. Symptoms of dopamine deficiency include an inability to concentrate, jaw and bone pain, receding gums, and loose teeth. Serotonin deficiency can cause the body to experience exaggeration of pain, mood swings and depression, insomnia, obsessiveness, compulsiveness, anxiety and paranoia, daytime sleepiness, carbohydrate food cravings, and obesity. These are the most important neurotransmitters in treating individuals with immune disorders. Other neurotransmittors that may be involved are glycine, GABA (gamma-aminobutyric acid), acetylcholine, and glutamate. Given the symptoms that a deficiency of these neurotransmitters can produce, it is no wonder that an allergy to them can be extremely important for individuals with immune disorders.

For example, once they have cleared serotonin, many patients with immune disorders report that their depression has lifted, they are sleeping better, and their mental clarity has improved. After all, many of these individuals have been taking antidepressants such as Prozac and Zoloft which are serotonin-reuptake inhibitors. Here we have a treatment that undermines the need for these drugs by making serotonin more available by clearing the allergy. Treatment for serotonin, in combination with the addictive substance, has also proved helpful in addictions such as smoking, alcoholism, and food addictions.

In addition to clearing the neurotransmitters, it is imperative that we also clear any allergy to the amino acids tryptophan and tyrosine from which the neurotransmitters are produced. Tyrosine is especially important in cases of thyroiditis.

Emotions

Another allergen to treat for in cases of immune disorders is emotions. Many reactions in the body are related to core emotions such as anger, fear, sorrow, grief, shame, disappointment, frustration, hopelessness, helplessness, self-sabotage, guilt, paranoia, and even joy. These reactions are often related to significant experiences in the person's life. I first discover what the core emotion or experience is by using the muscle-testing procedure, then have the patient feel the emotions or recall the experience while I treat him or her with NAET. When a patient experiences nausea and dizziness, or other extreme symptoms during the 25 hours following treatment for a particular allergen, there is usually an emotional component that also needs to be cleared.

In addition, I find that many children with attention deficit disorder, hyperactivity, autism, and behavioral problems respond well to treatments for their emotions. Performing these treatments can be an emotional experience for me as well because I find it extremely gratifying to see their lives turn around. To help maintain the progress they have made, I also teach their parents how to test and treat for these emotions.

Sometimes it is necessary to determine the particular incident that triggered the reaction. I narrow down the times in the patient's life by muscle response, testing for particular age ranges such as 0–5 years old, 5–10 years old, and so on. Then I check for any relation involved with the incident—mother, father, sister, brother, child—and the kind of incident experienced such as love, financial, business, or health. While patients recall the incident and feel the emotions, I treat areas on the spine related to the pathways or organs that are blocked. This treatment is inevitably successful. For example, one girl lost her voice when her singing teacher told her she needed to lower her voice and practice speaking more softly.

When we treated the girl for rage toward the teacher, her voice began to return.

Similar to material substances, emotions can be allergens and cause an electromagnetic disturbance in the body. Some emotions can cause an exaggerated response to another allergen or an allergy treatment, always an indication to me that there is an emotional allergy involved. This kind of emotional allergy occurs when something happens that ties an allergen, such as a food, to family members or friends, and an emotional component is stored in the body tied to this allergen. The body is not able to eliminate this allergen unless the emotion connected to it is treated as well. Within minutes after a treatment for an emotional allergy, patients generally feel better, look different, and can contact former allergens without problems. When treating for emotional allergies to foods, the 25-hour restricted diet is not always necessary.

Every individual with CFIDS that I have treated with NAET has needed emotional allergy treatments. Many of the foods, hormones, and infectants to which they are allergic are related to core emotions or emotional traumas. One young man I treated began having trouble with one of his teachers when he started high school. This manifested as chronic fatigue, a learning difficulty, and some behavior problems. I treated him for an emotional allergy connected to an incident between himself and his father that he had not remembered. Immediately after the treatment, his expression and bodily attitude changed, his learning difficulty went away, and his behavior improved.

In another case, a man with colitis who was responding well to NAET had a slight exacerbation of symptoms. We tried to understand the reason behind this, as it did not seem to be a food or an infectant. After some detective work, we found that he had a problem being joyful. When he succeeded at something, as he had recently at work, he would begin to sabotage himself and the outcome would be intestinal cramping and pain. When we treated him for self-sabotage and joy, his symptoms immediately dissipated. He was thrilled because he had always recognized the problem but had no idea how to remedy it. NAET solved the enigma.

COMBINATION ALLERGIES

Some people have combination allergies. In other words, they are allergic to one thing in combination with something else. After I have treated for an allergen, I always check to see if there is any combination to which the person may be allergic. There may even be more than one combination with a given allergen. For example, Vitamin C may be combined with DNA, meaning there is a genetic tendency to the sensitivity. The same person may also have a Vitamin C allergy in combination with a food, an organ, or an infectant. It often helps to make up a vial of the allergen for people with combination allergies, send it home with them, and have them treat themselves several times a day for a week or two, or until the combination clears. We do not need to know the other part of the combination, nor do they have to avoid it. Sometimes these allergies are so strong that it takes many acupressure self-treatment sessions to clear them. Clearing for the one allergen while doing the acupressure self-treatment described earlier eventually clears the combination. This self-treatment is effective, but only after people have been completely cleared of the original allergen (for example, Vitamin C). Otherwise, the self-treatment could aggravate some of the symptoms.

I recently treated Wendy, a young woman with eczema, severe itching, and lesions on her eyelids and neck whose symptoms increased around citrus foods. I treated her for ascorbic acid four times, and after the fourth treatment, thinking she was finally cleared, I had her self-treat with ascorbic acid at home. Two days later she reported that she was itching so severely she had drawn blood. She had noticed that the itching intensified when she treated herself. I had her come in immediately, retested her, and found she was still allergic to ascorbic acid and needed to be retreated. The fifth treatment held, and she was able to self-treat. Her symptoms quickly subsided, and now she eats citrus fruits with no problems.

DNA AND RNA

In my experience, anyone with a chronic illness will develop it again eventually unless it is cleared in combination with DNA and RNA which clears the genetic tendency. This clearing is often essential with certain immune disorders such as herpes, thyroiditis, colitis, and even candidiasis. When an allergen does not clear after a treatment or two, even though the person follows the directions, it usually needs to be treated in combination with RNA and DNA. Some doctors are using the DNA and RNA treatments in treating certain cancers and other chronic illnesses.

PHYSICAL ALLERGIES

The physical allergies to heat, cold, sun radiation, humidity, and dampness can play a major role in the health of individuals with immune disorders. I treat these allergies often and with great success. Many CFIDS sufferers have allergies to cold by itself or in combinations with other allergens which can cause discomfort with cold and feeling cold in the extremities. This is also a familiar problem for people with thyroiditis. People with herpes simplex I are often allergic to the sun and may get an outbreak when they are overexposed. Colitis sufferers have trouble with heat or cold in combination with foods and hormones. When treating for cold, the patient holds ice cubes, and when treating for heat, the patient holds very hot water or a towel that has been in the microwave for a few seconds. I use a humidifier for treating for humidity and dampness. After being treated for sun, one should not be around any radiation for 25 hours, including microwaves, computers, and televisions.

FLUORESCENT LIGHTS

An allergy to fluorescent lights can produce fatigue, chronic headaches, and nausea. These lights, which are often found in the workplace, place an especially heavy burden on people with immune disorders. Treating for fluorescents can be helpful for those who are exposed to them day after day.

ELECTROMAGNETIC CURRENT OR ELECTRICITY

Sometimes I have successfully treated individuals with chronic fatigue for electricity and electromagnetic current. The most common reactions to this ubiquitous allergen are fatigue and immune suppression. Once I actually had someone hold an electric wire while I treated them, and the results were gratifying: their fatigue improved considerably and a lingering virus disappeared.

NAET TREATMENT PROTOCOL FOR CHRONIC FATIGUE IMMUNE DISORDER SYNDROME (CFIDS)

Many people regard CFIDS as synonymous with the Epstein-Barr virus. Although other factors are usually also involved, I always test and treat for EBV after clearing the basics. Some 90 percent of the American population has been infected with EBV by the age of thirty, but most show no signs or symptoms. Therefore, one should wear a mask and not come into close contact with anyone for 25 hours after being treated for the virus. Otherwise, the treatment may fail. I always treat EBV with DNA and RNA as well to clear any genetic tendency toward a recurrence.

EBV can involve many combinations and may cause a variety of symptoms. I have seen it linked to hypertension, headaches, chronic runny nose and fevers in children, and, of course, chronic fatigue. Other viruses that are often linked with it in combination are cytomegalovirus (CMV), which can create fatigue, swollen lymph glands, and fever; human herpes virus-6 (HHV6), which targets both the B and T cells of the immune system and is believed to awaken EBV from its latent state; adrenoviruses, which can cause cold, fevers, and sore throats; enteroviruses and the coxsackie B virus, which are both known to cause sore throat, cough, and gastrointestinal upset; retroviruses; coronoviruses; and enteroviruses.

Research has discovered that CFIDS patients have altered levels of certain brain hormones including increased levels of ACTH (adrenocorticotropic hormone) and decreased levels of the steroid hormone cortisol. Cortisol is important for sugar metabolism and regulation of the immune system. When the adrenal cortex cannot produce enough hormones, the level of ACTH increases to help stimulate the adrenals. However, when the adrenals are fatigued, even an increase in ACTH will not increase the levels of cortisol, and the result will be symptoms such as low blood pressure, dizziness, slow pulse, nausea, pallor, blurred vision, and headaches which so closely match the symptoms of CFIDS.

Epinephrine and norepinephrine are secreted by the adrenal medulla, and a disturbance in the balance of these two can cause manic or depressive symptoms.

Testing and treating for allergies to cortisol, the adrenal cortex, the adrenal medulla, ACTH, epinephrine, and norepinephrine are important steps in the chronic fatigue protocol. In completing treatment of the adrenal gland, one should recheck these important minerals and trace elements: potassium, zinc, magnesium, calcium, and sulfur. They are vital to optimum adrenal function which includes carbohydrate metabolism and maintaining a proper pH balance.

Rechecking the amino acids, especially carnitine, is essential. Lysine and methionine are needed for carnitine synthesis. Deficiency of carnitine can cause muscle weakness and general fatigue. In addition, I always check the thymus and pancreas, both of which are important for immune function and metabolism.

Glutathione, a sulfur-containing molecule composed of glutamic acid, cysteine, and glycine, is abundant in human cells and plays an essential role in protein synthesis, leukotriene and prostaglandin metabolism, and proper immune function. Reduced levels of glutathione can be associated with numerous conditions including Parkinson's disease, myopathies, and chronic fatigue syndrome. Treatment for glutathione followed by supplementation can lead to improvements in these disorders and in individuals with drug toxicities, kidney dysfunction, and possibly also cancers. In healthy cells, glutathione is rapidly recycled back to the reduced state by glutathione reductase, a metabolic enzyme. This recycling is supported by the presence of certain antioxidants. Therefore, when treating for glutathione, I also check for allergies to various antioxidants and metabolites, including glutamic decarboxylase, alanine aminopeptidase, glutathione peroxidase, lysosyme, hesperidinase, and SOD (superoxide dismutase).

Other important items to test and treat for CFIDS sufferers include supplements like lecithin, acidophilous, evening primrose oil, and shiitake mushrooms; herbs such as *astragalus, echinacea, ginkgo biloba*, burdock root, dandelion, red clover, goldenseal, pau d'arco, licorice root, and St. John's wort; and foods, particularly fruits, vegetables, grains, nuts, seeds, turkey, fish, coffee, tea, and shellfish.

Phenylalanine is a natural metabolite that lowers serotonin levels and can be detrimental for chronic fatigue sufferers. The liver regulates how much phenylalanine is metabolized and how much stays in the bloodstream, where it can pass into the brain and be converted into the neurotransmitters dopamine and norepinephrine. These neurotransmitters stimulate the nervous system while lowering serotonin levels. Therefore, treating for phenylalanine can be critical in maintaining proper serotonin levels.

Another major aspect of phenylalanine is that the artificial sweetener aspartame contains it. But phenylalanine from aspartame is absorbed directly into the brain, bypassing the normal biological mechanisms that exist for regulating phenylalanine levels. This can be extremely toxic to the nervous system. Therefore, I always test and treat for artificial sweeteners, as well as for methanol (methyl alcohol, or wood alcohol), a dangerous element in these sweeteners that is metabolized into formaldehyde, a serious poison.

CANDIDIASIS—NAET PROTOCOL

Candidiasis and other fungal infections are a chronic problem. Normally, they are limited to the skin, the vagina, the bladder, and the mucous membranes of the gastrointestinal and upper respiratory tracts. Candida is controlled by the immune system and kept in balance by the normal, friendly bacterial flora. Implicated in every immune disorder discussed in this book, candidiasis deserves special attention because it is insidious and tenacious, and causes a variety of symptoms including bloating, fatigue, constipation, asthma, headaches, and depression.

Yeast organisms convert sugars to a chemical called pyruvate which is then converted to acetaldehyde and carbon dioxide. Human metabolism cannot convert acetaldehyde into anything useful for the body. When we are allergic to it, acetaldehyde can cause symptoms like hangovers, poor memory, lightheadedness, and lack of concentration. Carbon dioxide is one of the main culprits in bloating and gas. When I suspect a yeast infection, I generally test and clear carbon dioxide, acetaldehyde, and alcohol. Some scientific studies have shown that Candida albicans in the body produces enough ethanol to make the infected individual drunk. A list of the all the Candidas and funguses found in the body are included in the Resource Guide of this book.

Before I begin the treatment for Candida, I always recheck sugar, artificial sweeteners, and B vitamins, since Candida will never clear unless they have cleared completely. Sugars feed the yeast, and B vitamins reduce the craving for sugar. I then treat for all the Candidas together, separate from the other fungus, making sure that the patient follows the directions for the 25-hour restrictions, followed by the 10-day Candida diet. The rigorous 25-hour protocol requires that patients wear masks and gloves and live in virtual isolation, and I enforce this routine because I find that even the slightest exposure to any kind of fungus can nullify the treatment and cause a return of symptoms. The Candida infectants include *Candida albicans, Candida parapsilosis, Candida stellatoidea, Candida tropicalis, Candida guilliermondii, Candida lusitaniae, Candida pseudotropicalis,* and *Candida rugosa. Candida albicans* and *Candida tropicalis* are the most common and also the most persistent. Candida albicans prefers an acid pH and grows rapidly in a medium of sugars, biotin, and organic salts. The higher the biotin level, the more the yeast reproduces.

After clearing the Candida allergy, I do a complete fungus treatment with the same 25-hour restrictions, then follow up by clearing any allergies to mold. Next, I treat Brewer's and baker's yeast separately, both of which usually require only dietary restrictions during the 25 hours following treatment.

Candidiasis is an ever-increasing health problem, in part because of the widespread use of antibiotics which are commonly prescribed from an early age for bacterial infections, including teenage acne, and are ingested in the meat and poultry we buy. When there is evidence of candidiasis, I always clear for antibiotics with NAET. Tetracycline is cleared among the basics with eggs and chicken because it is an antibiotic used in chickens.

When a couple comes to see me and both have Candida, the one exhibiting symptoms is usually the one who is allergic. Although they may continue to transmit the Candida back and forth between them, however, the symptoms will not reoccur once the allergy has been successfully treated, because Candida's pathogenicity, or ability to do harm, is caused by an allergy, not by its inherent pathogenicity.

Even though it takes as long as two months to completely balance the intestinal flora, the 10- to 14-day diet is crucial. Candida overgrowth or allergy occurs in the human body when the defenses are locally impaired, such as in a disturbance of the gut flora caused by parasitic, viral, or bacterial infections. Therefore, clearing these infectants with NAET is imperative in dealing with candidiasis. Nutritional deficiencies, altered glucose metabolism, hypoglycemia, and diabetes can also be factors since poor sugar metabolism exacerbates the growth of Candida or fungus. Impaired immunity can also be caused by HIV infections, chemotherapy, radiation, genetic defects, toxic chemicals, high carbohydrate and sugar diets, pregnancy, menses, thyroid and adrenal deficiencies, cortical steroids, and oral contraceptives. Therefore, I treat for these items with NAET, if necessary, although in severe cases of vaginal Candida, abstaining from oral contraceptives seems to be the best and quickest alternative. When treating for stubborn yeast infections, especially in an immune-suppressed individual—for example, one who is on chemotherapy or has HIV—I often treat for the bodily fluids such as the blood, urine, vaginal secretions, and saliva.

Candida may require many combinations to clear. I commonly treat Candida in combination with sugars, grains, hormones, oxygen (when experiencing bloating), carbon dioxide, emotions, mercury and other metals, heat and cold, DNA, RNA, certain organs, fabrics, sanitary napkins, tampax, glands, and even pollens such as grass and flowers. (In one case, this combination cleared up a severe case of psoriasis and eczema.) ·

For example, a 12-year-old girl came to see me with severe eczema around her mouth. Her mother had taken her to dermatologists and pediatricians who offered her steroid creams and lotions, but nothing proved effective. In fact, her eczema had just gotten worse with each new remedy. When I inquired about the history of the rash, her mother recalled that it had appeared right after she had had braces put on her teeth. An orthodontist in my building was kind enough to give us all the necessary brace materials to test her, and we found that she was allergic to the rubber bands, plastic, metals, and cement in combination with fungus. First I treated her for fungus, and she followed the protocol for 11 hours (since she was only 12). Then I treated her for all the brace materials in combination with fungus. Within 48 hours her rash was completely gone. Her father, a physician, was amazed, and pleased. I could only wonder why none of the physicians she had seen had even asked her about the braces.

In any case, fungus can have many combinations, and I will often give the fungus or Candida vial to a patient to take home and self-treat for as long as two to three weeks, if necessary. Treatments for the various hormones in combination with Candida can be especially important, including estrogen, progesterone, pituitary, adrenal, and thyroid, since Candida can upset the receptor sites for these hormones in the body.

Another significant discovery has been the effect on candidiasis of NAET treatment for chromium. Chromium is an essential mineral that stimulates the activity of enzymes involved in the metabolism of glucose for energy. It also appears to increase the effectiveness of insulin and its ability to handle glucose, preventing hypoglycemia and diabetes. Chromium is difficult to absorb, and many people are allergic to it, causing sugar absorption problems and exaggerated candidiasis. Bloating especially is a major symptom. Treating for chromium on its own and in combination with sugar and Candida has proven to be a breakthrough for bloating and poor sugar metabolism.

The food allergens I commonly treat in combination with Candida are vegetables, especially corn, peas, and legumes; fruits, especially citrus; meats; wheat, rye, and corn; cheese; eggs; vinegars; red and white wine; beer; food coloring and food additives; chocolate; melons; potatoes; yams; and food combinations.

When undergoing treatment for candidiasis, including antifungal medication or dietary changes, many people have what is called a die-off reaction. This can usually be prevented with NAET treatments for Candida in combination with other allergens.

One man in his forties came to see me with chronic Candida infections. For years he had experienced fatigue, insomnia, bloating, and fogginess, and he had tried many alternative treatments with only occasional and temporary relief. The woman he was with was also diagnosed with Candida, and they were passing it back and forth. After clearing the basic allergies, we treated for Candida and some other fungi which took several sessions. Then he went on the special diet for 10 to 14 days, and I prescribed AllerZyme C containing probiotic microflora, cellulase, and magnesium, helpful in the detoxification of Candida (see enzyme formulas for Candida in the Resource Guide of this book). After treatments that stretched over a three-month period, he felt better, he was able to resume his sexual relationship, and he could eat the foods that had previously caused difficulties.

It is necessary to test all patients being treated for Candida for their specific medications as well as the supplements they will be taking for their Candida infection. In particular, many people are allergic to acidophilous and other probiotic microflora. As a result, they will not be able to utilize them well and may develop bloating, diarrhea, and gas.

Since most Candida infections are long-standing and well established, it is important to be persistent with the NAET treatments, the 10-day diet, and the supplementation designed to detoxify the body, curtail yeast growth, and establish a healthy flora. Although treatment length will vary from patient to patient, NAET is by far the best approach for clearing Candida. If a Candida infection is not taken care of immediately, it will continue to spread and create havoc for the immune system, setting the stage for more chronic health problems. Once Candida has been cleared, a renewed, energetic, healthy being shines through.

FIBROMYALGIA—NAET PROTOCOL

Fibromyalgia and chronic fatigue have many similar clinical features, and the chronic fatigue protocol can be applied to these. The distinguishing symptoms of fibromyalgia are unrelenting musculoskeletal pain and soft tissue swelling which require their own treatment approach.

Since the typical fibromyalgia patient I see is a woman in menopause, I usually begin the phase of treatment specific to this order by treating for hormones, especially estrogen, progesterone, testosterone, cortisol, DHEA, and the thyroid hormones. I will also look for several combinations, with heat, cold, DNA, RNA, nerve tissue, and emotions. After clearing the hormones, I frequently supplement with a progesterone oil or cream which can also be used topically for joint and muscle pain.

Digestion is a key factor in fibromyalgia, as is in all immune disorders. When digestion is poor, the CICs increase, causing autoimmune reactions, inflammatory processes, and suppressed healing. Good digestion protects the body from undigested food or antigens entering the bloodstream, a condition known as leaky gut. Therefore, it is crucial to test and treat for probiotic microflora and all the digestive enzymes: HCL, pepsin, ptyalin, lactase, pancreatin, protease, trypsin, chymotrypsin, bromelain, papain, amylase, lipase, ribonuclease, cellulase, and maltase. After these have cleared, I usually prescribe enzymes that contain these essential substances. Immune mediators are also important to test and treat to assure adequate protection against immune invaders such as parasites, bacteria, and fungus, which add to the immune stress caused by the CICs

Next, I will retest and carefully screen all the minerals and metals, especially magnesium. A deficiency of magnesium interferes with nerve and muscle impulses and can cause muscle twitching, tremors, and weakness. An allergy to magnesium can contribute to insomnia. I also retest Vitamin D, B_{12}, folate, Vitamin C, myoglobulin, malic acid, and niacin, all of which tend to be low in fibromyalgia patients.

Other allergens that may require treatment include serotonin, norepinephrine, dopamine, and tryptophan which correspond to symptoms of severe anxiety, depression, insomnia, and bowel irritability. Lyme disease and other bacteria, viruses, parasites, and fungi are also important to test and treat.

Some contactants such as plastics, chemicals, fabrics, silicon, tap water, metals, cold, and woods, may be implicated in fibromyalgia, and inhalants such as perfumes, dust, pesticides, pollen, radiation, and molds can play a major role in causing or exacerbating fibromyalgia symptoms.

Studies have indicated that abnormal carbohydrate metabolism may be a factor in FM, and this has been associated with decreased levels of lactate dehydrogenase (LDH), a muscular metabolic enzyme. Thus, I always test for LDH, as well as lactic acid, a byproduct of this anaerobic metabolic process. Oxygen can also be an important factor and frequently needs to be treated.

Organs, glands, and tissues I treat include muscles, ligaments, connective tissue, and all the components of circulation: arteries, veins, capillaries, and blood. Some studies have pointed to muscle abnormalities in fibromyalgia patients, but the results have been inconsistent. With certain patients, being treated for these organs has reversed the muscle fatigue to the point that they can begin to exercise, whereas with others the change has not been significant. Other chemicals worthy of testing and treating are ATP (adenosine triphosphate) and ADP (adenosine diphosphate), present in every cell and necessary for cell function. Levels of ATP and ADP can be depressed by the continuous contraction of muscle caused by tension, as well as by the body's allergic reaction to the individual ingredients of the ATP or ADP molecules adenosine, ribose, and phosphate radical. Lowered ATP production causes reduced energy for the cells. Uric acid, a result of the catabolism of ATP, usually needs to be treated as well because it can cause muscle and joint pain.

Common food allergens associated with fibromyalgia are nuts, spices, artificial sweeteners, animal fats, amino acids, essential fatty acids, alcohol, turkey (due in part to the tryptophan and serotonin naturally contained in turkey), food coloring, food additives, gelatin, gums, onion, garlic, yeast, modified vegetable starch, sulfites, solanine (a phenolic naturally contained in the nightshade family of vegetables, such as green pepper, eggplant, tomatoes, and potatoes), and caffeine and chocolate.

CROHN'S DISEASE AND ULCERATIVE COLITIS— NAET PROTOCOL

Crohn's disease and ulcerative colitis are both classified as inflammatory bowel diseases (IBDs) and involve similar symptoms relating to the inflammation of the digestive system. I refer to them together in this chapter on treatment procedures.

I have been treating IBDs for almost 20 years with a success rate that is remarkable, given that they are generally considered incurable by mainstream medicine. The problem usually stems from food allergies and an overabundance of sugar in the diet, coupled with poor digestion of sugars and starches. I generally begin with a full abdominal palpation examination and 24-hour urinalysis to assess dietary stress, food absorption, and bowel toxicity. The majority of these individuals demonstrate a severe sugar intolerance, accompanied by allergies to lactose, maltose, and glucose (predominantly present in those with Crohn's disease). They also appear to have poor absorption and assimilation of proteins, thus causing bouts of constipation and painful joints. (The calcium required by the bones needs good protein digestion to be absorbed.) My initial focus is to expedite digestion and absorption with digestive enzymes. Therefore, I test and treat with NAET for all the digestive enzymes, including bromelain, an effective anti-inflammatory. Enzyme supplementation can work wonders, especially for Crohn's disease (see AllerZyme IB section in the Resource Guide).

For example, a man in his late 20s came to see me with severe abdominal pain, diarrhea, bleeding stools, and weight loss. After being diagnosed with Crohn's disease, he was prescribed steroids and told to refrain from milk products. This last recommendation was helpful, but the long-term use of steroids posed enormous risks, and the prognosis was not satisfactory. He was referred to me for enzyme evaluation and allergy testing. After this procedure was completed, I found he was sugar and starch intolerant, and I recommended a digestive enzyme (pan) be taken before meals for complete sugar digestion and another for sugar absorption (srg) taken 2 hours after meals. We also treated him for a few of the basic allergens including B vitamins, calcium, and sugars. Since seeing me three years ago, he has not had any serious exacerbation of his Crohn's, and he enjoys a varied diet.

Again I want to emphasize the importance of repeatedly retesting the basic allergies to make sure they have cleared and that there are no combinations. Because diarrhea promotes the depletion of many minerals, retesting for zinc and magnesium is essential. Folic acid, which helps to regenerate tissue, is also important. Vitamin C can irritate the intestines when there is an allergy to it, so I always recheck it before suggesting supplementation. Many IBD patients also suffer from bleeding, so it is important to retest for an iron allergy, since this allergy can compound the severe anemia and resultant fatigue caused by the bleeding. Quercetin, a bioflavonoid and another basic, has been known to have a soothing effect on the intestinal wall, and I recommend it in combination with digestive enzymes containing bromelain once any allergy to it has cleared.

A man in his 40s came to see me for IBD, complaining of severe abdominal pain, cramping, and weight loss. In his own words, he was a "mess." He had sought out every therapy I had ever heard of, but nothing had worked, and he was at the end of his rope with frustration. He believed that food allergies were the underlying cause of his problem, and he hoped that NAET might be the answer at last. As the basics cleared, he improved dramatically. Now he could eat and not feel sick. He felt so good that he stopped coming to see me.

One year later, he returned with similar symptoms. The cramping was back, though not nearly as severe, and he noticed he needed to minimize his diet again. By doing some thorough testing and investigation, we learned that the B vitamin and sugar allergies had returned, but only on the emotional level. "What does that mean?" he asked. I explained to him that if one eats certain foods when experiencing intense emotions, an allergy to the food can return. This is called an emotional allergy. Once these emotions are treated and cleared with NAET, the foods that initiated the reactions will no longer be a problem. I explained that clearing the emotions linked to these basics would clear all the foods that contain them (and were cleared the first time we treated for them), which, in the case of B vitamins and sugars, was just about every food. That is precisely what occurred: the basics cleared and he could resume eating again. I have not seen him in many years, but I hear he is doing fine and continues to refer his friends to me.

With IBDs, after treating for the digestive enzymes, I then clear all the food allergies. Most of the allergies clear after the phenolics are desensitized, but some stubborn foods may remain, for example, gluten, and therefore wheat and other gluten-containing grains, fiber, artificial sweeteners, dairy, including milk, cheese, and yogurt, vegetables with a higher sugar content, such as peas, carrots, and potatoes, nuts and fruits, beans, animal and vegetable oils, fatty acids, alcohol, wine, and beer, chocolate, coffee, caffeine, tea, cocoa, carob, yeast, vinegar, food additives, food coloring, modified vegetable starch, sulfites, spices, acid and alkaline pH, alone and together, and amino acids such as L-glutamine, which has been known to help heal the gastrointestinal tract.

After clearing their food allergies, I caution individuals with IBD to incorporate certain foods into their diet gradually such as grains, fruits, dairy, beans, and alcohol as these foods tend to be the most irritating to their digestive system. I work with each individual differently, but I always work slowly and carefully to be certain they are free of acute intestinal inflammation. I perform a series of testing procedures on each patient to determine what foods should be introduced, when, how often, and in what quantities, and I encourage them to use their enzymes each and every time for digestion and absorption.

After the foods, I always clear the infectants, beginning with bacteria. For example, I often find allergies to *klebsiella, proteus*, and *pseudomonas*, but many other bacteria may also be involved. Then I clear parasites, with *blastocystis hominis* and *entamoeba histolytica* being among the most common. Fungus and Candida should also be completely cleared, since their problems with sugar predispose these patients to Candida infections, complicating their disease and causing other problems. Finally, viruses are important with all the immune disorders because a weakened immune system makes these people more prone to contract viral infections.

Other NAET treatments to consider are toothpastes because they have been known to set up inflammatory reactions in the intestines. Treating for any medications that have been taken, including steroids like prednisone, antibiotics, and other drugs, even aspirin and tylenol, is imperative, even if they are not presently being taken. I check and treat these individuals for everything they have ever ingested, as they could be suffering from long-lasting autoimmune reactions. When necessary, I treat for probiotic microflora including lactobacillus and bifidus, as well as for fiber products and supplements. I also test for all the vaccines and childhood diseases, especially measles, which has been proposed as a possible cause or link with IBD, causing the chronic inflammation of lymph tissue in the intestine. If there is an allergy, any one of the vaccinations, including the flu vaccine, can be deleterious to the body.

Testing and clearing for hormones, such as estrogen, progesterone, DHEA, adrenalin, gastrin, secretin, and thyroid, can help relieve fatigue and reduce stress.

The organs and glands I treat for with every IBD sufferer are the colon, small intestines, stomach, spleen, liver, ileum and cecum, jejunum, pancreas, and gallbladder. I also treat for the adrenal, thyroid, pituitary, thymus, and lymph glands, as well as the individual parts of the immune system as described in the general section on immune disorders. When necessary, I treat for the glands in combination with foods, fungus, DNA-RNA, prostaglandin, and emotions. Finally, I treat for the disease (Crohn's or ulcerative colitis) itself, alone and in combination with DNA-RNA and other allergens. These treatments are helpful for some of my IBD patients, but the foods and infectants are crucial.

Through the use of NAET, enzyme therapy, and individual dietary provisions, every person with IBD should be able to have a healthy, vital digestive system. I am a living example of the benefits of this approach, and the case histories in this book attest to it as well.

HERPES—NAET TREATMENT PROTOCOL

"Can you really help with the herpes virus?" I'm asked this question again and again, and my reply is always a confident "Yes." About 90 percent of the population in America and Europe is already infected with at least one of the six strains of herpes. These viruses are insidious and lie dormant in the body, waiting for an opportunity to become active. In particular, contact with allergens linked with this virus can awaken the virus and cause an outbreak. But NAET treatment for these allergies can permanently prevent this from happening.

Herpes simplex I (HSV-I) can begin as early as childhood. After the initial infection, the virus retreats into the fascial nerves, reemerging as the typical blisters around the mouth when an allergen is contacted. Many people remark that the outbreaks occur under stress. This may be true, but when the allergies are eliminated and the allergy load reduced, there should be no recurrence, even under the worst stress. The allergens that precipitate herpes outbreaks are mostly foods such as almonds and brazil nuts, high in the amino acids arginine, cheese, spices, chocolate, milk (Vitamin D in milk is often the culprit), yeast, sugars, and wines, as well as dental materials and anaesthesia, vitamin supplements, food additives, sulfites, and food coloring. The second most common cause is the sun, which can be successfully treated. When treating for sun, we recommend no contact with sunlight for 25 hours; therefore, it is preferable to treat on a rainy day.

With HSV-I, I have also treated successfully for materials in braces, toothpaste, lipstick, cigarettes, cigars, pipes and tobacco, plastics, tap water, and hormones, including melatonin, testosterone, estrogen, progesterone, and adrenalin. It is important to retest all the vitamins for combinations, including D, F (fatty acids), and all the Bs. Drugs too, both prescription and nonprescription, should be tested and treated, as they can be a major cause of outbreaks. I always treat for herpes I, alone and in combination, with DNA and RNA and certain other combinations. But each individual is different and needs individual testing and evaluation.

These herpes outbreaks may look the same on the surface, even though they occur on different parts of the body, but the diseases are different and should be respected as such. With all the herpes viruses, I give patients a vial to take home and use when they sense that they may be getting an outbreak. They can then stop the outbreak by self-treating for the vial using the accupressure points (see accupressure emergency treatment protocols in Chapter 5). This treatment should only be done if they have already cleared herpes by itself; otherwise, it can cause the opposite effect and enhance the virus's activity. We are essentially using the vial to help treat any combinations that may arise.

My son, Aaron, who is now 18, had outbreaks of oral herpes since he was a young boy. He detested the sores, and when I first learned about enzymes and NAET, Aaron became my first patient. I treated him with NAET for many foods, including sugars, dairy, food additives, and fruits, as well as the sun. I also prescribed certain enzymes for preventing outbreaks (AllerZyme H) and for eliminating them once they had appeared. He has not had an outbreak in seven years, and he no longer needs the enzymes.

Other treatments I usually need to do with herpes patients concern the viruses, bacteria, and Candida. People who develop common virus symptoms such as runny nose, sore throat, and flu-like symptoms tend to have outbreaks, possibly because their immune system has been compromised or because the viruses are linked with herpes. Emotions also play a role in this disorder and are important to treat, alone or in combination with the herpes virus or foods.

Although the frequency of occurrence may vary from person to person, with some people getting outbreaks as often as every few weeks, and others as infrequently as once every few years, herpes simplex II (HSV-II), or genital herpes, is still a worrisome, painful, and highly contagious disease. It has been implicated as a promoter of cervical cancer, and an infant delivered through the vagina of a woman with active lesions risks being born blind and brain-damaged. When herpes is treated with NAET, the outbreaks can be diminished in frequency or even eliminated entirely. Again, foods are the most important allergens to treat with NAET, especially those high in the amino acid arginine, such as chocolate, peanuts, sugar, alcohol, coffee, cashews, pecans, almonds, sesame seeds, and bleached white flour. I also treat for arginine itself and for the amino acid lysine, which has been known to reduce outbreaks, as well as for antibiotics, especially penicillin, which seem to induce outbreaks in some people.

As with HSV-I, it is essential to treat for viruses, bacteria, fungus, and parasites, when necessary. I also treat HSV-II sufferers for EBV, when appropriate, as the two viruses have been linked together. Contactants can be important, such as cotton and other fabrics, tampax, sanitary napkins, plastics, condoms, and any other allergy that causes a burden on the immune system. Many of the same allergy treatments used for herpes I also apply here, including hormones, emotions, and the herpes vial.

The herpes virus called shingles, or herpes zoster, also known as varicella zoster, requires special consideration. The virus first appears as chicken pox and produces an antibody-antigen reaction that can linger long after the initial outbreak is gone. The virus will replicate itself or part of itself in an altered form so that the body treats it as if it were another allergen. This chicken pox virus becomes linked with other allergens to form CICs that have a tendency to lodge on nerve cells. This sparks an autoimmune reaction, causing inflammation, damage to the cells, pain, the typical burning, itching blisters of shingles, swollen lymph nodes, and general fatigue. Enzymes (AllerZyme H) can be helpful in deactivating the virus and preventing it from damaging the nerve cells, but the treatment has to be initiated early in the virus' development. But NAET treatments can wipe out the shingles by breaking the links with other allergens and putting the virus to sleep permanently, with no side effects or further complications.

The most important allergy treatment with an individual with shingles, besides the basic allergies, is the treatment of the chicken pox, or varicella, virus. Children should definitely be treated with NAET as early as possible for this virus, to keep them from catching chicken pox, if possible, and to prevent them from contracting shingles later in life. Since many of the basic allergies, especially Vitamins C, B, and A, form combinations with herpes zoster, the disease may improve substantially after the basic allergies have cleared. After treating people with shingles for the varicella virus, I include the herpes zoster vial in every subsequent allergy treatment, whether with foods, infectants, contactants, or inhalants, to clear any possible combinations with these allergens.

Often, the onset of shingles is linked with an emotion, a flu virus, or a bacteria, and successfully clearing these allergens with the herpes zoster vial can cause a dramatic recovery. There may be many combinations with herpes zoster, including DNA, RNA, hormones, organs, and antibiotics, especially if the person has had shingles symptoms for more than five years. In any case, one should expect almost a complete recovery. Compared to the traditional medical approach, which is limited to pain-killers, the combination of NAET and enzyme therapy is a monumental advance in the treatment of shingles, offering drugless, noninvasive relief.

Herpes VI, formerly known as human B-lymphotrophic virus (HBLCV), infects as many as 30 percent of adult Americans and causes many of the chronic fatigue symptoms characteristic of EBV. Indeed, some researchers have speculated that it is merely a new strain of Epstein-Barr. Others have linked it to roseola, a virus found in infants. As with EBV, an allergy to HBLCV can be problematic. I treat this virus exactly the way I treat EBV, using the protocol recommended for CFIDS. I do not come across it in chronic fatigue sufferers as often as coxsackie, EBV, or CMV, but I have encountered a few cases in my practice. Again, it is important to strengthen the immune system through allergy elimination and enzyme therapy. Often, I will treat for the immune organs, glands, cells, and mediators, to strengthen them in their fight against infectants.

By the time this book is published, other virulent strains of herpes viruses may have been discovered. By freeing ourselves of allergies and metabolic imbalances and maintaining a healthy immune system, we can prevent these microorganisms from compromising our health.

NAET PROTOCOL FOR THYROIDITIS (HASHIMOTO'S THYROIDITIS)

When treating Hashimoto's thyroiditis, I follow a precise sequence of treatments. After clearing all the basic allergens, I recheck the trace mineral iodine to see if there are any combinations because iodine aids in the development and functioning of the thyroid gland and is an integral part of thyroxine. I have see many individuals progress dramatically in their struggle with this disease once they have cleared iodine and begun eating foods high in iodine. Such foods include seafood, kelp, garlic, lima beans, summer squash, mushrooms, Irish moss, and turnip greens. In addition, consuming 3.4 grams of iodine-enriched salt a day provides 260 micrograms of iodine.

Next, I use NAET to clear any allergy to their thyroid supplement, if they take one, whether it is synthetic or natural. After treating for the medication, I do muscle testing to determine dosage and times to take the medication. I consistently do this testing, as the dosage may change with each new clearing. In fact, I do this again after clearing each item on this protocol list because at some point, the patient may not need medication anymore. As I have mentioned before, I find that medications do not desensitize permanently but need to be tested and retreated at two- to six-month intervals. I have also found that the dosage for people on synthyroid, the synthetic thyroid medication, tends to remain more consistent over longer periods of time, whereas the dosages for other medications need frequent testing.

Then I treat for the thyroid gland itself. An allergy to the thyroid generally indicates that the gland is functioning abnormally, and NAET treatment can restore and strengthen it. Within 25 hours, patients will often remark how much more energetic they feel. After this treatment, I usually begin a regimen of supplementation that includes a natural glandular thyroid supplement and a thyroid enzyme (see AllerZyme thy in Chapter 20). The exact regimen depends on the results of the 24-hour urinalysis, the abdominal palpation, and the axillary basal temperature test.

I then treat for thyroglobulin, a glycoprotein secreted by the thyroid that contains sugars such as manose and glucosamine. The iodine of the thyroid combines with thyroglobulin to form the thyroid hormones which take shape within the thyroglobulin molecule. The synthesis of thyroglobulin is regulated by the hypothalamus and the adrenals, and the rate of secretion of thyroglobulin is regulated by TSH (thyroid stimulating hormone) secreted by the hypothalamus. When thyroid hormone levels are low, the secretion of TSH is increased, and more thyroglobulin is secreted. Therefore, a balance is important, and an allergy to thryoglobulin can upset the synthesis of thyroid hormones.

The next step in the protocol is to treat for the thyroid hormones, pituitary hormones, and thyroid releasing hormones including diiodothryonone (T_2), triiodothyronine (T_3), thyroxine (T_4), thyroid stimulating hormone (TSH) secreted by the anterior pituitary, and thyrotrophin releasing hormone (TRH). The thyroid releasing or inhibiting hormones control the secretion of the anterior pituitary hormones. I usually treat the thyroid hormones first, then the pituitary hormones and the releasing hormones. These treatments usually reverse many of the symptoms of low thyroid such as dry skin, hair loss, irregular periods, premenstrual and menopausal symptoms, and low energy.

Following the hormones I treat for Hashimoto's thyroiditis itself, then do a second treatment 25 hours later for Hashimoto's thyroiditis in combination with DNA and RNA. This clears any genetic tendency to the disorder and raises the basal temperature. Next I treat for the amino acid tyrosine, which, when combined with iodine, is a precursor to thyroxine, as well as the neurotransmitter norepinephrine which increases basal metabolic rate.

Most Hashimoto's patients test positive for an allergy to Candida, particularly Candida albicans and Candida tropicalis, and NAET treatment can be crucial. (A separate chapter of this book is devoted to Candida infection which is an immune disorder in its own right.) With thyroiditis, Candida can damage the body's receptor sites for thyroid and other hormones, resulting in a slowing down of the entire endocrine system.

Fluorine and fatty acids are two other allergens to treat next. Fluorine or its active form, fluoride, is present in all animal tissue. It increases the deposition of calcium and reduces the formation of acid in the mouth, thereby preventing tooth decay. Excessive amounts of fluoride, which can occur through ingesting too much fluoride, are definitely harmful, as well as an allergy to fluoride, because they can destroy the enzyme phosphatase, vital to metabolism. Natural sources of fluorine are fish and seafood, milk, cheese, meat, and tea. Fatty acids, essential in the daily diet and necessary for the elasticity of cells and the production of hormones, can help improve many of the symptoms related to thyroiditis such as eczema, high cholesterol, irregular periods, hair and nail problems, and premature aging.

When treating any immune disorder, I always check and treat for mercury and amalgams. Allergies to these can directly influence energy level and mood and can cause headaches, insomnia, memory loss, and pain in muscles and joints. Treatment can help clear many of the symptoms that plague the individual with hypothyroid and Candida.

The foods I regularly check with thyroiditis are vegetable and animal fat, grains, gluten, yeast, food additives, food coloring, and dairy.

An organism's immune system is designed to protect it against foreign substances and pathogens. However, the ability to distinguish between "self and not self" is compromised in autoimmune diseases, and all aspects of the immune system should be tested and treated for regulation and proper function. I always test for allergies to macrophages, lymphocytes, antibodies, immune mediators, in particular, antithyroid peroxidase (anti-TPO) antibodies, as well as the thyroid peroxidase enzyme itself. This enzyme catalyzes the synthesis of iodine and tyrosine in the thyroglobulin molecule to produce thyroid hormone. The anti-TPO antibodies, which inhibit this conversion, has been reported high in patients with Hashimoto's thyroiditis.

The amount of time it takes to treat a chronic ailment with NAET varies from patient to patient. Every individual is different, and every individual's program is different. In evaluating the program and making recommendations for different people, the practitioner must become familiar with the symptoms, history, immune response, and particular allergens. Everyone's response to NAET is influenced by these factors.

The healing inevitably takes time. For some it takes a couple of months, for others it could take as long as two years. Having worked with many hundreds of patients with a wide variety of problems, I know that with persistent NAET treatment, good digestion, and enzyme therapy, homeostasis will eventually be restored to the body. People with chronic immune disorders who pursue this approach will eventually find themselves feeling vastly improved. They should understand, however, that it takes some time.

For example, a fourth-grade boy, John, came to me with hay fever, allergies, chronic fatigue and asthma, and about twenty warts on each hand and arm. We went through all the basic allergies, some foods, and moved to the pollen and environmentals. He asked me if I could make his warts go away before the school year started. I told him I had very good results with warts and that we would treat the virus that caused them with NAET. We treated for many wart combinations and he treated himself at home. Nothing happened; not a single wart fell off. At that point, we took a break because it is often a good idea to give the immune system time to catch up with the treatments and to give the body time to detoxify. I talked to his mother about bringing him in for evaluation at the end of the summer but he did not come. One month after school started he walked into my office, and there wasn't one wart on his body. His skin was as smooth as silk, and the dark circles were gone from under his eyes. He told me what had happened. Seven weeks after we ended the treatment, he woke up in the morning and found that he could brush off the warts. Within one week all his warts were gone. He had no more problems with mold or pollen and has been around cats and other animals without any reaction. His mother was so impressed that she started treatment for herself.

The lists of allergens I have discussed in this chapter and others are simply examples. Patients should be tested and evaluated by a competent practitioner to find out exactly what their allergies and sensitivities are. Then they should observe responses, test possibilities, and research their own bodies.

C h a p t e r

18 | STAMINA

the "who" of me   is not defined by this body I live in.
Yet live in it I must.   And so must come to a breaking
away,   the breathing in and breathing out   of resistance
and letting go   Opening to the winds   The airing out
of what has been held onto   too long.
                    —from "Meridians of Longing"

Debbie

Debbie, 47, complained of bouts of chronic fatigue, including
sore throat and itching, that occurred every four months and
lasted for a few weeks. She was baffled by these attacks for
which she had tried a number of alternative therapies including liver cleanses and homeopathic remedies.

She also experienced hay fever and food allergies, particularly to peaches and potatoes.

On the fasting part of the abdominal diagnostic enzyme
evaluation exam, which was done in June at the end of one
of her bouts of itching and severe fatigue, I found a possible
thyroid reflex, but a basal temperature test showed up normal. I also found a positive reflex related to circulation, indicating that there might be a circulatory problem supported by
the fact that she had had trouble with hemorrhoids in the
past. I immediately prescribed an enzyme to enhance circulation (circ). An upper right quadrant inflammation suggested
liver toxicity, even though she had just completed a liver

cleanse. She also had trouble absorbing sugars, a calcium deficiency which indicated a possible allergy to calcium, an adrenal deficiency (which I suspected, with her chronic fatigue and itching), and slight irritability in the lower right colon suggesting constipation and possibly a Vitamin E deficiency and allergy.

On the nonfasting portion, I found that she was having trouble digesting fats, proteins, and sugars. The only foods she seemed to digest at all well were the complex carbohydrates. She did not experience any digestive problems per se; she simply noticed these cyclical bouts of fatigue.

I prescribed an enzyme for the complete digestion of fats, proteins, and sugars (hcl) and a liver enzyme for toxicity (lvr). I also considered prescribing an adrenal enzyme when we cleared B vitamins and a calcium enzyme when we cleared calcium, if she was allergic to it. On the urinalysis evaluation, I found an inability to digest sugars, a problem with fat or a slight excess of fat intake (which coincided with what I found on the palpation), a bicarbonate deficiency which again indicated a problem with sugars and starches, a Vitamin C deficiency, and a trace of protein and some positive nitrates in her urine which denoted either a kidney problem (although the kidneys looked fine) or the possibility that she had not refrigerated her sample adequately. Calcium was also quite low, which I had suspected.

Debbie turned out to be allergic to all the basic allergens except chicken and eggs. After we cleared the basics, I found some other important allergens that were relevant to her symptoms. The first was fungus which I always suspect when someone comes in with itching or skin problems. Debbie was allergic to about 50 molds and fungi, more than anyone I had ever worked with before. Most people have an allergy to an infectant like fungus, bacteria, or virus, which their body is constantly struggling with and which can create autoimmune problems including low-grade infections, fatigue, and arthritis. I also found her to be allergic to certain chemicals, weeds and shrubs, miscellaneous pollens, wheat, nuts and seeds, yeast,

herbs and spices, oils and fats, food additives, shellfi
some bacteria. Our goal was to clear these and then che
see how she was doing.

After a hiatus of about a month, when she was away on
vacation, I did some further testing and allergy elimination.
First I treated her for wheat, checking the whole wheat, wheat
germ, wheat bread, and white flour separately, as I always do.
Then I treated her for herbs and spices including stimulants
like garlic, and oils and fats. Next, I treated her for mold and
fungus which involved the usual precautions and the 10-day
follow-up diet. It took three treatments to clear them all. Then
she took a break from our work for another month. When she
returned, she reported that she had not had a single bout of
fatigue and related symptoms during that time. We still do not
know why she had the bouts of fatigue every four months, but
the important thing is that they stopped.

Fatigue is often the result of allergy reactions, poor digestion, and a buildup of toxins that slow the body down.
Most people react to low energy levels by drinking coffee, eating sugar, smoking cigarettes, or relying on other
drugs that give them a boost of energy. These short-term
solutions make the real problem worse, cause complications, and aggravate chronic health problems. The maintenance of high levels of energy is achieved by
eliminating allergies, improving digestion, absorption,
and assimilation, removing toxins from the body, and increasing nutrients. Good energy levels, stamina, and a resistance to aging are all by-products of optimum health
and homeostasis.

ENERGY LEVELS

There are many things that hinder the maintenance of
healthy energy levels. To determine the cause of low energy, I use an abdominal diagnostic palpation exam, an

enzyme evaluation exam that includes the twenty-four hour urinalysis, and muscle response testing. Many factors relating to energy levels show up on these tests.

Digestion

The first indicator is the efficiency of digestion and absorption of nutrients into the body. People can eat the best foods but if they do not digest or absorb them properly, they cannot benefit from them because they are not getting the vitamins and minerals necessary for the metabolic functions of the body and a healthy immune system.

Digestion is the key to high energy levels, and problems with digestion differ from individual to individual. Some people are sugar intolerant, some are fat intolerant, and some are complex carbohydrate intolerant. These intolerances show up in the urinalysis and palpation exams and can be treated with enzymes.

Impaired Thyroid Function

The next indicator is impaired thyroid function that can cause a decrease in energy because the thyroid influences many other metabolic processes, hormonal processes, and tissue function in the body. Impaired adrenal function can have similar effects. More will be discussed in the section on Thyroiditis.

Deficiencies and Allergies

Other possible causes of low energy levels include vitamin and mineral deficiencies resulting from poor absorption, allergies to foods and other allergens, poor liver function, an overgrowth of yeast, bacteria, or parasites in the gastrointestinal system, lack of sleep, insufficient exercise, and mental and emotional illnesses and imbalances. Fatigue can also be caused by other medical problems and serious pathologies. All possibilities should be checked.

In dealing with food and environmental allergies, it is helpful and appropriate to remove the allergenic foods from the diet and the environmental toxins from the patient's surroundings. Because some allergens are extremely difficult to avoid, however, treating with NAET is an important alternative to permanent avoidance. Often, the foods people are allergic to are the ones they like best. Food cravings are frequently connected to food allergies or to a deficiency of some nutrient. If the body is lacking in B vitamins, for example, the individual might crave grains and meat high in B vitamins.

By eliminating the allergies, often the cravings are eliminated as well. Over time, allergic reactions can inhibit good immune system function and impair energy levels and stamina. When the allergy is eradicated, the process of toxicity and immune system damage ends. Feeling tired after eating a particular food is a common experience that signals an allergy to that food. When a food allergy is cleared, a person feels a change of energy either immediately or within ten days.

Good digestion is critical to high energy levels. When undigested food gets into the bloodstream, it creates possible autoimmune reactions, autoaggressive disease, and severe immunosuppressive response that, in turn, causes vulnerability to infection. It also consumes essential metabolic enzymes needed to complete the process of digestion. The extra energy used in this process reduces the amount of energy gained from the food. This is one of the main causes of severe chronic fatigue.

DETOXIFICATION

Toxic buildup in the body is another common cause of fatigue. The toxins come from chemicals in our environment, food and environmental allergens, and by-products of the body's everyday metabolism. Smog and pesticides, food additives, alcohol, drinking water, medications, and drugs can poison our systems. Sometimes these toxic buildups occur because the organs of elimination—skin, colon, lungs, and kidneys—are not working properly. Detoxification requires healthy digestion and elimination and an awareness of what is put into the body. NAET can be a lifesaver for the detoxification process. Effective detoxification can be achieved through a combination of desensitization to environmental allergens, reduction in consumption of foods grown with pesticides, fungicides, and herbicides, and elimination of rancid fats, refined carbohydrates, and chemically prepared fats and margarine. Rancid oils, margarine, and fried foods contain partially hydrogenated oils that can interfere with the production of ATP, a substance in cellular metabolism that helps produce energy at the cellular level. Partially hydrogenated oils can also toxify the liver. Smoking and exposure to secondhand smoke should be avoided and water should be filtered to remove chemicals such as chlorine, fluorine, and other toxins. Finally, stimulants such as caffeine and sugars that lower energy, deplete vitamins and minerals such as potassium and weaken the immune system should be avoided.

The liver is an important organ in maintaining good energy levels and detoxifying the body. Good digestion, allergy elimination, and good nutrition keep the liver working optimally. In addition, the liver should be cleansed at least once or twice a year. I recommend the "Ultra Clear" program developed by Jeffrey Bland, one of the most thoroughly researched products of this type.

A liver detoxification program works particularly well after a person has been treated for the ten basic allergies. When those allergies have been cleared, the person experiences fewer side effects such as detoxification symptoms and the cleansing is quicker and more effective. Liver cleansing is highly recommended for anyone with energy and stamina problems and for those with chronic infections or degenerative diseases.

EXERCISE

Exercise is one of the most important factors in increasing energy levels because it brings more oxygen into the body through increased circulation. Higher oxygen levels help burn off sugars and fats in the body which, in turn, can increase energy levels. Exercise also increases circulation to the brain and stimulates the lymphatic system that removes toxins and aids digestion. Daily exercise can be revitalizing. People should develop their own exercise routines that work for them and not overdo it or overstimulate the body. The point is to stay in balance and thereby maintain good energy levels.

SKELETAL ALIGNMENT

Skeletal alignment is also a factor in maintaining energy levels. As a chiropractor I have had a lot of experience treating people for structural problems by aligning vertebrae and bones that are out of alignment. Misaligned bones affect nerve function and tissue and good muscle tone is essential for optimum energy. When a muscle is inflamed or a vertebra is out of alignment, there is an impeded flow of nerve impulses to the brain and back to the specific muscles, ligaments, and organs as well as poor circulation in that area. This reduces the amount of energy available in the body, no matter how healthy the diet, or how well the liver is cleansed. If there is a structural imbalance or abnormality, the energy does not flow through the body the way it should and it is impossible to exercise well. Correction of problems and proper maintenance through chiropractic care can restore good alignment and a healthy nervous system, basic necessities in achieving good energy levels.

YEAST, BACTERIA, FUNGI, AND PARASITES

Yeast, bacteria, fungi, and parasites in the intestinal system and bloodstream can overload the immune system and prevent it from dealing with other kinds of infections and illnesses. Two of the many symptoms of Candida or candidiasis (yeast infection) are fatigue and insomnia (refer to Chapter 10).

Sugar, simple carbohydrates, and alcohol all fuel the growth of this yeast; merely taking acidophilus, a bacteria that aids digestion, without changing the diet does not help with Candida infections. Using enzymes without NAET treatment does not work either. Both are essential and effective.

It is important to understand the importance and seriousness of these infections. Both sexes are capable of succumbing to them, and the infections—viral, bacterial, and fungal—can be passed back and forth sexually.

SLEEP

Sufficient and restful sleep are all important for good energy maintenance. Many people overwork and do not get enough rest. A great deal of repair work occurs during sleep: hormones are manufactured, glands are rejuvenated, and toxins are removed. When people do not get enough sleep, they use more stimulants to compensate for the insufficient rest. They need to understand, however, that the body cannot endure long hours of work and overstimulation forever.

Sleep is essential. When we are deprived of it, aging is accelerated and we burn out. Burnout can happen over a long period of time or in one day. People come into my office and say they used to be able to go, go, go, and thought nothing could happen. They were immune to the physical problems other people had. Overnight, they were suddenly unable to get out of bed and have been unable to function well for years. Or they might say they cannot work anymore and have no appetite.

Not everyone needs eight or nine hours of sleep a night, but people know what rest they need. When people wake up naturally, without an alarm clock, they have had the sleep they need. If they have to use an alarm to wake up, they probably need more sleep.

Some people are now using melatonin to help them sleep. I find that many people are allergic to the melatonin produced in their own bodies. Released during sleep, melatonin is thought to be an antiaging and antioxidant chemical. When treated for melatonin sensitivity, people can use their own melatonin rather than taking it orally. If there is no allergy, the body should be producing enough melatonin and other antioxidants and there should be no need to take an excessive amount. I prefer to have all nutrients, hormones, and other metabolic chemicals absorbed from the food of a good diet and from the body's natural production rather than from using supplements. By taking large amounts of supplements they are allergic to, people may do more harm than good.

MENTAL HEALTH

Mental health is important for all age groups because it is a product of homeostasis and freedom from allergies. When energy levels are low, people are more vulnerable to physical, mental, and emotional problems. When they are tired, it is difficult to relate, hard to function properly, or deal with everyday stresses. I know from experience, that by strengthening digestion, eliminating allergies with NAET, adjusting the diet, exercising, and receiving good chiropractic care, we can not only strengthen the body, but also reduce the impact of mental and emotional stresses. It is easier to have a positive point of view when one feels rested and energized.

When allergies are cleared, digestion and nutrition are improved, the body is detoxified, and the patient gets enough rest stable energy levels are generally easy to maintain. Some people need some forms of supplementation such as enzymes or thyroid or adrenal supplements. They might also use a green drink such as spirulina or blue-green algae that is not toxic to the system. When used in moderation, supplementation of this kind is helpful in conjunction with a good diet and efficient digestion.

Energy levels sometimes improve dramatically; more often they change slowly. After bodies have been abused with coffee, alcohol, and smoking, it takes time to restore adequate energy levels. I prefer to see the energy rebound slowly in order for the body to heal in its own time. I always do a post-treatment abdominal exam and allergy testing and there are usually remarkable changes, especially seen in the urinalysis.

Depression and feelings of anxiety ease as energy levels rise and the body detoxifies itself. With detoxification, stable energy levels can be established and maintained. Each person must pursue health on every level to maintain abundant energy throughout his or her life.

IV | ADJUNCTIVE THERAPY

19 | ENZYME THERAPY

If I returned to Italy, maybe I could swing in the breeze on the clothesline. Between my grandmother's nightgown and my great grandfather's socks. Swing from clothespins against a cloudless Mediterranean sky.
                                        —from "Café Venezia"

Sharon

Sharon, 46, had multiple sclerosis, and her symptoms included autoimmune problems, intermittent fatigue, and extreme periods where she was unable to get out of bed. She also experienced headaches, numbness, fainting spells, dizziness, low back pain, and heart palpitations, and she knew that she was intolerant to certain foods. Her primary concern was fatigue.

On the abdominal diagnostic enzyme evaluation exam, I noted some positive reflexes related to the liver and gallbladder area. A positive upper left quadrant reflex indicated that she had trouble absorbing sugars, and a positive kidney reflex corresponded to her low back pain. Many people with MS have concurrent back and disk problems, and many suffer from similar low back pain, sciatica, or leg weakness. I also found a positive reflex in the ascending and descending colon.

She suffered considerable abdominal swelling, suggesting a systemic yeast or fungus infection.

On the nonfasting part of the exam, I found her unable to tolerate sugars and proteins which would tend to cause problems with calcium absorption, a weakened immune system, yeast and fungus infections, and hypoglycemia. I prescribed three enzyme formulas: one for the digestion of proteins and sugars (hcl); another to support the spine which can be beneficial for people with disk problems (ivd); and a fungus reduction formula (AllerZyme C) to help relieve the abdominal swelling.

A 24-hour urinalysis corroborated many of the findings of the palpation exam. I found an alkaline pH, which can indicate chronic pain, difficulty with digesting and absorbing protein, poor absorption of sugars, and an inability of the kidneys to concentrate the urine properly. Because she needed to acidify her body slightly and activate the kidneys, I prescribed a kidney enzyme and an a enzyme to help digest protein since proper protein digestion helps restore urine to its normal pH.

Next, I began treating her for the basic allergies, in addition to doing some chiropractic work for her low back. After we completed calcium, I prescribed enzymes for calcium, Vitamin C, B vitamins, and minerals. After clearing the basics, I proceeded to treat her for certain other foods. Then I prescribed an adrenal enzyme to help with the absorption of sugars. I did some retesting and continued to treat for food allergens including animal and vegetable fat, coffee, caffeine, and vegetables. After we cleared some of the foods, her abdominal swelling diminished and her digestion improved remarkably. Her low back pain disappeared, and her spine became more flexible. Although she still had periods of fatigue throughout the day, her overall stamina began to increase.

In my research on MS, I learned that certain allergens are generally involved such as nuts, fats, chemicals, lactic acid, pesticides, certain fabrics, and heavy metals like mercury. Research has emphasized the importance of having MS patients get their mercury amalgams removed. However, I believe it is important to treat for mercury prior to removing it so the toxicity released into the body during the removal process does not deplete the person's energy. Most MS patients also tend to have problems with heat or other forms of radiation as well as vaccinations and antibiotics. We treated for mercury, heat, vaccinations, fabrics, lactic acid (found in milk), and certain other foods that tend to cause joint and muscle pain after exercising. Treating for lactic acid can eliminate this pain almost immediately.

Then I reviewed the basics, the foods, and a few other items and found that she was allergic to beans, some beverages, food additives, food coloring, fish, bacteria, fungus, and parasites. We treated for these in that order, and about a month after we cleared the infectants, I prescribed specific enzymes for fungus and a liver cleanse. Finally, we treated for MS itself. When we treated her for MS, we did so alone and in combination with DNA-RNA which allowed us to attack the genetic makeup of the disease. Then I checked to see if there was any other combination that needed to be treated. With women, hormones are often involved, and with MS there are often combinations with muscle and connective tissue.

Treatments like this do not get rid of MS, AIDS, or whatever other chronic problem is being addressed, but they help the body cope with the problem without being overwhelmed. This can be an ongoing process, and Sharon comes back every few months for a check-up. If there is nothing else to be treated, we do something to strengthen her body to cope with the MS. She has been doing very well, although she does have occasional periods of fatigue. With the help of her enzymes and certain supplements, she can resist infections, work a full day, and eat pretty much what she wants.

After many years of working with others, I am delighted to be able to share my own story. At forty-seven I am healthier now than I was twenty years ago. I owe this feeling of well-being to Dr. Howard Loomis who changed my life, my health, and my practice as a healer and taught me many mysteries and miracles of the human body.

Above all, he taught me about balance, homeostasis, and a healthy immune system.

MY PERSONAL EXPERIENCE WITH ENZYMES

For as long as I could remember, I suffered from digestive problems. I was constipated, bloated, tired, and depressed, especially at the end of a day of eating. No matter what I ate or when, how, or with whom, I would end up feeling as if I was three months pregnant. As a result, I always wore loose clothing with an elastic waist. When I was young, both my father and grandmother had complained of digestive problems. I assumed it was an inherited condition I would have to live with for the rest of my life.

In the seventies I became involved in healing with an emphasis on massage and polarity therapy. I went on to study homeopathy and nutrition with various doctors including Dr. Bernard Jensen at his ranch in Escondido, California. Refusing to believe that my problem and other digestive problems were all inherited, I was determined to find a solution. I studied every book about natural healing available at the time. I tried every vitamin, explored homeopathy, and experimented with diets including fasting. But nothing ever changed my digestive abnormalities. At times I despaired of ever finding the answer I was seeking.

After years of studying nutrition on my own, I decided to get a degree in chiropractic. My twin brother had gone into conventional medicine, but I was drawn to a more natural approach. Unlike medical school, chiropractic college offered a good course in diet and nutrition. I enrolled in 1972.

During my first year there, probably because of the stress of the study, my symptoms worsened. Everything I ate aggravated my digestion and I became severely constipated and bloated. At the chiropractic clinic affiliated with the school, I had X rays, barium studies and various blood tests, and I proceeded to do colonics, fasting, and food rotation. I remember doing a grape fast for almost three months. When I fasted, my symptoms seemed to improve slightly but I would relapse after I began to eat regular foods. I tried different chiropractic treatments, homeopathy, and other new diets. Nothing seemed to help.

After graduating from chiropractic school and practicing for a number of years, I decided to enroll in a three-year post-graduate chiropractic orthopedics training program. This course changed my life, my health, and my professional practice forever. It was here that I was introduced to enzyme therapy by one of my instructors and the work of Dr. Howard Loomis, a chiropractor and biochemist.

At my first seminar with Dr. Loomis I took exhaustive notes that I still read over from time to time. He began the seminar by saying, "The most profound thing we do every day is eat." He went on to explain that the body's ability to maintain homeostasis, crucial for the life of every cell, is based on its ability to digest what it eats. A twenty-four hour urinalysis examines how well the body digests and metabolizes food by looking at what the body discards and keeps. The body strives to resist change and withstand disease by maintaining its internal environment relatively constant. It does this, Loomis said, by keeping the intracellular fluid within certain narrow limits of temperature, volume, pH, and concentrations of various solutes. Laboratory tests can detect deviations from normal homeostasis.

"By definition," Loomis explained, "if blood chemistries are not normal, homeostasis has already been compromised and the body is evidencing exhaustion or an inability to adapt to an excessively strong or persistent stimulus. In order to prevent disease, this process must be identified before deviations in blood chemistry are evidenced."

Loomis told us that studies showed that significant digestion from salivary enzymes alone occur in the stomach before hydrochloric acid and pepsin begin their work. In fact, thirty-five to forty-five percent of starches can be digested before HCl is secreted. The problem is that we do not chew our food long enough to allow this to happen.

Loomis said, "Since the resting pH of the stomach is between 5.0 and 6.0, many nutritional and physiological tests do not consider predigestion in man to be significant. The enzymes in plants will work in a pH environment of 3.0–9.0 and continue digesting until inactivated in the stomach when the pH reaches 3.0. Therefore plant enzymes play a significant role in predigesting food, offering a solution to many acute and chronic digestive disorders, and a means of delivering food past an incompetent digestive system."

After his talk, Dr. Loomis performed an abdominal palpatory diagnostic evaluation and a twenty-four hour urinalysis on some of the doctors in the seminar, including me. The next day I helped him to analyze the urine so I could learn the lab work myself, and he helped me evaluate the test and compare it with the abdominal palpation exam. The purpose was to uncover enzyme and nutritional deficiencies and specific food intolerances. We discovered that I was carbohydrate intolerant, a poor assimilator of sugar, and that I was unable to digest foods containing sugars and other carbohydrates including grains and breads. We also saw that I had moderate bowel toxicity that showed I had some fermentation and putrefaction in the bowel and probably constipation. I was **hypoadrenal** and presented with a slight inflammation of the liver, and I was deficient in calcium, potassium, magnesium, and Vitamin C.

Dr. Loomis recommended I take an enzyme consisting of disaccharidase, cellulase, maltase, sucrase, and lactase to help me digest sugars and carbohydrates. He also recommended I take an enzyme for calcium, minerals, and Vitamin C and a bowel cleanser to help with the bowel toxicity. Two weeks after beginning the enzymes, the bloating and constipation I had experienced my whole life disappeared and they have never returned. It was miraculous!

After this total regeneration of my digestive system, I studied enzymes and enzyme therapy extensively with Dr. Loomis and began to utilize his work in my practice. I performed an abdominal palpation on each patient along with a twenty-four hour urinalysis. I then recommended enzymes and created diets for each individual based on their specific food intolerances. These diets can be found in Part VI of this book.

After careful study, trial, and error, I developed a sugar-intolerant diet for myself. I have found that eighty percent of the people who come to see me are sugar intolerant. Aside from bloating and constipation, sugar intolerance can lead to diabetes, adrenal dysfunction, asthma, hyperactivity, attention deficit, depression, fatigue, poor assimilation of foods, obesity or malnutrition, frequent sore throats, ear infections, and colds. Sugar intolerance can be responsible for **Crohn's disease**, an inability to tolerate lactose (milk sugar) and for **celiac disease**, an inability to tolerate gluten. Furthermore, it can also be responsible for chronic yeast infections and chronic food and environmental allergies. I suffered from many of these problems myself, and the sugar-intolerant diet I developed has changed my life. This diet is low in carbohydrates, grains, fruits, and sweet vegetables and high in protein. I recommend this diet for all sugar-intolerant people.

This regeneration occurred almost fifteen years ago and I continue to be grateful to Dr. Loomis' research and his enzyme formulas. Since I seem to have inherited this sugar intolerance, I will always need supplementation for the predigestion of sugars. Therefore, these enzymes are essential to my health and the health of many of my patients. Indeed, I believe enzymes have saved my life and made me a happier and healthier person. We will hear more and more about enzymes and their miracles in the twenty-first century. This book is only the beginning, and *Winning the War Against Asthma and Allergies* is only the beginning.

WHAT ARE ENZYMES?

Enzymes are complex proteins in the body that cause chemical changes in other substances in order to provide the labor force and energy necessary to keep us alive. They are energy catalysts that are essential to the successful occurrence of over 150,000 biochemical reactions in our bodies, particularly involving food digestion and the delivery of nutrients to the body. Enzymes help convert food into chemical substances that pass into cell membranes to perform all of our everyday life-sustaining functions. By supporting normal function, enzymes keep our immune system strong enough to fight off disease. Enzymes help to nourish and clean the body, making possible the human body's miraculous capacity for self-healing. They also make available the energy needed for a normal body to burn hundreds of grams of carbohydrate and fat every day. Without enzymes, life could not be sustained.

Enzymes perform so many important functions in the body that they have been called the basis of all metabolic activity. Some of their responsibilities are as follows:

1. Transform foods into muscles, nerves, bones, and glands.

2. Help to store excess nutrients in muscles or the liver for future use.

3. Help to rid carbon dioxide from the lungs.

4. Metabolize iron for utilization by the blood.

5. Aid in blood coagulation.

6. Decompose hydrogen peroxide and liberate healthful oxygen.

7. Attack toxic substances in the body so they can be eliminated, essential for patients with chronic health problems.

8. Help convert dietary phosphorus to bone.

9. Extract minerals from food for use.

10. Convert protein, carbohydrates, fats, vitamins, and nutrients for the body's use.

In other words, enzymes deliver nutrients, break down and carry away toxic waste, digest food, purify the blood, deliver hormones, balance cholesterol and triglyceride levels, feed the brain, build protein into muscle, and feed and fortify the endocrine system. They also contribute to immune system activity. White blood cells are especially enzyme-rich in order to digest foreign invading substances.

While one of the advantages of enzymes is that they can cause a chemical reaction without being destroyed or changed in the process, the number of enzymes we can produce is limited. Every person is born with an enzyme potential or number of enzymes he or she can produce in a lifetime. This number is determined by the DNA code. In addition, each enzyme can only perform a certain amount of work before it becomes exhausted and must be replaced by another. Along with digesting processed food, enzyme supply can be diminished by caffeinated and alcoholic beverages, colds and fevers, pregnancy, stress, strenuous exercise, injuries, and extreme weather conditions. If we do not eat an enzyme-rich diet, we deplete our enzyme potential without replenishing it. This is why supplementation and a good diet are essential. When all enzyme activity stops, the body stops functioning and the person dies. However, humans have the capacity to store external food enzymes to ensure the body's ability to metabolize the needed nutrients. This explains an abundance of new enzyme health products and the recommendations from experts that people supplement their diet with raw foods and manufactured food enzymes.

Enzymes save peoples lives by restoring energy and homeostasis, reversing the aging process, turning a dysfunctional digestive system into a healthy one, and strengthening the immune system. In my fifteen years of working with enzyme therapy, I have witnessed enormous success with a variety of illnesses. The most noticeable and immediate change in each case has always been in the energy level. Patients no longer feel that "crash" after meals, especially after lunch, the most common time.

Enzymes also have been utilized by many industries in various products and processes including laundry detergents, skin care, meat tenderizers, agricultural processes, and waste conversion.

WHAT IS THE FUNCTION OF ENZYMES?

When I began the study of enzymes many years ago, I encountered the phrase "acid-base balance." I did not really understand it until I met Dr. Howard Loomis and learned about the urinalysis and its nutritional evaluation. One of the first evaluations done on urine is the pH level, the degree of a solution's acidity or alkalinity. An alkaline pH is 7.0 or above; an acid pH is below 6.5. To maintain homeostasis, the blood has to have a neutral pH of 7.5. The body keeps it from becoming too alkaline or too acid by buffering it with hydrogen or bicarbonate ions. In doing this, it can rob the digestive system of substances necessary to digest foods or perform other tasks efficiently.

For example, an alkaline urine indicates that the blood does not have adequate quantities of hydrogen and chlorine to aid digestion in the stomach in the form of hydrochloric acid. This condition is called hypochlorhydria, or HCl deficiency, and is characterized by difficulty digesting protein and severe bloating immediately after eating. The opposite is true when the urine is acid: the blood is not capable of supplying enough bicarbonate ions to the pancreatic secretion for proper digestion of starches and fats.

Individuals with immune disorders usually have a chronically acid urine that leads to flatulence and bloating two hours after a meal. A twenty-four-hour urinalysis determines how the body compensates to maintain homeostasis. The pH is calculated over the twenty-four hour period because if urine is checked over the course of a day, the pH varies with waking and after meals. The twenty-four hour catch indicates the overall pH for an entire day and gives more accurate information on the compensations the body is presenting. This incredible tool provides information on tendencies toward certain illnesses and imbalances including respiratory problems, diabetes, anxiety, chronic bowel problems, and poor thyroid and adrenal function.

Stanley, a professional pilot, came to see me a few years ago suffering from chronic fatigue and chronic allergies that greatly affected his performance. He loved to fly but was afraid he would fail the physical and lose his job. I did a thorough evaluation and prescribed an enzyme for digestion and carbohydrate absorption. Within two weeks he had so much energy that his coworkers were amazed. He passed his physical easily. In fact, his physician said his health was better than it had ever been. By predigesting foods, enzymes save the body's energy to perform other metabolic functions effectively.

The pH is one aspect of the useful information the urinalysis provides. The urine pH also reflects a person's diet and basic dietary imbalances. For example, an alkaline pH is usually representative of a vegetarian who eats mostly vegetables and fruits and is perhaps deficient in grains, meats, eggs, and proteins. An alkaline urine can also represent more serious problems including insomnia and anxiety. On the other hand, an acid urine usually reflects an excess of protein in the diet and possibly a deficiency of vegetables and fruit. An acid urine causes sluggishness and lethargy. Respiratory acidosis, emphysema, and asthma produce a persistently acid urine by interfering with respiration and causing an accumulation of carbon dioxide in the body (pH below 6.0). Carbon dioxide becomes carbonic acid and the excess acid causes a loss of hydrogen in the urine. The body holds bicarbonate to buffer the acidity, and the loss of hydrogen limits HCl production for proper digestion. If it is possible to discover this aspect of the nutritional makeup early on, a person can be given enzymes that prevent chronic diseases. We treat people both to prevent and to heal existing immune disorders.

For example, when the pH of the urine is high or alkaline, it seems that hydrogen is being lost in the urine or it is low, and the body is in a state of alkalosis. This occurs because of inadequate protein digestion or low intake of protein, commonly seen in vegetarians. This metabolic situation can cause tetany or muscle cramping, nervousness, anxiety, and insomnia. It also can mimic an autoimmune reaction, possible symptoms similar to fibromyalgia. Enzyme therapy, to help the body digest protein, is paramount.

Bob, age fifty-three, came to see me recently for chronic insomnia. He had been on medication for over nine years. Because of the severe side effects of the medication, he went to see an Asian physician and herbalist in New Mexico who helped him to get off drugs and detoxify his body. Unfortunately, his insomnia slowly returned, and with one to two hours sleep a night, he became weaker and more depressed each day. Palpation showed poor protein and fat utilization and digestion as well as low levels of calcium. A urinalysis revealed a pH of 8.1, metabolic alkalinity, indicating a nervous individual with possible insomnia. We put him on enzyme supplements to lower his pH, raise his calcium, and help digest protein and fats. Within two to three weeks he began to sleep five to six hours a night. Today he sleeps six to seven hours without interruption and is able to function with clarity and peace of mind.

WHY DO WE NEED ENZYMES?

Enzymes enable our bodies to digest the food we eat. They break down the various foods we consume—proteins, fats, carbohydrates, vitamins—into smaller compounds that the body can absorb. They are absolutely essential in maintaining optimal health.

Enzymes are present naturally in raw foods but are destroyed in the cooking process. It is important to eat as much raw food as possible, to subject food to as little heating as possible, and to chew food well because enzyme production begins in the mouth. Because we often fail to follow these guidelines, we do not receive all the enzymes we need to do the job of digestion. Enzyme supplements provide the missing pieces.

Maintaining the body's enzyme levels is critical today when so much of the food in a typical American diet is processed or cooked, as much as eighty-five percent according to recent studies. Enzymes are only found naturally in raw foods such as vegetables and fruits that contain the very enzymes needed to digest them. Food enzymes are extremely heat sensitive, especially at or above temperatures of 118 degrees Fahrenheit. When raw foods are processed or heated in any way (steamed, baked, boiled, stewed, fried, microwaved, canned), they may lose one hundred percent of their enzyme activity and up to eighty-five percent of their vitamin and mineral content. Even the raw food we eat could be enzyme deficient if it was grown in nutrient-lacking soil. In addition, enzyme deterioration begins the moment the food is picked or killed. For all these reasons, supplementing with enzymes is crucial to achieve a more efficient digestive process and better utilization of our food's nutrients.

When digestion is not properly completed, partially digested proteins putrefy, partially digested carbohydrates ferment, and partially digested fats turn rancid. These toxins remain in the body, harming the system. Fermented toxins in the digestive tract can be absorbed into the blood and deposited as waste in the joints and other soft-tissue areas.

The results of enzyme deficiency include digestive disturbance, fatigue, headaches, constipation, gas, heartburn, bloating, colon problems, excess body fat, and problems as serious as cardiovascular or heart disease. Enzyme deficiencies have been linked to premature aging and degenerative diseases as well. Research has also shown that white blood cells are increased to compensate for an enzyme-deficient diet. Making use of the immune system to aid in digestion whenever enzymes are lacking compromises the body's ability to defend itself from disease.

Digestion has first priority on the limited number of internal enzymes available; metabolic enzymes must be satisfied with whatever is left. When food enzymes are introduced from outside the body, the body does not need to manufacture as many digestive enzymes, allocating more of the enzyme potential toward the production of the metabolic enzymes needed for growth, maintenance, and repair. Studies have shown that diets deficient in enzymes cause a thirty percent reduction in animal life span and low enzyme levels are associated with old age and chronic diseases. Cancer research has discovered that certain enzymes are completely lacking in the blood and urine of cancer patients.

When we eat food that is devoid of enzymes, the body must draw on its own internal supply of enzymes, both metabolic and digestive. Eventually we deplete our limited reserves, forcing the immune system to aid in digestion instead of rebuilding the body and fighting illness. The pancreas, salivary glands, stomach, and intestines all might contribute the enzymes needed for digestion, robbing the body of metabolic enzymes needed for muscles, nerves, blood, and other glands.

Enzyme supplements help create more energy, promote faster and easier digestion, and encourage superior nutrient absorption. It is the responsibility of our digestive system to release the nutrients that are trapped in our food by breaking the food down. But our digestive system works best when enzyme supplements assist in setting the nutrients free for the body to absorb and use. Receiving all the nutrients in the food we eat is critical, because these nutrients are needed to build and repair the body's tissue, produce energy, and maintain a strong immune system.

In my practice I see many patients with chronic food intolerances. For example, people can inherit or develop intolerances to proteins, sugars, fibers, complex carbohydrates, or fats. These patients lack the enzymes they need to break down the food that causes them trouble. Through palpation examination and testing (described at the end of this chapter), I am able to ascertain which foods a person cannot tolerate and which enzymes they should take as supplements to restore homeostasis. With the proper enzyme supplements, these patients regain the ability to digest their food properly and thoroughly. Human saliva contains the necessary factors needed to activate plant enzymes in the food we eat but because we fail to chew foods well, we are unable to digest foods. We need to chew each mouthful at least seventy times for complete predigestion!

Protein Intolerance

People who do not digest proteins crave sugars. They tend to experience anxiety, osteoporosis, edema, eye or ear inflammation, endometriosis, or bone spurs. Many of these patients also have an allergy to calcium that further promotes osteoporosis. When one is allergic to particular minerals or vitamins, he or she is usually low in those same minerals or vitamins.

Carla, age fifty, came to see me with a family history of osteoporosis and arthritis. Two years ago she was screened for osteoporosis and the results suggested she might have already developed the disease. She was advised to eat dairy products and take 1,500 mg. of calcium daily. After two years she was tested again and the results were even worse. She also complained of bloating and indigestion. Worried, upset, and afraid, she came to me for a nutritional consultation. An abdominal diagnostic enzyme exam, twenty-four hour urinalysis, and complete allergy test were performed. The results showed that she was deficient in calcium and allergic to calcium and the dairy products she had been eating. After putting her on an enzyme for the digestion of sugars that would help ease the dairy allergy, I treated her with NAET for calcium and dairy and prescribed calcium supplements with her enzymes. In one year her test results were significantly better. I often wonder how many of the millions of women taking calcium supplements to prevent osteoporosis and arthritis are allergic to it.

Sugar Intolerance

People who are sugar intolerant tend to crave protein and suffer from depression, malabsorption, bloating, acute food allergies, hyperactivity, Crohn's disease, asthma, chronic ear infections, and constipation. They usually are very allergic to B vitamins as well.

Starch, Fiber, or Fat Intolerance

People who are starch and fiber intolerant tend to crave fat and suffer from spastic colons, high blood fats, obesity, irritable bowel, ulcerative colitis, and occasionally constipation. People who are fat intolerant tend to crave sugar and suffer from eczema, liver and gallbladder disease, and toxicity.

TYPES OF ENZYMES

There are three main categories of enzymes: metabolic, digestive, and food.

Metabolic Enzymes

Metabolic enzymes are produced internally and are responsible for running the body at the level of the blood, tissues, and organs. They are required for the growth of new cells and the repair and maintenance of all the body's organs and tissues. Metabolic enzymes take protein, fat, and carbohydrates and transform them into the proper balance of working cells and tissues. Metabolic enzymes also remove worn-out material from the cells and keep them clean and healthy.

Digestive Enzymes

Digestive enzymes also are produced internally and deal with the digestion of food and the absorption and delivery of nutrients throughout the body. The most commonly known digestive enzymes are secreted from the pancreas into the stomach and small intestine. Each enzyme is specific to a particular compound which it can break down or synthesize. The three most important enzymes for digestion are protease, amylase, and lipase. They digest protein, carbohydrate, and fat, respectively.

Food Enzymes

Food enzymes, the only ones produced externally, are derived solely from raw fruits, raw vegetables, and supplements. They help the digestive enzymes break down food. Food enzymes must also have the presence of vitamins and minerals, called coenzymes, for proper functioning. Unlike raw enzymes, coenzymes are not completely destroyed by cooking. Because raw food enzymes become useless after heat processing, coenzymes in our diet are not utilized to their full potential.

Enzymes perform best at a certain pH. For example, animal enzymes perform best at a pH of 6.5–9.0. On the other hand, plant enzymes have a broader pH range of 3.0–9.0. I prefer to use plant enzymes because they can survive transport through the acid pH of the stomach (pH 2.0) and can be used in the pancreas and small intestine to further digestion.

Some of the reported benefits of consuming food enzymes are the elimination of:

- heartburn
- bloating
- gas
- constipation or loose bowels
- colon problems
- overweight and underweight problems
- headaches
- food allergies
- hay fever
- fatigue after meals
- stress
- weakened immune system

Some people have claimed that supplemental enzymes cannot survive the strong acids in the stomach. However, manufacturers reply that these enzymes might disintegrate when mixed with acid in a laboratory test tube but not in a living human body. The stomach normally allows salivary, food, and supplementary enzymes to digest food for up to an hour after eating. When they have finished their job of performing predigestion, food and supplementary enzymes that function at a low pH continue digestion of protein, carbohydrate, and fat for a longer time than salivary or pancreatic enzymes. As the stomach acid level increases, the acid enzyme pepsin continues the digestion of protein where the others left off. This information has been elicited after the stomach and upper intestinal contents have been pumped out and examined at various intervals following meals.

Some of the products on the market have a natural enteric coating to protect the enzymes from stomach acids thereby allowing them to pass through the stomach into the small intestines for assimilation. Taking enzymes on an empty stomach minimizes the presence of damaging stomach acids.

The following list contains the names of the main digestive enzymes that are used therapeutically to help restore the body's homeostasis and strengthen the immune system, along with a brief description of each enzyme's function:

Protease breaks down protein into amino acids; acts on pathogens such as bacteria, viruses, and cancer cells; works best in the high acidity of the stomach; also found in pancreatic and intestinal juices.

Amylase breaks down carbohydrates (starches) into simpler sugars such as dextrin and maltose; found in our saliva, pancreas, and intestines; secreted by the salivary glands and the pancreas.

Lipase along with bile from the gallbladder, breaks down fats into glycerol and fatty acids and the oil-soluble Vitamins A, D, E, and F; helpful in losing weight and for cardiovascular conditions.

Cellulase   breaks down fiber and cellulose found in fruits, vegetables, grains, seeds, and plant material; increases the nutritional value of fruits and vegetables; foods high in cellulose must be chewed well to allow cellulase to do its work to prevent putrefaction, bloating, and gas.

Pectinase   breaks down pectin-rich foods such as citrus fruits, apples, carrots, potatoes, beets, and tomatoes.

Lactase   breaks down lactose, the complex sugar in milk products; ideal for lactose-intolerant individuals; production usually decreases with age; NAET treatment for lactose combined with lactase enzyme effectively takes care of lactose intolerance.

Cathepsin   breaks down meat from animals.

Antioxidant enzyme   protects us from the negative effects of free radicals, highly reactive compounds that can damage almost any cell in the body.

Bromelain   breaks down food protein into smaller peptones by hydrolysis; helps the body to fight cancer, improves circulation, and treats inflammation; after a musculoskeletal injury it can reduce inflammation as well as, or even better than, any anti-inflammatory drug; said to improve the effect of some antibiotics; assists in the absorption of nutrients from foods and supplements; reduces swelling after dental surgery and helps in dysmenorrhea; increases tissue permeability; prevents the narrowing of arteries that contributes to heart attacks.

Papain   breaks down food protein into smaller peptones by hydrolysis; aids the body in digestion.

Glucoamylase   breaks down maltose (the sugar in all grains that may cause cravings for breads and carbohydrates) into two glucose molecules, allowing greater absorption of this energy-giving sugar.

Invertase helps to assimilate and utilize sucrose, a sugar that contributes to digestive stress if not properly digested.

Catalase breaks down hydrogen peroxide to water and oxygen. It is found in almost every cell. Catalase plays an important role in immune function. It destroys any hydrogen peroxide that forms in the cell. Hydrogen peroxide is formed during energy production. If one is deficient in catalase, hydrogen peroxide builds up and is very toxic to the cell.

Some herbs also aid digestion. Aloe vera provides relief from peptic ulcers and helps with constipation, and slippery elm is good for hiatal hernias and acid reflux. Both are common symptoms in asthmatics.

THERAPEUTIC USE

One of the most common complaints I hear from my patients is "I don't have enough energy." Before I discovered enzymes, I had no response. Now I know they can change the situation immediately. For the most part, low energy occurs because people are not digesting their food properly and they cannot benefit from the energy that food provides. Instead of deriving the needed enzymes directly from the food itself, the body has to borrow enzymes from metabolism. Energy is required to accomplish this. In fact, digesting food without an adequate amount of enzymes actually uses more energy than the food provides. Reversing this situation can free up the body's energy for other tasks because the stealing of enzymes from other parts of the body causes certain metabolic dysfunctions as the enzymes are distributed among other organs and tissues. Chronic degenerative diseases, as well as energy depletion, can be the result of metabolic dysfunction.

The regular consumption of enzyme supplements brings numerous positive benefits in terms of ongoing general health, including:

- the prevention of toxic waste buildup in the intestines

- more efficient assimilation of fats and proteins in the body

- more comfortable and efficient absorption of nutrients

- more comfortable digestion of large amounts of carbohydrates

- accelerated digestive process because of catalyzation from enzymes

According to Dr. Edward Howell who researched the effect of enzymes for more than fifty years, it is very likely that every degenerative disease could have its origin in a raw food enzyme deficiency. In response to this research, enzyme advocate William E. Frazier, M.H.P, N.C. remarked, "Not to realize that most, if not all, degenerative diseases are traceable to a common denominator, and that common denominator being the food that we eat for nourishment, is an insult to human intelligence." In my fifteen years of practice with enzyme therapy, I have seen many different illnesses helped by the addition of enzymes.

Digestive Aids

After a large meal, one might notice a sudden feeling of sluggishness and energy loss. The body is faced with an overload of calories and nutrients to break down and deliver to the bloodstream. If the food eaten was cooked, there are no enzymes included to assist in the energy-consuming task of digestion. If an enzyme supplement is taken at the beginning of a meal, the body is armed and prepared to handle the new food entering the digestive system. Without this additional supply of enzymes, it can take the body up to sixty minutes to gather the needed enzymes, sometimes borrowing them from other metabolic processes. When supplemental food enzymes are used, time and energy is conserved, allowing for more complete absorption of nutrients from the food consumed. When enzymes are taken between meals, they are absorbed into the bloodstream and distributed throughout the body instead of being used for digestion.

ENZYMES AND THE IMMUNE SYSTEM

Enzymes play a vital role in building and strengthening a healthy immune system, one of my major goals when working with patients. A strong immune system enables a body to be less vulnerable to viruses, bacteria, parasites, and other toxic invaders. It also helps the body stay healthy during times of stress or when a complete and balanced diet is not followed.

Circulating Immune Complexes (CICs)

According to the theories of Dr. Anthony Cichoke, a well-known enzyme therapist, when digestion is poor and substantial amounts of food remain undigested, these undigested food residues seep into the bloodstream. There they are viewed as antigens and quickly become attached to tiny antibodies and form antigen-antibody complexes known as circulating immune complexes (CICs). These tiny immune complexes float freely in the blood or the lymph until they are eaten by the large macrophages, the "Pac Men" of the body. If these CICs are overlooked by the macrophages, or if chemotherapeutic drugs, steroids, or excessive antibiotics suppress the macrophages, the CICs grow in size and latch themselves onto body tissue. Then the backup immune defense system, T and B cells produced by the bone marrow, start destroying their own tissue cells in an attempt to destroy the CICs. Unfortunately, the body's noble effort backfires and an autoimmune response occurs, creating inflammation, redness, and swelling. Glomerulonephritis, colitis, arthritis, fibromyalgia, migraines, asthma, and Hashimoto's thyroiditis are examples of autoimmune activity at work. Certain enzymes, especially protease, can break up the CICs. When I put an individual on protease (trauma), the immune system is enhanced and there is an immediate decrease in chronic bacterial, viral, and fungal infections.

Inflammation

Characterized by heat, redness, swelling, and pain, inflammation has a variety of possible causes from a minor cut or sunburn to a major infection such as appendicitis. All inflammatory conditions respond well to enzyme therapy. Inflammation is a sign that many bodily processes are occurring in sequence. The first is the body's fight against the infection, the second is the reparation of the destructive tissue, and the third phase of the inflammation process is the clearing and cleaning up of debris and dead tissue.

Whenever there is an injury, there is an invasion of white blood cells to repair and clean up the area. These white blood cells circulate in the blood and lymph all the time. During the dynamic process of inflammation and repair, blood flows to the area, causes blood clots, and obstructs blood flow that, in turn, causes swelling and oozing. A barrier of fibrin is formed to encircle the area of inflammation.

Supplemental enzymes such as proteolytic enzymes (trauma enzyme) and amylase can help bring more oxygen to the area and reduce swelling by breaking up the fibrous tissue and eating up the dead and infected tissue. This speeds healing and reduces pain. Enzymes remove foreign bodies such as bacteria, viruses, and other microorganisms and help to clean up the area so new nerve tissue and new cells can be formed.

Both acute and chronic inflammation are helped with the use of enzymes. Taking high amounts of amylase (mscle enzyme) with bromelain reduces inflammation. Many acute inflammatory processes such as colitis can become chronic when there are repeated cycles of damage and repair. Enzymes, by restoring digestion, cleansing the area, and preventing the formation of circulating immune complexes and autoaggressive reactions, can be beneficial to sufferers of colitis, Crohn's disease, and irritable bowel syndrome. In conventional medicine, cortisone therapy is often used to treat chronic inflammatory problems such as Crohn's. Cortisone helps stop inflammation but in the long run, makes the situation worse because it blocks the body's natural immune function. Bacteria, parasites, fungi, or other pathogens cause irritation and continue to destroy and invade the body, but the immune system is paralyzed by the cortisone and unable to fight. Even though the inflammation is curtailed, the pathogenic process still prevails and can worsen, causing more irritation and other autoimmune problems. Unlike cortisone, enzymes do not inhibit the immune system. Instead, they promote the healing process by attacking the pathogens and ultimately reducing swelling and inflammation. Enzyme preparations can be used to treat a wide variety of chronic inflammatory conditions including candidiasis, bronchitis, asthma, bacterial infections, kidney infections, ear infections, sinusitis, herpes zoster, and herpes simplex 1 and 2.

Asthma

Antioxidant supplements and enzyme therapy have been used to strengthen the immune system of asthmatics. Dr.

Howard Loomis and I have both observed that most children are sugar intolerant, not surprising given that the annual sugar consumption in the United States is now 150 pounds per capita. In fact, recent studies indicate that eighty percent of the population is sugar intolerant. Sugar intolerance involves all sugars including sugars found in fruits, vegetables, and grains and artificial sugars such as sorbitol, Equal®, NutraSweet®, and mannitol. Chronic fatigue syndrome (CFIDS) is frequently characterized by a B vitamin deficiency, caused by an overabundance of sugar and an allergy to B vitamins.

Linda and Neil, eight-year-old twins with chronic ear infections, came to see me a few years ago. A thorough enzyme evaluation indicated they were sugar intolerant. I took them off all refined sugar, limited their intake of grains and fruits, and prescribed large amounts of amylase and protease. Their chronic bouts with ear infections almost disappeared entirely, and their wheezing and coughing stopped completely.

Arthritis

Osteoarthritis is a degenerative joint disease characterized by pain, heat, and swelling. Rheumatoid arthritis is a systemic disease of unknown origin with similar symptoms.

Rheumatoid arthritis is thought to be related to the invasion of the joints by circulating immune complexes and the autoimmune reactions that occur as a result. By interrupting the immune complexes and causing their elimination from the body, enzymes—particularly protease, bromelain, and lipase—can be extremely beneficial in reducing symptoms and restoring a balanced life.

Enzyme therapy, in conjunction with NAET treatments for allergies, can also benefit those with osteoarthritis. In particular, I focus on allergies to foods that have an acid by-product such as meats, nightshade family vegetables, certain fruits, and sugars. I also treat bacteria as an allergy in working with arthritis and other joint problems. Enzymes that digest proteins and sugars can also be helpful as can lipase (for fats) and protease. Lipase also helps soothe the inflammation.

Jan, a woman in her fifties, came to see me with chronic severe hip pain and stiffness. She had tried everything from anti-inflammatory drugs to homeopathy and acupuncture with no relief. Reluctant to depend on drugs, she decided to see me for nutritional and enzyme evaluation. My examination revealed that she was sugar intolerant, hypothyroid, deficient in the essential minerals potassium, phosphorus, calcium, and magnesium, deficient in Vitamin C, and very acidic (low pH). I immediately gave her a sugar-digesting enzyme and created a diet low in sugar and acid forming foods. I treated her with NAET for calcium, Vitamin C, and acid from the acid-producing foods. Within days of rigorously adhering to the diet and taking the enzymes, she was free of stiffness and pain and looked ten years younger. Needless to say, she was elated.

After one year, she is doing quite well. Because her hip joint had already degenerated, she might have to have it replaced. But in the meantime, she can continue to work and enjoy participating in her children's activities without distraction.

Hypoglycemia

Hypoglycemia (low blood sugar) has a number of causes and eating protein is not always the answer. In fact, the most common cause of hypoglycemia is a problem with protein consumption. Fifty percent of the protein we consume is converted to sugars in the body to provide nourishment and energy. When intolerant of or allergic to protein, the body cannot utilize the amino acids needed to make sugar, and we become hypoglycemic. We must digest and tolerate protein in order to make use of the amino acids. Although elimination of the allergy or intolerance to protein is crucial, enzymes, particularly protease, can also be helpful.

Sugar intolerance or allergy is also important in understanding hypoglycemia. If one cannot digest and absorb the sugars, then hyperglycemia (high blood sugar) and hypoglycemia can develop. When blood sugar levels are too high as a result of overconsumption and poor digestion of sugar, the pancreas secretes too much insulin that brings blood sugar levels crashing. Ultimately, this can exhaust the pancreas and cause diabetes.

Cathy, a twenty-six-year-old aerobics instructor, came to see me for severe hypoglycemia. She had moments of low energy during the day that created difficulties conducting her classes. She turned out to be both protein intolerant and protein deficient. I prescribed an enzyme high in protease and treated her for her allergies to sugar and amino acids. Her hypoglycemia disappeared, her day-to-day energy level was restored, and those dark circles under her eyes vanished.

Environmental Toxins

Toxins in our environment, chemotherapy treatment, radiation, and unhealthy lifestyles contribute to the breakdown of the immune system. Enzymes interrupt the damage and inflammation to the immune system that go along with these stresses.

Prevention of Aging

By observing my patients, I have come to believe that enzymes help retard the aging process by breaking up the circulating immune complexes and restoring energy and vitality. People feel more vibrant and have more clarity after working with enzymes. I can see changes almost immediately when my patients begin enzyme therapy. A healthy diet not properly assimilated cannot benefit the body and keep it vital.

Women's Health

Enzymes play a role in many health issues affecting women such as PMS, unpleasant symptoms of menopause, vaginal infections, fibrocystic breasts, endometriosis, menstrual irregularities, and infertility.

The Endocrine System

Enzymes play an important role in maintaining normal, healthy adrenal and thyroid glands by reducing autoimmune reactions and conserving the metabolic enzymes needed for glandular function.

Other Systems

Enzymes help maintain a proper electrolyte balance by regulating the retention of water. Enzymes are excellent for reducing swollen lymph nodes and the fatigue related to lymphatic congestion. Enzymes also prevent the formation of kidney and gallstones by breaking up the oxalic acid that is the most common cause. In this case, NAET can be used as a complimentary therapy to help desensitize a person to oxalic acid and calcium. When a person is allergic to these nutrients, their absorption ability is reduced and there is a crystallization of calcium and oxalates and a formation of stones.

Intestinal Toxemia

Intestinal toxemia causes many symptoms, among which are fatigue, allergies, asthma, arthritis, nervousness, gastrointestinal conditions, impaired nutrition, skin disturbances, low back pain, sciatica, and many more. By restoring proper digestion, enzymes prevent intestinal toxemia and help restore normal intestinal flora.

A diet high in protein causes a predominance of proteolytic putrefactive bacteria in the intestine that produce toxic compounds, some of which are absorbed. If these compounds are incompletely detoxified by the liver, they enter the systemic circulation and cause or aggravate many diseases. The products of the putrefactive flora include indole and skatole from tryptophan, phenol from tyrosine, and hydrogen sulfide from the products of protein breakdown. A widely used measure of intestinal putrefaction is the amount of indican (a form of indole) in the urine. Skatole formed from bacterial action on tryptophan causes bad breath.

Histamine, another toxic decomposition by-product of tryptophan, causes headaches, head congestion, nervous depression, and nausea. Tyramine, a toxin decomposed from tyrosine, can cause high blood pressure.

When I was a young student of nutrition, I studied with Dr. Bernard Jensen. His lectures always included a discussion of intestinal toxemia (bowel toxicity) which he believed was the cause of many chronic health problems. Because the intestines were the hub of the body, he taught, a toxic colon could leak toxins into the bloodstream and cause anything from arthritis to early aging and cancer.

A seventy-year-old friend of mine named John came to see me about five years ago with frequent urination, pain, and burning associated with urination. A complete twenty-four hour urinalysis and abdominal diagnostic exam revealed that his pH was 4.5 and his indican level was 14, the highest I had ever seen. The indican measure usually represents a value that has been there for many years. His bowel toxicity had been poisoning his system for a long time and I suspected he had bladder cancer. Because he had other serious problems beyond my level of expertise, I referred him to another practitioner. He died a year later of bladder cancer. I always wonder had we done the test earlier and corrected his condition with enzymes, would things have turned out differently? Bowel toxicity is usually an inherited condition but it can certainly be reversed with enzymes and dietary changes.

A twenty-four hour urine test is a useful nutritional assessment of chronic enzyme deficiencies and digestive intolerances. It is effective in evaluating intestinal toxemia and excess protein, sugar, or fat in the urine that reflect poor digestion. It analyzes assimilation, calcium and vitamin deficiencies, as well as kidney, adrenal, and thyroid activity. With all these clues to a person's nutritional makeup, we can detect a predisposition to diabetes, heart disease, osteoporosis, and thyroid and adrenal dysfunction. The supplementation of enzymes to a proper level can help prevent these chronic problems in the future.

When the integrity of the bowel itself becomes compromised through bowel toxicity and fermentation, it allows foreign toxins and antigens to "leak" through the gut into the circulation and lymphatic system. This condition is called "leaky gut syndrome." This syndrome can lead to the formation of CICs, and produce inflammatory immune response and autoimmune diseases. For example, it can lead to chronic fatigue and fibromyalgia. Therefore, a primary matter in working with immune disorders is to prevent a "leaky gut," as well as repair one. Digestive enzymes are truly the most important preventative and healing tools for this problem. More will be discussed about this problem in the chapter on NAET.

Parasites

Enzymes help the body rid itself of parasites. With the addition of magnesium and other herbs, parasites can be eliminated as well as prevented.

Herpes and Other Viruses

I have used protease in treating children's illnesses such as runny nose, sore throat, and flu-like symptoms. Early detection and treatment with enzymes eliminates trouble-some viruses, including herpes, and prevents recurrence. Because enzymes prevent infections, my family and I take protease every day.

Whenever a child or an adult reports any symptoms of infection, I immediately give them high doses of protease every half hour until their symptoms subside. I also recommend NAET treatment with their own saliva every two to five hours (refer to the Self-Treatment section of Chapter 5). This usually eliminates the symptoms and prevents further complications or the progression of the infection.

Skin and Joint Problems

Enzyme therapy controls and treats psoriasis, eczema, joint swelling, and back problems. As a chiropractor, I have seen how enzyme therapy (protease, bromelain, lipase) speeds up recovery when used to treat sprains, strains, misalignments, swelling, and inflammation.

Margo, a woman in her twenties, came to see me for severe psoriasis, a condition she had been plagued with her whole life. After a thorough enzyme evaluation, I found that her pH was very acid (indicating an inability to digest fats and oils), chronic Candida, and another fungus. I recommended an enzyme (bil) for digesting fats (high lipase), a liver enzyme (lvr), and an acidophilus enzyme (sml) with cellulase for Candida, fungi, and intestinal toxemia. After eight months her psoriasis had almost completely disappeared. She has been on enzymes for years now and her condition is hardly noticeable. She would never be without her enzymes. They changed her life.

Chronic Diseases

Autoimmune diseases such as Crohn's disease, colitis, lung disorders, and systemic Candida infections all react to enzyme therapy. Enzymes restore digestion and free up a compromised immune system. Then those living defender cells can do their job fighting organisms and maintaining a clean inner environment, one that is not involved with diseases such as heart disease, malignancies, skin problems, low and high blood sugar, stomach and colon pains, eye trouble, and headaches. Enzymes destroy toxins and free radicals and antigens in the liver and bloodstream.

Research has found that the impaired ability of an enzyme to protect against free radicals may lead to damage to motor neurons in the brain and spinal cord. This research sheds some light on nervous systems disorders such as Parkinson's disease and ALS (Lou Gehrig's disease). Researchers now report early promise in treating a devastating childhood immune deficiency disease with injections of a manufactured form of the missing enzyme that causes the disease. In addition, recent research in Germany has found that MS can be held in check and in some cases improved through the use of enzyme therapy. Children previously treated unsuccessfully for acute lymphoblastic leukemia have achieved complete or partial remission with a newly developed enzyme: one hundred percent of the young patients responded favorably to treatment.

Allergies

Many allergies today are actually related to a lack of certain enzymes needed to digest the substance that causes the allergic reaction. Joint pain and gout often result from undigested proteins, fats, and minerals that form uric crystals that get caught in the joints. Yeast and fungal growth starts with undigested foods in the bloodstream and can be compounded by the white flour and sugar we eat. Extreme fatigue might be a consequence of an inability to digest proteins and fats that cause poor circulation. When blood cells clump together, they cannot carry as much oxygen which leads to slow and muddled thinking. It is also more difficult for white blood cells to travel where they are needed.

Proteolytic and lipolytic enzymes found in some supplements help break down unwanted toxins and irritants partially responsible for allergies and inflammation. The enzymes break the toxic substances into smaller, more manageable components that are then eliminated from the body.

Higher Energy

About half of the body's energy is spent digesting food. Studies find a definite correlation between the amount of enzymes a person has and their energy level. For example, athletes who take enzyme supplements have been able to work out more often with greater intensity and require less recovery time.

Obesity

There is a connection between eating a diet full of cooked, enzyme-deficient food and problems with excessive weight. Raw foods rich in enzymes aid the body in reaching and maintaining its normal weight and firmness. I have had wonderful results with enzyme therapy. Correcting digestive intolerances with enzymes and adjusting the diet based on the specific food intolerances help with either weight reduction or weight gain, whichever is desired.

Doctors throughout the United States have been researching the effects of plant enzymes on various clinical conditions including poor digestion, malabsorption, pancreatic insufficiency, celiac disease, lactose intolerance, arterial obstruction, and thrombotic disease. Results have shown that enzymes are effective for treating a wide range of conditions.

THE VALUE OF ENZYMES AND ANTIOXIDANTS

According to Hippocrates, "Man is not nourished by what he swallows, but by what he digests and uses." With the increasing pollution and depletion of healthy soil, the foods we eat today have only a fraction of the nutrition our ancestors consumed in centuries past. At the same time, we now have an advanced technology that allows us to replenish the nutrients we lose through food processing by producing enzyme supplements to be taken with every meal. Once known only to alternative health professionals, enzyme therapy has achieved such amazing results (measured by patient evaluations as well as by microscopic blood analysis) that the treatment has recently excited even the medical mainstream.

Superoxide Dismutase (SOD)

Superoxide dismutase (**SOD**), a copper/zinc-containing enzyme found in all body cells, is a primary defender against free radicals. SOD eliminates destructive superoxide molecules, a common free radical produced in the body, and soaks up free radical oxygen molecules in the bloodstream. Reactive oxygen molecules, or oxygen radicals, can destroy healthy tissue. Normally, the body makes enough SOD to hold oxygen radicals in check. But when the immune system destroys bacteria or other infectants and invaders, the surge in the number of white blood cells or antibodies triggers a rapid proliferation of oxygen radicals. In many autoimmune diseases, the white blood cells or immune reactors identify certain tissues as foreign and attack them. SOD scavenges the free radicals and interrupts the progress of this autoimmune reaction.

SOD also inhibits fats in the cells from becoming rancid which helps prevent premature aging. It also helps wounds to heal and alleviates symptoms related to radiation sickness. People deficient in this enzyme should use a supplement. The food sources of SOD are green vegetables, yeast, sprouted seeds, and grains.

Coenzyme Q₁₀

Coenzyme Q$_{10}$ is important for the production of energy by all cells because they help activate enzymes. For example, copper, iron, and other minerals and vitamins, including the B complex, are coenzymes. We need to absorb those important vitamins from our foods so that our enzymes and coenzymes can function optimally. Coenzyme Q$_{10}$, which occurs naturally in the body, has been found useful for heart problems, high blood pressure, diabetes, cancer, obesity, tumors, and Candida. Athletes take CoQ$_{10}$ for increased endurance.

Streptokinase is an enzyme that, according to recent research, helps establish blood flow to the heart. Administered as an injectant into the patients coronary artery, this enzyme acts to dissolve clots and has contributed to an encouraging survival rate among heart attack victims.

Enzymes help the body to build new muscle tissue, nerve cells, skin, and glandular tissue. For example, one enzyme assists in converting dietary phosphorous into bone. Other enzymes aid in digestion, regulate respiration, facilitate better elimination, and stimulate the immune system. There is another enzyme used for burn patients that helps reduce scarring and blood loss. The enzyme acts on dead tissue to expose tissue better able to accept skin grafts.

Flavonoids

Flavonoids, also called Vitamin P, are very significant as antioxidants. They include quercetin, catechin, rutin, anthocyanidin, khellin, asculetine, luteolin, apiin, kampferol, astragelin, and hesperidin. They all have anti-inflammatory and anti-oxidant properties. The anti-oxidant effect can prevent the formation of free radicals and neutralize immune mediators such as leukotrienes and histamines. They also increase the body's use of corticosteroids and lower blood sugar levels by helping with metabolism or carbohydrates. Flavonoids also help stimulate antibody production while helping to inhibit the activity of toxins produced in the body. They can also increase red blood cells, strengthen capillaries, and promote the formation of connective tissue. They have also proven to be antispasmodic, and can have a sedative-like effect.

ABDOMINAL PALPATION AND TWENTY-FOUR HOUR URINALYSIS

The abdominal palpation examination that I learned from Dr. Howard Loomis is based on the recognition of superficial pain or tenderness found in the muscular abdominal wall. When palpated or stretched, these muscles elicit a reflex contraction in the body. This contraction is measured through applied kinesiology or postural deviation, indicated in pelvic leg measurement and leg length discrepancy. These are all reflexes used by chiropractors and health practitioners in many fields to determine and correct areas of imbalance.

Each area of the abdomen, when stretched or palpated, relates to a specific organ or tissue function by means of sensory nerve affiliation. When the palpated area elicits a reflex, a possible inflammation, deficiency, or imbalance is evident. These areas and a brief description of symptoms are discussed below:

The *epigastrum* refers to the stomach, esophagus, and duodenum. A positive reflex in this area indicates gastritis with symptoms that include heartburn and bloating immediately after eating, reflux, and acid indigestion.

The *upper right quadrant* of the abdomen represents the liver and gallbladder. Symptoms include possible gallstones, pain onset several hours after eating a large meal, and poor digestion of fat.

The *upper left quadrant* refers to the jejunum. A positive reflex here can indicate celiac disease, gluten intolerance, or problems arising from poor digestion and absorption of sugars. Symptoms include bloating, diarrhea, chronic fatigue, asthma, and weight loss or gain.

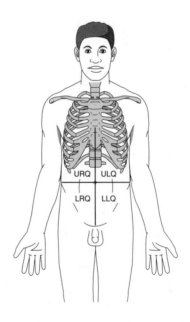

Figure 19–1 Abdominal Diagnostic Palpation Exam developed by Dr. Howard Loomis to determine specific dietary stresses and intolerances. When a trained practitioner palpates the different quadrants, a positive reflex usually is indicative of dietary stress or intolerance.

The *lower left quadrant* is related to the colon, particularly the sigmoid colon. Symptoms include irritable bowel, diarrhea, poor digestion of complex carbohydrates and fiber foods, obesity, and the over-consumption of fats, leading to high levels of triglycerides and cholesterol in the blood.

A positive reflex in the *lower right quadrant* represents acute appendicitis or poor protein digestion evidenced by a high urinary indican level. Symptoms include bloating, pain in the ileocecal valve that connects the small intestine to the large intestine, and possibly calcium deficiency with poor digestion of protein. Palpation of this quadrant can elicit a strong reflex and severe pain on even superficial pressure.

I use this palpation examination with patients to help me decide on the appropriate enzyme to aid them in the digestion of their food. As discussed earlier in this chapter, good digestion is the key to health. If digestion is poor, undigested food residues are deposited in the blood and lymph, creating an immune reaction that leads to the creation of CICs. These immune complexes inhibit the immune system from working adequately and they

Abdominal Palpation Reference Chart	
Positive Reflex in:	*Problem:*
epigastrum	excess acidity or alkaline deficiency
upper right quadrant	fat intolerant
upper left quadrant	sugar intolerant
lower right quadrant	protein intolerant
lower left quadrant	fiber intolerant

inhabit tissue and organs of the body that cause autoimmune reactions including inflammation, swelling, pain, and increased activity of pathogenic organisms in the body. Health declines, the liver overworks, and stress is internal as well as external.

Every one of our patients is prescribed a digestive enzyme formula to predigest food. I determine the appropriate formula by using the abdominal diagnostic enzyme evaluation. For example, many individuals with CFIDS elicit a reflex related to the upper left and lower left quadrants meaning they are unable to digest sugars and fibers. Much of the fatigue and bloating is caused by the improper digestion of sugars and starches. The diets of most people are made up largely of sugars including dairy products (lactose), fruit (fructose), pasta (maltose), breads, crackers, rice (rice sugar), and other grains. With this information, I put the individual on an enzyme that helps digest and utilize sugars and starches and that includes cellulase, sucrase, lactase, disaccharidase, amylase, protease, and lipase. I also put the person on a diet low in sugars and starches since he or she is intolerant to these foods (refer to Part VI for specific diets).

In combination with the abdominal palpation examination, I employ a twenty-four hour urinalysis laboratory exam developed by Dr. Howard Loomis to evaluate inherent food intolerances and dietary excesses, bowel toxicity, and other critical areas such as kidney function and vitamin deficiencies. The kidneys help the body maintain blood homeostasis by filtering the blood and discarding excess waste in the urine. Careful monitoring of the urine reveals what the body is holding and throwing away in its efforts to maintain homeostasis.

For example, the body regulates the pH of the blood by discarding excess acid and base. The inability to do this adequately is revealed in the urine which reflects the many stresses and strains the body experiences. Analysis of the urine can point out sick individuals whose bodies are struggling to cope better than can an analysis of the blood because the body maintains the homeostasis of the blood at all costs. The urine reveals dietary excess in the form of precipitated fat, carbohydrate, and protein that indicates poor digestion of, and/or overreaction to, these foods. The urine shows mineral deficiencies, anxiety, respiratory stress, sugar problems, prediabetic tendencies, gallbladder problems, bowel toxicity, and sluggish or overworked kidneys. With this evaluation and the abdominal palpation, we are able to recommend the appropriate diet and digestive enzymes to better serve an individual's homeostasis and to reinforce or maintain a healthy immune system.

V | RESOURCE GUIDE

20 | RESOURCES

NAET TREATMENT RULES

Treatment failures are a result of:

- *breaking the NAET Treatment Rules*
- *not following the NAET twenty-five hour restrictions*
- *coming within four to five feet of the treated allergens*

1. Do not wear any perfume, perfumed powder, strong-smelling deodorant, or aftershave lotion when you have a treatment or in the clinic where the treatment occurs.

2. Do not smoke before the treatment. It's important that one's clothes and hair do not smell of smoke.

3. Wash your hands before and after the treatment.

4. Do not expose yourself to extreme hot or cold temperatures after the treatment and do not exercise for six hours after the treatment.

5. Take a shower before coming for a treatment. Do not shower or bathe for 6 hours after the treatment.

6. Do not eat, chew gum, or smoke during treatment.

7. Do not cross your hands or feet during the treatment.

8. Do not read or touch other objects for twenty minutes following the treatment.

9. Check the previous treatment with the doctor to ensure that treatment passed before proceeding to the next treatment. Do this after the twenty-five hours, and within one week, or no later than two weeks.

10. Do not expose yourself nutritionally or physically to the allergen for which you are being treated for twenty-five hours. Stay four to five feet away or the treatment could fail immediately, sometime in the future, and symptoms could reoccur. *Be careful and prepare for each treatment ahead of time.*

11. Maintain your own treatment record.

12. Wear plastic gloves and masks when being treated for environmental allergens. These allergens include metals, pollen, grasses, leather, chemicals, smog, and so forth.

13. Eat a healthy meal prior to the treatment unless other instructions are given by your doctor because many treatments require restricted diets.

14. Do not eat heavy meals immediately after allergy treatments. Try not to eat anything to which you are allergic for twenty-five hours after treatment.

15. Drink plenty of water after the treatment. Distilled water is preferable unless otherwise instructed.

16. NAET treatments do not conflict with any medications and it is not necessary to stop taking them

unless advised otherwise by your doctor. Individuals should continue taking their medications unless other recommendations are given by their physicians. Additionally, NAET treatments do not interfere with other treatments you might be receiving.

17. Check the ingredients of any supplements (vitamins, enzymes, and so on) you are taking to ensure they do not contain the allergen for which you are being treated (brewer's yeast, mint, parsley, etc.).

TWENTY-FIVE HOUR NAET RESTRICTIONS

The following section contains a list of NAET restrictions divided into two parts. The first part entitled Basic Allergens is organized in the order in which they are treated. The second part, Other Allergens, lists them in alphabetical order. These lists cover the allergens most common for individuals with chronic health problems. These dietary and physical restrictions should be followed strictly for a twenty-five hour period after the NAET treatment. They were developed after several years of clinical research at my clinic and are responsible for the high rate of success I have in treating allergies.

I have found it is important to both physically and nutritionally avoid the allergen for the entire twenty-five hours. A four- to five-foot distance should be maintained from the allergen. If that distance cannot be maintained, I recommend wearing gloves and in certain cases, a mask as well. One of the easiest ways to fail is to smell an allergen (from hot or cooking foods, for example). Again, I recommend wearing a mask when cooking to avoid losing the treatment. If you expose yourself in any way, you not only lose the treatment but also could experience severe symptoms immediately such as an acute asthma attack, fainting, migraine, and so forth. Or, symptoms might recur over time.

The fingertips are the most sensitive part of the body and you should wear gloves whenever your hands come closer than four to five feet from an allergen. With many of the allergens (calcium, minerals, bacteria, parasites), you should use distilled water. If you have to use distilled water, we recommend no showers or baths and do not wash your hands in anything but distilled water. Use caution when attending to toilet needs. We recommend wearing gloves because the allergen could be present in the water. It is important to prepare for every treatment in order to avoid having to go into grocery or convenience stores to purchase foods or other items after the treatment. It is virtually impossible to avoid many of the allergens when going into a store or restaurant. Again, when you are undergoing treatment and have to prepare food for your children or pet, wear plastic gloves and a mask because the steam from food could cause the treatment to fail. Avoid going into a restaurant during the twenty-five hours after treatment.

The dietary and physical restrictions included in the following pages give a most complete list. In creating this list, I made sure there was not a trace of the particular allergen. In certain cases (Vitamin B, for example), I had to list foods such as Jell-O® that I would not normally recommend because they have no nutritional value. Whenever possible I recommend that my patients eat fresh organic produce, grains, poultry, fish, and meats.

If you have any doubt about a particular food or substance, don't eat or touch it. The golden rule is "when in doubt, abstain!" Many people ask me if they can have black coffee or tea. If it is free of the allergen, I include it. When I was in doubt, I excluded it. If a food or beverage is not included, I recommend avoiding it. It is so easy to drink or eat something that contains the allergen when you consume prepared, processed, or restaurant food. Therefore, I prefer that my patients prepare meals from scratch for themselves or eat foods in their original form. In all cases I recommend abstaining from alcohol consumption for the twenty-five hours following the treatment.

Children eight years old or younger only need to avoid the allergen for six hours after the NAET treatment. The diet and every other rule applies. When treating an infant for breast milk and formula, it might be difficult to avoid milk for six hours. Try for two to three hours. The allergy might need to be treated two or three times but eventually it will completely clear.

To be successful be careful, read the rules over and over again, and prepare for each treatment by reading the restrictions ahead of time. It is always better to have a game plan than to risk failing a treatment by handling a forbidden substance. If you must handle a product that might contain the allergen, minimize the risks of failing the treatment by wearing gloves and a mask.

ADDITION TO THE NAET SELF-TREATMENT

In certain patients, I recommend that a spouse or parent learn how to perform NAET treatment to help clear the many allergens from which the asthmatic individual suffers. In addition to emergency self-treatment, I teach individuals how to do the NAET treatment including muscle response testing for certain allergies. This expedites allergy elimination and accelerates healing. I do this only after a person has cleared their basic allergies because that is critical to clearing other allergens and establishing the foundation of their immune strength and support. After the basics are finished, I do extensive testing to see what allergens remain. I then work closely with each individual to see what allergens are to be cleared next and work out a plan. I educate and teach the spouse or parent and supply them with certain allergen vials for four to five treatments. I tell them emphatically they must see me every two weeks to see if they passed the treatments or if any combinations exist. Self-treatments should only be done under a *doctor's supervision.* I feel it is up to each individual doctor and patient to decide if self-treatment is the road upon which they want to embark. Many parents are delighted with this opportunity to treat their child because it allows them to participate in the healing process and when they see the progress, they are ecstatic.

Supervision by a doctor is mandatory; therefore, I do not describe the treatment in this book. If a doctor does recommend these home treatments, he or she should teach NAET to the patient and family member.

I have included all the 25-hour restrictions for almost all the allergens included in this book for the various protocols. If there it nothing recorded for a particular allergen, it is because there is no restriction or perhaps I could not find any in my research. It is advisable to ask your NAET practitioner for further guidance.

BASIC ALLERGENS

EGG MIX   egg yolks, egg whites, chicken, feathers, tetracycline
Eat only: Steamed rice (white or brown), pasta (without eggs), vegetables, fruits, dairy, oils, beef, pork, fish.
Drink only: Coffee, tea, juice, water, soft drinks.
Do not eat or touch: Eggs or products containing eggs, chicken or products containing chicken (READ LABELS!) feather pillows, shampoo, or other such products containing eggs (refer to the listing of "Foods and Materials Containing Eggs" in Part VI).

CALCIUM MIX   Cal-Carbonate, Cal-Gluconate, Cal-ascorbate, raw milk, cow's milk, goat's milk, milk-casein, milk-albumin
Eat only: White basmati rice, olive oil, salt, rice cakes with no calcium.
Drink only: Distilled water, (not mineral or spring), black tea made with distilled water (no milk).
Wash only: With distilled water.

VITAMIN C MIX   ascorbic acid, chlorophyll, rose hips, rutin, hesperidin, or bioflavonoids; oxalic acid; citrus (oranges, lemons, grapefruits); berry mix (strawberry, cranberry, boysenberry, raspberry); fruit (bananas, papayas, apples, grapes, peaches, nectarines); vegetable mix (green beans, cauliflower, broccoli, brussel sprouts, cabbage, asparagus); vinegar mix (white vinegar, apple cider, rice vinegar).

Eat only: Steamed rice (white, brown, wild), eggs, baked chicken, white breads, tofu (plain), miso, shitake mushrooms, red meat (not processed), boiled beans (white, black, or lima), rice cakes, salt.
Drink only: Water, black tea, black coffee, plain soy milk.

B-COMPLEX MIX B_1, B_2, B_3, B_5, B_6, B_{12}, B_{13}, B_{15}, B_{17}, biotin, choline, inositol, folic acid, PABA
Eat only: Minute Tapioca® (cooked in water only), Jell-O® gelatin (all flavors except those with natural fruit juice), Cool Whip® topping, imitation sour cream. You can use fructose or refined sugar with Jell-O® or tapioca.
Drink only: Water, Crystal Light® berry blend drink (from powder).

SUGAR MIX   maltose, glucose, dextrose, lactose, brown sugar, honey, corn sugar, raw sugar, molasses
Eat only: Eggs, red meat, poultry, oils, fish.
Drink only: Water.
Do not eat or touch: Alcohol, milk products, toothpaste (refer to "Foods and Materials Containing Hidden Sugars" in Part VI).

IRON MIX   ferrous sulfate, ferrous gluconate, beef, pork, lamb, gelatin
Eat only: White basmati rice (no iron), salt, peanut oil.
Drink only: Distilled water (not mineral or spring).
Wash only: With distilled water. READ ALL LABELS!
Wear: Gloves (plastic) when near or touching iron door knobs, and the like.

VITAMIN A MIX   fish, shellfish, betacarotene
Eat only: Steamed rice (white, brown, wild), pearl barley, millet, boiled white beans, boiled turnips, boiled parsnips, boiled red kidney or lima beans, onions, mushrooms, fresh ginger root, fresh garlic, salt, tamari, plain dry almonds or almond butter (pure), plain dry roasted peanuts or peanut butter (pure), cooked spaghetti or macaroni.
Drink only: Water, black tea (no milk).

MINERAL MIX   antimony, barium, boron, beryllium, bromide, cesium, chlorine, cobalt, copper, europium, fluorine, gadolinium, gallium, germanium, gold, holmium, iodine, lanthanum, lithium, manganese, molybdenum, neodymium, nickel, niobium, palladium, rubidium, ruthenium, samarium, scandium, selenium, silver, strontium, thulium, thorium, tin, titanium, tungsten, uranium, vanadium, yttrium, zinc, zirconium.
NOTE: Sulfur, magnesium, chromium, potassium, and phosphorus are not in the general mineral mix. They need to be treated separately.
Eat only: Jello-O® without any natural fruit juice (1 mg. of potassium), tapioca made with distilled water (2 mg. potassium, 1 mg. phosphorus).
Drink only: Distilled water (not mineral or spring).
Wash only: With distilled water.
Wear: Plastic gloves when handling metals.
NOTE: *Rice has large amounts of potassium and phosphorus.*

SALT MIX, CHLORIDES   sea salt, rock salt, table salt, iodized salt, sodium, chloride
Eat only: Rice (brown, white), nonsodium rice cakes (READ LABELS to ensure there is no salt) olive oil, sugar, chives, raspberries, plums, peaches, nectarines, apples without skin, fresh cherries, blackberries.
Drink only: Distilled water (not mineral or spring).
Wash only: With distilled water.
Wear: Mask and gloves when outside if one lives near the ocean.

OTHER ALLERGENS

CORN MIX   blue corn, yellow corn, white corn, corn-starch, corn silk, corn syrup
Eat only: Steamed vegetables, steamed rice, chicken, meat, fish.
Drink only: Water, black tea, black coffee.
Do not eat or touch: Blue corn, yellow corn, white corn, cornstarch, corn oats, corn syrup, corn oil, baking soda, baking powder, starched clothing (shirts, linen), ointments, powders or talcums, lozenges, supplements or other products that contain corn.
Read labels: Soft drinks, breads, toothpaste, shampoos, deodorant (refer to the listing of "Foods and Materials Containing Corn" in Part VI).

ACETYLCHOLINE (follow the guidelines for amino acids)

ACID
Eat only: Steamed or raw vegetables, cooked dried beans, fruits (refer to the listing of "Alkaline-Forming Foods" in Part VI).
Drink only: Water, milk.
Do not eat, drink or touch: Starches, grains, meat, coffee.
Avoid: Acid-forming foods (refer to the listing of "Acid-Forming Foods" in Part VI).

ACIDOPHILUS
Eat only: poultry, meats, vegetables, oils, fruits, grains.
Drink only: water,coffee, and tea.
Do not eat, drink, or touch: yogurt, acidophilus milk.

ALCOHOLS   beer, hops, red wine, white wine, cham-pagne, rubbing alcohol, plant alcohols
Eat only: Cooked or steamed (not raw) vegetables, meat, fish, eggs, chicken.

Drink only: Water, black tea, or coffee (no milk).

Do not eat or touch: Fruits, grains, alcoholic beverages, vanilla extract, sugar, starches, foods prepared with wine, medicines containing alcohol (cough syrup), shampoos, hair products, cosmetics, makeup containing alcohol, any extract with alcohol, any homeopathic or herb preparation containing alcohol. READ ALL LABELS!

Avoid: Eating in restaurants or eating catered foods during the twenty-five hour period.

AMINO ACID 1   lysine, leucine, threonine, valine, tryptophan, isoleucine, phenylalanine

Eat only: Lettuce.

Drink only: Water.

Do not touch: Protein products for external use.

AMINO ACID 2   alanine, arginine, aspartic acid, carnitine, citrulline, cysteine, cystine, glutathione, glutamic acid, glycine, histidine, ornithine, proline, serine, taurine, glutamine, tyrosine

Eat only: Lettuce.

Drink only: Water.

Do not touch: Protein products for external use.

ANIMAL EPITHELIALS and DANDERS

Do not touch: Animals, their saliva, hair, dander, and any other products made from animals or used by animals. If you have a pet, make arrangements to stay away from him or her for twenty-five hours.

ANIMAL FATS   butter, lard, pork or pork fat, beef or beef fat, chicken or chicken fat, lamb or lamb fat, fish or fish oil

Do not eat or touch: The above items and any foods fried with or containing animal fat, refried beans, chili beans, skin lotions made with animal fat, pet food.

ARTIFICIAL SWEETENERS
Do not eat or touch: Saccharine, Equal®, Sweet'N Low®, NutraSweet®, aspartame, sorbitol, or any products containing artificial sweeteners.
Read all labels: Soft drinks, sweet relish, pickles, cookies, toothpaste.

ASPARTAME
Eat only: Grains, vegetables, fruits, meat, poultry, fish, dairy, and beans.
Do not drink or eat: Soft drinks, sweet relish, pickles, cookies, toothpaste. READ ALL LABELS!

VITAMIN B$_1$ thiamine, thiamine mononitrate, thiamine hydrochloride
Eat only: Rice cakes, egg whites, oysters, angel food cake, gingersnap cookies, black olives, radishes, pickles (dill, bread and butter, kosher, and rennin only), tapioca, dried apples, lychees, butter, corn margarine, carob powder, aspartame powder.
Drink only: Water, apple juice, Hawaiian Punch® brand fruit juices (Hawaiian Punch® Fruit Punch^K Fruit Juicy, apple, cherry, grape), Kool-Aid® (sugar powder and sugar free), Country Time® (sugar and sugar free), Crystal Lite® (powder only), Tang™, black coffee.
Do not eat, drink, or touch: Dried yeast, pork, most vegetables, bran, milk, brewer's yeast, wheat germ, wheat bran, rice polishings, most whole grain cereals, milk products, leafy green vegetables, meat, liver, nuts, legumes, potatoes.

VITAMIN B$_2$ riboflavin, Vitamin G
Eat only: Baked, broiled, or poached snapper, oysters, butter, corn margarine, shallots, black olives, pickles (dill, bread and butter, rennin only), fruit leather rolls, Cool Whip®, Dream Whip®, gingersnap cookies, tapioca.
Drink only: Water, Hawaiian Punch® brand fruit juices

(Fruit Juicy, apple, cherry, grape), Kool-Aid® (sugar powder and sugar Free), Country Time® (sugar and sugar free), Crystal Lite® (powder only), black coffee, Coffee Mate® nondairy creamer.

Do not eat, drink, or touch: Milk, cheese, whole grains, brewer's yeast, wheat germ, almonds, sunflower seeds, liver, leafy vegetables, kidney, fish, and eggs.

VITAMIN B$_3$ niacin, nicotinic acid, niacinamide
Eat only: The following cheeses: cheddar, Colby, cream, Edam, Gouda, Gruyere, mozzarella, Muenster, Neufchatel, Parmesan, provolone, Romano, Swiss; processed American or Swiss cheese. Fruit leather rolls, shallots, watercress, black olives, pickles (dill, bread and butter, rennin only), tapioca, gingersnap cookies, Cool Whip®, butter, corn margarine, aspartame powder.

Drink only: Water, lemon and lime juice, Hawaiian Punch® (Fruit Juicy, apple, cherry), Kool-Aid®, Country Time®, Crystal Lite®, Coffee Mate® nondairy creamer.

Do not eat or touch: Lean meat, fish, eggs, roasted peanuts, brewer's yeast, wheat germ, rice bran, rice polishings, nuts, sunflower seeds, whole wheat products, brown rice, green vegetables, liver, white meat of poultry, avocados, dates, figs, prunes.

VITAMIN B$_5$ pantothenic acid, calcium pantothenate
Eat only: Ham, corn tortilla, instant maple and brown sugar oatmeal, mozzarella cheese, Parmesan cheese, eggplant, chili peppers, red peppers, radishes, pickled herring, air-popped popcorn, almond butter, corn margarine, cocoa powder, aspartame powder, tapioca, soybean protein powder, Coffee Mate® nondairy creamer, Cool Whip®, Dream Whip®, honey.

Drink only: Water, lemon or lime juice, Kool-Aid®, Country Time®, Crystal Lite®, black coffee, Tang™.

Do not eat or touch: Brewer's yeast, wheat germ, wheat bran, whole grain breads and cereals, green vegetables, peas and beans, liver, egg yolks, crude molasses, dried lima beans, raisins, meat, cantaloupes, kidneys, hearts, nuts, chicken.

VITAMIN B$_6$ pyridoxine, pyridoxal, pyridoxamine
Eat only: Black olives, tapioca, egg whites, butter, corn margarine, Arrowroot™ baby cookies, infant oatmeal, Coffee Mate® nondairy creamer, aspartame powder, Cool Whip®, Dream Whip®.
Drink only: Water, Kool-Aid® (sugar powder and sugar Free), Country Time® (sugar and sugar free), Crystal Lite® (powder only), honey, black coffee.
Do not eat or touch: Brewer's yeast, bananas, avocados, wheat germ, wheat bran, soybeans, milk, egg yolks, liver, green leafy vegetables, green peppers, organ meat, legumes, kidneys, heart, cantaloupes, cabbage, molasses, beef.

VITAMIN B$_{12}$ cobalamin, cyanocobalamin
Eat only: Fruits, vegetables, beans (except refried), nuts, seeds, cracked wheat, Aunt Jemima® whole wheat pancakes, instant oatmeal, instant maple and brown sugar oatmeal, banana chips, corn chips, corn nuts, fruit leather rolls, air-popped popcorn, caramel/peanut popcorn, potato chips, pretzels, rice cakes, plain tortilla chips, tapioca, cheese soup, onion soup, tomato or tomato rice soup (no cream tomato soup), gelatin consomme, minestrone soup, vegetarian vegetable soup, gazpacho soup, defatted peanut flour, soy flour, soybean protein powder, canned spaghetti or tomato sauce, tomato paste, tamari soy sauce, vinegar, Arrowroot™ baby cookies, baking powder, aspartame powder, dry cocoa powder, fruit pectin, Coffee Mate® nondairy creamer, Cool Whip®.
Drink only: Apricot nectar, cranberry juice cocktail, grape juice, peach nectar, pear nectar, pineapple juice, prune juice, tangerine juice, carrot juice, Kool-Aid® (sugar powder and sugar Free), Country Time® (sugar and sugar

free), Crystal Lite® (powder only), black coffee, Postum®, Tang™.
Do not eat, drink, or touch: Milk, eggs, aged cheese, liver, meat, pollen, pork, kidneys.

VITAMIN B$_{13}$ orotic acid
Do not eat or touch: Milk whey (the liquid portion of soured or curdled milk; READ LABELS for all dairy products), root vegetables.

VITAMIN B$_{15}$ pangamic acid, calcium pangamate
Do not eat or touch: Whole grains, seeds, nuts, whole brown rice, brewer's yeast, pumpkin seeds, sesame seeds.

VITAMIN B$_{17}$ nitrilosides, amygdalin, laetrile
Do not eat, drink, or touch: Fruits with seeds, vegetables, raspberries, cranberries, blackberries, blueberries, mung beans, lima beans, flaxseeds.

BACTERIA MIX
Do not eat, drink, or touch: Uncooked foods, sugar, any water or beverages except distilled water.
Wear: plasticor cotton gloves at all times.

BAKING POWDER
Eat only: Fresh fruits, vegetables, meat, chicken, fish, fats.
Drink only: Water, black coffee, black tea.
Do not eat or touch: Baking powder, baking soda, baked goods, medications, toothpastes, deodorants and antiperspirants, talcum powders, soaps. READ ALL LABELS!

BAKING SODA
Eat only: Fresh fruits, vegetables, meat, chicken, fish, fats.
Drink only: Water, black coffee, black tea.
Do not eat or touch: Baking powder, baking soda, baked goods, medications, toothpastes, deodorants and antiperspirants, talcum powders, soaps. READ ALL LABELS!

BASE
Eat only: Starches, breads, meat, poultry, fish, all dairy products except milk and yogurt, and any of the foods on the list of "Acid-Forming Foods" in Part VI.
Do not eat, drink, or touch: Vegetables, beans, milk, fruit.
Avoid: Alkaline-forming foods (refer to the listing of the "Alkaline-Forming Foods" in Part VI).

BEET SUGAR
Avoid: Beets and any products containing beet sugar; READ ALL LABELS!

BERRY MIX   Strawberries, blueberries, blackberries, raspberries, loganberries, cranberries, wild berries, gooseberries
Eat only: Vegetables, grains, meat, breads, poultry, fish, dairy products.
Do not eat, drink, or touch: Berries, jams, fruits, and fruit juices made from berries.

BIOFLAVANOIDS   citrin, hesperidin, rutin, quercetin
Eat only: Meat, grains, poultry, vegetables, beans, dairy products.
Do not eat, drink, or touch: Garlic, onions, lemons, limes, grapes, plums, black currants, grapefruits, apricots, buckwheat, cherries, blackberries, rose hips, and oranges.

BIOTIN   vitamin H, coenzyme R
Do not eat, drink, or touch: Brewer's yeast, unpolished rice, soybeans, liver, kidneys, milk, molasses, nuts, fruits, beef, yolks.

BROWN SUGAR
Eat only: Grains, meat, vegetables, fruits, poultry, fish.
Do not eat or touch: Anything that contains brown sugar. READ ALL LABELS!

CAFFEINE   coffee, tea, tannic acid
Eat or drink: Anything that contains no caffeine or chocolate.
Do not eat, drink, or touch: Coffee, tea, chocolate, caffeinated drinks, leather goods, tannic acid. (Do not even smell coffee brewing.)

CANDIDA MIX
Eat only: All protein (poultry, fish, meat, eggs, cooked or steamed vegetables), oils, tofu and beans for vegetarians.
Do not eat, drink, or touch: Simple sugars, grains, fruits, dairy, yeast products (breads, beer, wine), vinegar, hops, malts, peanuts, mushrooms, condiments (soy sauce, catsup) (refer to the listing "Foods and Materials Containing Yeast" in Part VI).
Prior to treatment: Buy new clothes, socks, underwear, toothbrush, hairbrush, sheets, towels, etc. Anything you put on your body should be new and never worn before. Scrub shower stalls and bathtubs and remove mold from house. Shower and wash hair.
After treatment: Change into new clothes, socks, and shoes. No skin-to-skin contact or sexual contact. Wear gloves for twenty-five hours. Do not touch animals or makeup. Wear gloves when attending to personal hygiene following toilet use. Start the 10-day Candida yeast avoidance diet listed in Part VI.

CANE SUGAR
Eat only: Fruits, meat, poultry, fish, vegetables.
Do not eat, drink, or touch: Anything with cane sugar. READ ALL LABELS!

CAULIFLOWER
Eat only: Fruits, meat, poultry, vegetables, fish, grains, beans.
Do not eat, drink, or touch: anything with cauliflower (for example, vegetable juice).

CELERY MIX
Eat only: Grains, meat, fruits, vegetables, poultry, beans, dairy products, salt, pepper.
Do not eat or touch: Anything with celery and celery salt such as sauces, dressings, vegetable juices, spice mixes, seasonings, and so forth.

CHEESE MIX   American, cheddar, jack, Parmesan, mozzarella, cottage, and the like.
Eat only: Grains, vegetables, poultry, fruits, beans.
Do not eat, drink, or touch: Anything made from dairy products.

CHEMICALS
Do not eat or drink: Water or any foods cooked in tap water.
Do not touch: Soaps, detergents, cleaning chemicals, chlorine, bleach. If your water supply is chlorinated (city water), do not wash with tap water. Use spring or distilled water.

CHICKEN   white/dark meat chicken, chicken feathers
Eat only: Vegetables, meat, fish, fruits, dairy products, beans.
Do not eat or touch: Chicken, eggs, chicken feathers, anything with eggs, egg whites, egg yolks, or feathers.
Avoid: Down pillows or cushions, down comforter, down couches, down coats. Do not go into a linen, furniture, or clothing store for twenty-five hours following the treatment.

CHOCOLATE MIX   cocoa, cocoa butter, chocolate, carob
Eat or drink only: Anything that has no caffeine or chocolate.
Do not eat, drink, touch, or smell: Coffee, tannic acid tea, chocolate, caffeinated drinks, leather goods.

CHOLINE

Eat only: Fruits, dairy products, vegetables (except peas and green leafy vegetables), fish, poultry, meat.

Do not eat or touch: Brewer's yeast, wheat germ, egg yolks, liver, green leafy vegetables, legumes, peas, beans, brains, heart, lecithin.

CHROMIUM

Eat only: White rice, pastas, cauliflower, potatoes, salt.

Drink only: Water, black coffee, black tea (no milk).

Do not eat, drink, or touch: Meat, chicken, liver, whole grains, wheat germ, corn oil, brewer's yeast, mushrooms, sugar, shellfish, clams.

CITRUS MIX grapefruits, lemons, limes, oranges (all types), tangerines, pineapples

Eat only: Meat, poultry, fish, fruits other than citrus, beans, grains, dairy.

Do not eat, drink, or touch: Grapefruits, lemons, oranges and orange juice, pineapples, tangerines, mandarin oranges, and limes.

COBALT

Eat only: White rice, pastas, cauliflowers, potatoes, fruits, noniodized salt.

Drink only: Water.

Do not eat, drink, or touch: Green leafy vegetables, meat, liver, kidneys, figs, buckwheat, oysters, clams, dairy products.

COFFEE MIX coffee, tea, tannic acid, caffeine

Eat or drink only: Anything that has no caffeine or chocolate.

Do not eat, drink, touch, or smell: Coffee, tea, chocolate, caffeinated drinks, leather goods, tannic acid.

COLD (use ice when treating)
Eat only: warm cooked foods
Drink only: warm liquids
Do not eat or touch: ice cubes, cold drinks, cold water, cold objects, avoid cold air, use gloves and socks at all times. Protect all parts of the body from cold.

COPPER
Eat only: White rice, pastas, cauliflower, potatoes, fruits, noniodized salt.
Do not eat, drink, or touch: Tap water, almonds, green beans, peas, green leafy vegetables, whole grains, whole wheat, prunes, raisins, dried beans, liver, seafood.
NOTE: *Use only distilled water for cooking or steaming foods and for washing.*

CORN SUGAR
Eat only: Vegetables other than corn, grains other than corn, dairy products, fruits, beans, meat, poultry, fish.
Drink only: Water, coffee, tea, fresh squeezed juices.
Do not eat, drink, or touch: Corn sugar or anything with corn sugar. READ ALL LABELS! Foods can contain corn sugar in processed, store prepared foods, or restaurant foods such as soups, sauces, stews, and so forth.

CORTISOL (refer to hormone guidelines)

CRUDE OIL
Do not touch or smell: Gasoline or crude oil products, products made of plastics such as computer key boards, telephones, pens, vinyl chairs, book covers, toothbrush, hairbrush, and the like.
Wear: Cotton or leather gloves; wear mask when outdoors.

CUCUMBER MIX
Do not eat or touch: Fresh cucumbers, pickles, soups, salad dressings, skin products that contain cucumber.

VITAMIN D
Eat only: Poultry, meat, fruits.
Drink only: Water, black tea, black coffee (no milk).
Do not eat, drink, or touch: Egg yolks, dairy products, fish or fish oil, sprouted seeds, mushrooms, sunflower seeds or oil.

DEXTROSE
Eat only: Poultry, meat, fish. Follow same diet as sugars mix.
Do not eat or touch: Vegetables, fruits, dairy products, grains. Follow same diet as sugar mix.

DIGESTIVE ENZYMES   amylase, protease, lipase, cellulase, maltase, pepsin, hydrochloric acid
Eat only: cooked foods of any type.
Drink only: water, coffee.
Do not eat, drink or touch: raw food, house plants, soil.

DNA
Eat only: Lettuce.
Drink only: Water, black coffee, black tea.
Do not eat or touch: Proteins such as meat, fish, poultry, dairy products, grains, vegetables, fruits.

DOPAMINE
Eat only: vegetables, poultry, meats, oils, beans, grains
Drink only: water, coffee, tea
Do not eat, drink or touch: pineapple, banana, plantain, avocados

---

DRIED BEAN MIX   blackeyed peas, black beans, white beans, pinto beans, soybeans, peas, red beans, mung beans, kidney beans, lima beans, lentils, garbanzo beans, navy beans
Eat or drink only: Anything that does not contain beans, peas, or bean oil including rice, fruits, meat, chicken, fish, and fresh vegetables.

Do not eat or touch: Chips, crackers, baked goods, and mayonnaise made with soybean oil.

DUST MIX AND DUST MITES
Avoid: Dusty areas. Clean up the living and sleeping areas before the treatment and do not come in contact or touch dusty areas.
Wear: A mask and plastic gloves for twenty-five hours.

VITAMIN E
Eat only: Fresh fruits, carrots, potatoes, poultry, meat.
Drink only: Water, black coffee, black tea.
Do not eat or touch: Wheat germ or wheat germ oil, vegetable oils, soybeans or soybean oil, green vegetables, flours, grains, eggs, nuts, raw or sprouted seeds, fish.

EGG WHITE/EGG YOLKS   follow the same restrictions for eggs listed under Basic Allergens

---

EPINEPHRINE (adrenalin):   (refer to hormone guidelines)

EQUAL®
Avoid: All products which contain Equal®. READ ALL LABELS! Soft drinks, sweet relish, pickles, cookies, toothpaste, and so forth.

VITAMIN F (fatty acids)
Do not eat or touch: Vegetable oils, wheat germ oils, linseed oils, sunflower oils, safflower oils, soybean oils, peanuts or other nuts, peanut oils, flax seeds or oil, evening primrose oils, breast milk.

FABRIC MIX
Avoid contact: With the fabrics that are being treated. Do not touch home furnishings such as couches, upholstered furniture, curtains, towels, sheets, and so on. Be careful to wear socks and/or shoes if you walk on rugs.

Do not go into stores or be in close proximity to others who might be wearing the fabrics being treated.

Wear: Gloves if in proximity to the treated fabrics (closer than four to five feet).

NOTE: *Treat one kind of fabric first. Then wear the allergy-cleared item when treating for the fabric mix.*

FIBER
Do not eat: Raw foods
Eat only: Cooked vegetables, dairy, meats, poultry, fish.

FISH MIX   crappie, red snapper, cod, tuna, sardine, catfish, anchovies, sea bass, halibut, petroli, orange roughy, shark, mahi mahi, salmon
Do not eat or touch: Any fish products or any oils made from fish. Do not lick or touch stamps and envelopes. Wear plastic gloves to handle pet food.

FLUORIDE
Eat only: Fruits, yellow vegetables, potatoes, cauliflower, meat, chicken, white rice.
Drink only: Distilled water (not mineral or spring), fresh squeezed juices, black coffee or black tea made with distilled water only.
Wash only: With distilled water.
Do not eat, drink, or touch: Tap water, gelatin, sunflower seeds or oil, milk, cheese, garlic, almonds, green vegetables, carrots, fish.
NOTE: *Use only distilled water for cooking or steaming foods.*

FLOWER MIX
Avoid: Flowers, pollen, and perfumes.
Wear: A mask outdoors.

FOLIC ACID   pteroylglutamic acid, folate, folacin
Eat only: Ham, salami (beef or pork), concord grapes,

shredded coconut, Chex party mix, pork rinds, Chinese cabbage, iceberg lettuce, pickled herring, corn margarine, tapioca, Coffee Mate®, Cool Whip®, Dream Whip®.

Drink only: Water, hot chocolate (from a mix, with water), Kool-Aid® (sugar powder and sugar Free), Country Time® (sugar and sugar free), Crystal Lite® (powder only), black coffee, apple or cherry juice.

Do not eat, drink, or touch: Dark green leafy vegetables, broccoli, asparagus, lima beans, Irish potatoes, brewer's yeast, wheat germ, mushrooms, nuts, liver, carrots, tortula, yeast, egg yolks, cantaloupes, apricots, pumpkin, avocados, beans, whole wheat and dark rye flour, dairy products.

FOOD ADDITIVES   calcium sulfate, calcium phosphate, sodium sulfate, sodium nitrate

Eat only: Fresh vegetables or fruits, freshly cooked grains, eggs, fresh fish, chicken; READ ALL LABELS!

Drink only: Water, milk, home-squeezed juices.

Do not eat, drink, or touch: Any store-prepared, processed, frozen or restaurant foods such as hot dogs, sausages, prepacked meat, soups, crackers, candies, cookies, salad dressings, sauces, premixed powdered spice, ice cream, chewing gum, soft drinks.

FOOD COLORING

Eat only: Fresh vegetables or fruits, rice, white pasta, eggs, chicken, fish.

Drink only: Water, milk, home-squeezed juices.

Do not eat, drink, or touch: Any store prepared, processed, frozen, or restaurant foods such as hot dogs, sausages, prepacked meat, soups, crackers, candies, cookies, salad dressings, sauces, premixed powdered spices, ice cream, chewing gum, soft drinks (refer to the listing of "Foods and Materials Containing Artifical Colors" in Part VI).

FORMALDEHYDE

Avoid: New buildings or buildings with recent remodeling, new clothing, newspapers, paints, pressed woods (refer to the listing of "Foods and Materials Containing Formaldehyde" in Part VI).

Wear: A mask and cotton gloves for twenty-five hours.

FREON

Avoid: Air-conditioned areas, supermarkets, soft plastic products, refrigerator and freezer.

Wear: A mask and gloves if you must take food in and out of the the refrigerator and freezer. Treat for cold first.

FRUCTOSE

Eat only: Grains, vegetables, dairy, poultry, meat, fish.

Do not eat, drink, or touch: Fruits, or anything containing fructose, for example, high fructose corn syrup in drinks and sugared foods. READ ALL LABELS!

FRUIT MIX   bananas, papayas, apples, grapes, peaches, nectarines

Eat only: Grains, vegetables, fish, poultry, meat.

Do not eat, drink or touch: Fruits or anything containing fruits.

FUNGUS   see entry for Candida and follow the same guidelines but wear a mask as well as gloves

GABA (follow guidelines for amino acids)

GELATIN

Eat only: Vegetables, rice, grains.

Drink only: Water, black coffee, black tea.

Do not eat or touch: Chicken, meat, apple skins, hard skin of other fruits, pectin (READ LABELS for jam), Jell-O®, gelatin capsules, puddings with gelatin, sticky candy, dairy products.

PART V: *Resource Guide*

GERMANIUM
Eat only: Fruits, vegetables, vegetable oils, dairy, poultry, meat.
Do not eat or touch: Whole grains, sprouts, breads.

GLUCOSE   follow the sugar mix restrictions

GLUTATHIONE
Eat only: chicken, fish, beans, eggs, grains
Do not eat or touch: vegetables, plants, fruits, yeast, liver, and kidney

---

GLUTEN
Avoid: Gluten-containing grains such as barley, buckwheat, oats, rye, and wheat.
Eat only: Corn flour, corn meal, corn starch, gluten-free wheat starch, lima bean flour, potato flour, rice, rice flour, soy flour.

GOLD
Do not touch: Gold jewelry and gold fillings in your teeth. Use plastic gloves when eating or brushing teeth to avoid touching fingertips to the gold fillings.

GRAIN MIX   wheat, millet, oats, rye, rice, wheat bran, oat bran, wild rice
Eat only: Meat, chicken, raw or cooked vegetables, and fruits.
Drink only: Water, milk, black coffee, black tea.

GRASS MIX
Avoid: Being outdoors or in contact with grass products.
Wear: A mask and gloves outdoors.

GUM MIX
Eat only: Rice, pastas, vegetables, fruits without skin, meat, chicken, eggs, fish.

Do not eat, drink, or touch: Soft drinks or carbonated drinks, chewing gum, cream cheese, glues (do not lick stamps or envelopes). READ ALL LABELS!
Heat: treat with using hot water
avoid hot drinks, hot food and anything hot to the touch.

HISTAMINE
Do not eat, drink, or touch: Meat, poultry, fish, shellfish, black beans, cow's milk or milk products, goat's milk, breast milk, wines.

HONEY
Eat only: Vegetables, fruits, meat, poultry, fish, grains, beans.
Do not eat, drink, or touch: Anything with honey. READ ALL LABELS!

HORMONES
Do not eat or touch: Meat, poultry, dairy products, eggs, hormone supplements, soy products, herbal products.
Use only: Distilled water, no regular water.

HUMIDITY
Do not treat on a humid day. Treatment procedure requires using a humidifier to simulate humid conditions.

HYDROCARBONS (see hydrocarbons in the Resource Guide, pg. 526)

INOSITOL
Do not eat or touch: Brewer's yeast, wheat germ, lecithin, unprocessed whole grains, nuts, milk, citrus fruits, liver, lima beans, beef, brains, heart, raisins, cantaloupes, unrefined molasses, peanuts, cabbages.

INSECT MIX bees, ants, spiders, fleas
Avoid: Touching any insects.

IODINE
Eat only: White rice, pastas, cauliflowers, potatoes, fruits, noniodized salt.
Drink only: Water.
Do not eat or touch: Kelp, seafood, iodized salt, onions.

VITAMIN K
Eat only: Fruits, rice, potatoes, poultry, meat.
Do not eat or touch: Green vegetables, kelp, alfalfa, soybean oils, safflower oils, egg yolks, cow's milk, yogurt, liver.

LACTOSE (milk sugar)
Eat only: Grains, vegetables, meat, poultry, fish, fruits, beans.
Do not eat, drink, or touch: Anything with dairy products such as milk, cheese, yogurt, kefir. READ ALL LABELS! Lactose is often used as a preservative in ketchup and sauces.

LATEX: avoid toys, pacifiers, tires, rubber gloves, garden hoses, rubber bands, balloons, bandages, medical tape, socks, and underware with elastic. Also, tennis rackets, bananas, avocados, chestnuts, papaya, kiwi, milk, pineapples, potatoes, tomatoes.

LEAD
Eat only: White rice, pastas, cauliflowers, potatoes, fruits, noniodized salt.
Drink only: Distilled water (not mineral or spring).
Do not eat, drink, or touch: Tap water, almonds, green beans, peas, green leafy vegetables, whole grains, whole wheat, prunes, raisins, dried beans, liver, seafood, any products that may contain lead.
Avoid: Old buildings that might have lead paint.

NOTE: *Use only distilled water to cook or steam food.*

LECITHIN
Eat only: White rice, cauliflowers, potatoes, fish, poultry, meat, fruits, vegetables.
Drink only: Water, black tea, black coffee.
Do not eat or touch: Lecithin products, cookies, candy bars, vitamin supplements.

MAGNESIUM
Eat only: White rice, potatoes, cauliflowers, eggs, chicken, meat, fruits.
Drink only: Water, fresh-squeezed juices.
Do not eat or touch: Nuts or seeds, soybeans, green leafy vegetables, whole grains.

MALATHION (see also PESTICIDES)
Eat only: Cooked grains, cooked organic vegetables, cooked fruits.
Drink only: Water.
Do not eat or touch: Fresh vegetables, fruits, meat, poultry, insecticides, herbicides, spices, and herbs.

MALTOSE   grain sugar
Eat only: Fruits, vegetables, meat, poultry, fish and beans, dairy products.
Drink only: Water, fresh fruit juices, black coffee, black tea.
Do not eat or touch: Grains, breads, cereals, pastas, avoid malt and malt products.

MANGANESE
Eat only: White rice, pastas, cauliflowers, potatoes, fruits, noniodized salt.
Drink only: Water.
Do not eat or touch: Green leafy vegetables, beets, blueberries, oranges, grapefruits, apricots, nuts and grain bran, peas, kelp, raw egg yolks.

MAPLE SUGAR
Eat Only: Fruits, grains, poultry, meat, fish, vegetables, beans.

Do not eat or touch: Anything with maple sugar. Keep away from maple trees or wood.

MEAT MIX red meat, beef, lamb, veal, liver
Eat only: Fish, vegetable, fruits, beans, grains, breads, poultry.
Do not eat or touch: Red meat or anything with meat in it. READ ALL LABELS and ask chefs how their soups, stocks, and sauces are made.

MELON MIX crenshaws, watermelons, cantaloupes, honeydews
Eat only: Grains, vegetables, poultry, meat, fish, beans, and dairy.
Do not eat or touch: All types of melons.

MERCURY AMALGAMS
Do not eat or touch: Fish and fish products, mercury products. USE GLOVES when eating or brushing teeth to avoid close contact with mercury in the mouth from tooth fillings.

MILK MIX cow's milk, goat's milk, breast milk
Eat only: Vegetables, grains, poultry, meat, fruits, fish, and beans.
Do not eat or touch: All milk products including yogurt, cheese, and kefir. READ ALL LABELS! Watch out for milk solids (refer to the listing of "Foods and Materials Containing Milk" later in Part VI).

MODIFIED STARCH
Eat only: Vegetables, meat, eggs, beans, fish, poultry.
Drink only: Water, fresh fruit juices, black coffee, black tea.
Do not eat or touch: Table salt, refined grain products, sauces, vitamin supplements, prescription drugs, starch products including starched shirts or garments. READ ALL LABELS!

MOLD MIX   see entry for Candida and follow the same guidelines and use a mask. There is no need to go on the 10-day Candida diet.

MOLYBDENUM
Eat only: White rice, pastas, cauliflowers, potatoes, fresh fruits, noniodized salt.
Drink only: Water.
Do not eat or touch: Whole grains, brown rice, brewer's yeast, legumes, dark green leafy vegetables.

MSG, HVP, NF, and other food additives
Eat only: Follow same restrictions as food additives.
NOTE: *MSG can be added to food under different names: HVP (hydrolyzed vegetable protein), autolyzed yeast, NF (natural flavors), sodium caseinate, calcium caseinate, hydrolyzed milk protein. READ ALL LABELS!*

NEWSPAPER
Do not touch: Any newspapers or magazines.

NEWSPAPER INK
Do not touch: Newspapers or magazines.

NOREPINEPHRINE
Eat only: meat, poultry, fish, vegetables except those listed below, oils, beans, grains.
Drink only: water, coffee, and tea.
Do not eat, drink or touch: bananas, oranges, plums, potatoes, sweet potatoes.

NUT MIX 1   peanuts, black walnuts, English walnuts
Do not eat or touch: The above and oils or butters made from them.

NUT MIX 2   cashews, almonds, pecans, brazil nuts, hazelnuts, macadamias, pistachios, sunflower seeds

Do not eat or touch: The above and oils or butters made from them.

ONION MIX   brown, red, white, green onions
Eat only: Fruits, vegetables, grains, meat, poultry, fish, dairy products, and beans.
Do not eat or touch: Onions and products made with onions.

VITAMIN P
Do not eat or touch: Citrus fruits, green peppers, grapes, apricots, strawberries, black currants, cherries, prunes, rose hips, buckwheat.

PABA MIX   para-aminobenzoic acid
Do not eat, drink, or touch: Brewer's yeast, whole grain products, milk, eggs, yogurt, wheat germ, molasses, liver, kidneys, whole grains, rice, bran, sunscreen products containing PABA.

PARASITES MIX
Drink only: Boiled water or beverages made with boiling water.
Do not eat or touch: Uncooked or raw food, plain tap water. Wear gloves when attending to personal hygiene following toilet use.

PEPPER MIX   red, green, black, yellow, Mexican, Italian, Indian peppers
Eat only: Vegetables, poultry, meat, grains, fish, dairy products, fruits, and beans.
Do not eat or touch: All peppers and any foods made with peppers.

PERFUME MIX
Avoid: Perfumed soaps, makeup products, hair products, flowers. You may have to wear a mask to avoid the scent.

When being treated, wear shower cap so hair doesn't smell like perfume and change into new clothes after treatment.

PESTICIDES
Eat only: Cooked organically grown grains, cooked organic vegetables, organic fruits, organically raised meat or poultry.
Do not eat, drink, or touch: Meat, uncooked foods, insecticides, coffee, tea.
Wear: A mask outdoors if the temperature is above freezing.

PHOSPHORUS
Eat only: Potatoes, cauliflowers, fresh fruits, fresh vegetables, vegetable oils.
Drink only: Water.
Do not eat or touch: Whole grains, seeds, nuts, legumes, dairy products, egg yolks, fish, corn, dried fruits, poultry, meat.

PHENOLICS following are the phenolics to which individuals with immune disorders are commonly allergic. If one is treated for all phenolics, one needs to fast. Avoid all foods and drink only water.

Acetaldehyde

Eat only: Rice, and all grains, vegetables, oils, fish, beans
Drink only: Water.
Do not eat, drink, or touch: Perfumes, rubber, gelatin, wood, apples, broccoli, berries, butter, chocolate, apples, cheese, grapes, grapefruit, grape juice, chicken, beef, pineapples, pears, peaches, oranges, ice cream, chewing gum, propane and butane.

Alanine

Eat only: Vegetables, fruits, fish, oils, grains, and beans.
Drink only: Water, coffee, tea.
Do not eat, drink, or touch: Chicken, turkey, pork, cottage cheese, ricotta cheese.

Androsterone

Eat only: Fish, vegetables, meat, poultry, fish, and beans

Drink only: Water, coffee, tea.

Do not eat, drink, or touch: Liquors, soda water, syrup, butterscotch, caramel, fruit and nut flavoring, gums, ice cream, and ices.

Caffeic acid

Eat only: Fish, poultry, meat, grains, oils, beans.

Drink only: Water.

Do not eat, drink, or touch: Asparagus, yam, potato, tomato, lettuce, fruits, tobacco, green tea, and coffee.

Carnitine

Eat only: Grains, vegetables, fruits, oils, beans.

Drink only: Water, coffee, tea, and juice.

Do not eat, drink, or touch: Avocado, milk, and meat.

Coumarin

Eat only: Vegetables and fruits other than those mentioned below.

Drink only: Water.

Do not eat, drink, or touch: Rice, barley, corn, soy, cheese, beef, eggs, lavender oil, sweet clover, cow's milk, albumin, apples, bananas, barley, beer, beets, beet sugar, celery, chicken, cinnamon, cocoa, lemons, lettuce, peanuts, black pepper, sweet potatoes, sage, tomatoes, tuna fish, turkey, vanilla, wheat bran, whole wheat, yeast, plants.

Ferrous fumerate

Do not eat: salt.

Gallic acid

Eat only: Other than mentioned below, turkey, meat.

Drink only: Water.

Do not eat, drink, or touch: Food coloring, cream of tartar, maple syrup, beer, tea, sumac trees, tannins, apples, apricots, bananas, barley, basil, bay leaf, lima beans, navy beans, pinto beans, red beans, soybeans, string beans, blackberries, blueberries, brussel sprouts, cantaloupes, cow's milk casein, cashew nuts, chicken, cocoa, coconuts, crabmeat, cucumbers, eggs, garlic, ginger, grapes, hops, olives, papayas, peaches, peanuts, pears, pineapples, plums, potatoes, sweet potatoes, prunes, pumpkins, quinces, raisins, rhubarb, rice, strawberries, tomatoes, vanilla, walnuts, watermelons, whole wheat, yeast.

Glutamine

Eat only: Poultry, grains, fruit, oils, and beans.

Drink only: Water, coffee, and tea.

Do not eat, drink, or touch: Sugar beets, carrots, radishes, celery root, gelatin, milk.

5 hydroxytryptophan (follow instructions for serotonin)

Hypericin (no restrictions necessary)

Lactic Acid

Eat only: Vegetables, except for those mentioned below, beans, rice, oils.

Drink only: Water.

Do not eat, drink, or touch: Sour milk, any dairy, apples, tomato juice, beer, pickles, sauerkraut, wines, whey cornstarch, potatoes, molasses.

Malvin

Eat only: Rice, meat, fish, barley, grains.

Drink only: Water.

Do not eat, drink, or touch: Chicken, corn, eggs, soy, fruits, vegetables, dairy products, nuts, spices, honey, mustard seeds, black-eyed peas, green peas, tomatoes, walnuts, watermelons.

Menadione

Eat only: Rice, meats, fish, and vegetables except those mentioned below.

Drink only: Water, coffee, and tea.

Do not eat, drink, or touch: Green leafy vegetables, fruits, cauliflower, kelp, alfalfa, soy, and egg yolks.

Nicotine

Eat only: Poultry, fish, vegetables except those mentioned below, fruits, beans, oils.

Drink only: Water.

Do not eat, drink, or touch: Beef, tobacco, potatoes, tomatoes, bananas, milk and cheese, cocoa, barley malt, yeast.

Oxalic acid

Eat only: Grains, fruits, vegetables except those mentioned below, poultry, meats, fish, oils, and dairy.

Drink only: Water.

Do not eat, drink, or touch: Beet leaves, spinach, rhubarb, turnips.

Phytic acid

Eat only: Meats, fish, poultry, fruits.

Drink only: water.

Do not eat, drink, or touch: Chlorophyll, grains, seeds, plants, wheat, rye, oats, peas, beans, barley, rice, flax seed, soybeans, peanuts.

Piperine

Eat only: Fish, vegetables, except those mentioned below, fruit, beans, oils.

Drink only: Water, coffee, and tea.

Do not eat, drink, or touch: Beef, beet sugar, cheese, chicken, eggs, lamb, milk, tuna, turkey, yeast, black pepper, tomatoes, potatoes, chili powder, cucumber, black, green, and red pepper, vanilla, yeast.

Proline

Eat only: Poultry, fish, vegetables, fruit, beans, oils, rice.

Drink only: Water, coffee, and tea.

Do not eat, drink, or touch: Gelatin and wheat.

Threonine

Eat only: Fish, vegetables, fruits, oils, beans, meat.

Drink only: Water, coffee, and tea.

Do not eat, drink, or touch: Eggs, milk, gelatin, oats, wheat, ricotta and cottage cheese, pork, chicken, turkey.

Uric acid

Avoid: foods high in uric acid (refer to the listing on page 547).

Indol and skatol

Eat only: Meats, fish, poultry, vegetables except those mentioned below, fruits, oils, and beans.

Drink only: Water.

Do not eat, drink, or touch: Oranges, flowers, green vegetables, perfumes, dairy products.

Rutin   follow list of restrictions for bioflavanoids.

Uric Acid

Avoid: Foods high in uric acid (refer to the listing later in Part VI).

Drink only: Water.

PHENYLALANINE

Eat only: Vegetables, fruit, except those below, grains, except wild rice and barley.

Drink only: Water, coffee, and tea.

Do not eat, drink, or touch: Wild rice, beef, eggs, milk, chicken, fish, soybeans, cottage cheese, baked beans, bananas, peanuts and almonds, potatoes, sweet potatoes, barley, coconut, codfish, crabmeat, gelatin, grapes, chocolate, cocoa, ginger, hops, black-eyed pea, green peas.

PLASTICS

Avoid: Crude oil and plastic products such as computers, telephones, pens, toothbrushes, hairbrushes.

Wear: Cotton or leather gloves.

POLLEN MIX

Avoid: Being outdoors; use a mask and gloves outdoors.

POTASSIUM
Eat only: White rice, pastas, cauliflowers, chicken, meat, eggs.
Do not eat or touch: Vegetables, oranges, bananas, cantaloupes, tomatoes, mint leaves, watercress, potatoes, whole grains, seeds, nuts, cream of tartar.

POTATO MIX   russet, white, red, sweet, yam
Eat Only: Vegetables except potatoes, fruits, meat, poultry, fish, dairy products, grains, and beans.
Do not eat or touch: All types of potatoes and the products made from potatoes.

PROSTAGLANDINS (refer to hormones and follow the same restrictions).

RADIATION
Avoid: Sun, television, microwave, X rays, computers. Treat on a rainy day or at night and stay indoors.

RED WINE   follow list of restrictions for alcohol

RNA
Eat only: Lettuce.
Drink only: Water.
Do not eat or touch: Proteins such as meat, poultry, fish, nuts.

RICE SUGAR
Eat only: Fruits, vegetables, poultry, meat, dairy products, fish, beans, cane sugar.
Drink only: Water, black coffee, tea.
Do not eat or touch: Rice, or anything with rice sugar.

SACCHARINE
Eat Only: Grains, fruits, poultry, meat, vegetables, fish, cane sugar, dairy products and beans. READ ALL LABELS!

Drink only: Water, tea, coffee.

Do not eat, drink, or touch: Products with sacchrine, soft drinks, sweet relish, pickles, cookies, toothpastes.

SELENIUM

Eat only: White rice, pastas, cauliflowers, potatoes, chicken, fruits, salt.

Drink only: Water.

Do not eat, drink or touch: Seafood, milk, eggs, whole grains, beef, beans, bran, onions, tomatoes, broccoli, garlic, mushrooms, brewer's yeast, wheat germ, kelp, sea water, sea salt.

SEROTONIN

Eat only: Grains, chicken, meat, rice, cauliflowers, eggs, apples.

Do not eat, drink or touch: Dairy products, oranges, turkey, potatoes, soy, yeast, avocados, bananas, cocoa, pineapples, plums, tomatoes.

SHELLFISH MIX   shrimp, crabs, lobster, crayfish, abalone, clams, oysters, mussels

Do not eat or touch: Any of the shellfish listed above.

SILVER

Do not eat or touch: Fish, fish by-products, items containing silver (jewelry, coins, pens, flatware) and mercury. USE GLOVES.

SMOKING

Avoid: Smoke from cigarettes, clothes, and substances that have been in contact with cigarette smoke. Wear a mask for twenty-five hours if necessary. Treat with a shower cap and change into new clothes after treatment.

SORBITOL

Eat only: Fruits, meat, poultry, fish, vegetables, cane sugar, dairy products, grains, and beans.

Drink only: Water, tea, coffee.

Do not eat, drink, or touch: Products containing sorbitol such as soft drinks, sweet relish, pickles, cookies, toothpastes. READ ALL LABELS!

SOYBEAN
Eat only: Dairy products, vegetables, meat, poultry, fish, fruits.
Do not eat, drink or touch: Tofu, soy milk, soy oil, soy lecithin, any soy product; (refer to detailed listing "Foods and Materials Containing Soybeans" in Part VI).

SPICE MIX 1   ginger, cardamom, cinnamon, cloves, nutmeg, garlic, cumin, fennel, coriander, turmeric, saffron, mint
Do not eat or touch the above: READ ALL LABELS! Also included are toothpastes, massage oils, and toiletries.

SPICE MIX 2   black pepper, red pepper, green peppers, 20 different peppers, jalapenos, onions, oregano, chives, chervil, mace, marjoram, rosemary, anise seeds, caraway seeds, basil, bay leaf, fenugreek, cream of tartar, dill, horseradish, MSG, mustard, paprika, poppy seeds, parsley, sage, sumac, vinegar
Do not eat or touch the above: READ ALL LABELS! Also included are toothpastes, massage oils, and toiletries.

SULFITES
Eat only: Poultry, meats, eggs, vegetables except those below.
Drink only: Water.
Do not eat, drink, or touch: Avocados, baked products, beet sugar, dried fruits, fresh shrimp, fruit drinks, gelatin, wine, beer, potatoes, starches, vegetables, salads, cider, and cellophane. Sulfites can be used in the manufacture of drugs and asthma aerosols.

SULFUR
Eat only: White rice, pastas, cauliflowers, potatoes, fruits, noniodized salt.
Drink only: Water.
Do not eat or touch: Meat, fish, eggs, dried beans, cabbages, soybeans, watercress, string beans, celery, onions, turnips, radishes.

SWEET'N LOW®
Eat only: Fruits, vegetables, meat, poultry, grains, cane sugar, dairy products, fish, and beans.
Drink only: Water, coffee, tea.
Do not eat, drink, or touch: Products that contain Sweet'N Low® such as soft drinks, sweet relish, pickles, cookies, toothpastes. READ ALL LABELS!

VITAMIN T
Do not eat or touch: Sesame seeds, egg yolks, vegetable oils.

TOMATO MIX green, yellow, and red tomatoes
Eat only: Vegetables other than tomatoes, meat, fruits, dairy products, fish, poultry, grains, and beans.
Do not eat or touch: Tomatoes of all kinds and products made from tomatoes such as soups, sauces, and stews.

TREE MIX
Avoid: Being outdoors.
Wear: Mask, gloves, socks, and shoes outdoors.

TURKEY turkey, milk products, tryptophan, Vitamin B_1, B_3, B_6
Do not eat, drink, or touch: Turkey, milk products, tryptophan, and all items that contain the B vitamins listed above (refer to the detailed listing of foods under Vitamin B_1, B_3, and B_6 earlier in Part VI).

VANADIUM
Do not eat or touch: Fish, seafood.

VEGETABLE FAT   almond oil, palm oil, flax seed oil, canola oil, cottonseed oil, safflower oil, sesame oil, super-heated vegetable fats, olive oil, corn oil, Crisco Oil, coconut oil, peanut oil, linseed oil, sunflower oil, mustard oil
Eat only: Steamed vegetables, steamed rice, meat, eggs, chicken, butter, animal fats, fruits.
Do not eat or touch: Oils listed above or products containing them, products for external use containing these oils.

VEGETABLE MIX   green beans, cauliflowers, broccoli, brussel sprouts, cabbages, asparagus
Eat only: Fruits, meat, dairy, fish, poultry, beans, grains, eggs.
Do not eat or touch: Vegetables of any kind.

VINEGAR MIX   white, apple cider, and rice vinegar
Eat only: Grains, vegetables, meat, poultry, fish, and dairy products.
Do not eat, drink, or touch: Vinegar, rice, apples, salad dressings with vinegar, condiments such as mustard, mayonnaise, and ketchup. READ ALL LABELS!

VIRUS MIX
Avoid: Contact with sick or infected persons for twenty-five hours. Wear a mask to be safe. Use clean sheets, pillowcases, new toothbrush, and sterilized telephone.

WEED MIX
Avoid: Being outdoors.
Wear: A mask and gloves outdoors.

WHEAT MIX   red, white, buckwheat
Eat only: Rice, vegetables, fruits, poultry, meat, fish, dairy products, and beans.

Do not eat or touch: All wheat products, (refer to "Foods and Materials Containing Wheat" later in Part VI).

WHEY
Eat only: Rice, vegetables, fruits, meat, poultry, fish.
Do not eat, drink, or touch: Dairy products, or products containing whey. READ LABELS! Also included are crackers and french breads.

WHITE WINE   follow restrictions for alcohol

WHITEN ALL   sulfites
Eat only: Cooked vegetables, pastas, rice, meat, fish, chicken, eggs.
Do not eat or touch: Uncooked or frozen vegetables, canned foods, potato salads, fruit salads, potatoes any style (baked, french fried, or the like), sauces, dips, condiments, wines, wine vinegar, fruits (especially grapes), restaurant prepared or catered foods, foods from salad bars.

WOOD MIX
Avoid: Contact with woods and items made with woods.
Wear: Gloves.

WOOL
Avoid: Wool.
Wear: Gloves and cotton socks when walking on a wool rug.

YEAST MIX   baker's yeast, brewer's yeast, tortula yeast
Eat only: Vegetables, chicken, fish, extra virgin olive oil, canola oil, sesame oil.
Do not eat or touch: Dairy products, yeast products (breads, beer, wine), vinegar, hops, malts, peanuts, mushrooms, simple sugars, condiments (soy sauce, catsup), fruits (refer to the listing "Foods and Materials Containing Yeast" in Part VI).

YOGURT   yogurt, cheese; products from whey, yogurt, or cheese

Eat only: Rice, vegetables, fruits, meat, poultry, fish.

Do not eat, drink, or touch: Dairy products such as yogurt or cheese and products containing whey as well as dairy.

ZINC

Eat only: White rice, pastas, cauliflowers, potatoes, chicken, salt.

Drink only: Water.

Do not eat or touch: Green leafy vegetables, pork, beef, lamb, fish, brown rice, eggs, milk, brewer's yeast, mushrooms, onions, peas, dried beans, seeds, wheat bran, wheat germ, herring, oysters, mustard.

FOODS AND MATERIALS CONTAINING KEY ALLERGENS
Foods Containing Artificial Colors and Flavors

TO BE AVOIDED

Bakery Goods:
All manufactured cakes,
  cookies, sweet rolls, pastries,
  doughnuts
Frozen baked goods
Many packaged baking mixes
Pie crusts

Beverages:
All instant-breakfast drinks
All quick-mix powdered drinks
Beer
Cider
Diet drinks
Prepared chocolate milk
Soft drinks
Tea, hot or cold
Wine

Candies:
All manufactured types,
  hard or soft

Cereals:
All cereals with artificial colors
  and flavors
All instant-breakfast
  preparations

Desserts:
All dessert mixes
All powdered puddings
Flavored yogurt
Manufactured ice creams unless
  the label specifies no synthetic
  coloring or flavoring

PERMITTED

Bakery Goods:
All commercial breads except
  egg bread and whole wheat
  (usually dyed)
All flours
Any products without artificial
  color or flavor; most bakery items
  should be prepared at home

Beverages:
Grapefruit juice
Guava nectar
Homemade lemonade or limeade
  from fresh lemons or limes
Milk
Pear nectar
Pineapple juice
Seven-Up®

Candies:
Homemade candies, without
  almonds

Cereals:
Any cereals without
  artifical colors or flavors, dry or
  cooked

Desserts:
Commercial ice cream stating no
  artificial flavor or color
Homemade custards and puddings
Homemade gelatins from pure
  gelatins with any permitted
  natural fruit or fruit juices
Homemade ice cream without
  artificial coloring or flavoring
Plain yogurt

TO BE AVOIDED

(continued)

Fish:
Fish sticks that are
  dyed or flavored
Frozen fish fillets that are dyed
  or flavored

Luncheon meats:
Bologna
Frankfurters
Ham, bacon, pork*
Meat loaf
Salami
Sausages*

Miscellaneous Items:
All mint-flavored items
Barbecue-flavored potato chips
Catsup
Chili sauce
Cider vinegar
Cloves
Colored butter
Colored cheeses
Commercial chocolate syrup
Margarine
Mustard
Soy sauce, if flavored or colored
Wine vinegar

Poultry:
All barbecued types
All turkeys with prepared
  basting (self-basting)
Prepared stuffing

Sundry Items:
All cough drops
All mouthwashes
All pediatric medications and
  vitamins that contain artificial
  color and flavors when

PERMITTED

Desserts: (continued)
Tapioca

Fish:
All fresh fish

Luncheon meats:
All fresh meat

Miscellaneous Items:
All cooking oils and fats
All natural (white) cheeses
Distilled white vinegar
Homemade chocolate syrup for all
  purposes
Homemade mayonnaise
Jams or jellies made from
  permitted fruits and not artificially
  colored or flavored
Mustard prepared at home from
  pure powder and distilled vinegar
Sweet butter, not colored or flavored

Poultry:
All poultry except stuffed

TO BE AVOIDED

Sundry Items: (continued)
medications are required, a
physician should be consulted.
Most over-the-counter medications
contain aspirin as well as artificial
flavors and colors (Aspirin,
Bufferin®, Excedrin®, Alka-Seltzer®,
Empirin®, Empirin Compound®,
Anacin®)
All throat lozenges
All toothpastes and toothpowders†
Antacid tablets
Perfumes

*If a product is colored or flavored, it is usually indicated on the package

†A salt and soda mixture can be used for cleaning teeth; Neutrogena® soap (unscented) can be substituted for toothpaste or powder

Foods and Materials Containing Corn

Adhesives
Ale
American brandies
 apple
 grape
Aspirin and other tablets

Bacon
Baking Mixes
 Aunt Jemima® Pancake Mix
 Bisquick®
 Complete Pancake Mix®
 Doughnuts
Baking Powders
Batters for frying meat, fish, fowl
Beers
Beets, Harvard
Beverages, carbonated
Bleached wheat flours
Bourbon and other whiskies
Breads and pastries

Cakes
Candy
 Box candies, all grades
 Candy bars
 Commercial candies
Carbonated beverages
Catsups
Cheerios®
Cheeses
Chili
Chop suey
Coffee, Instant
Confectioner's sugar
Cookies
Corn
 flakes
 flour
 meal
 oil (Mazola®)
 parched
 popped

soya
starch
sugars
  cerelose
  dextrose
  dyno
unripe
  canned
  fresh
  fritters
  frozen
  roasting ears
  succotash
Cough syrups
Cream pies
Cream puffs
Cups, paper

Dates, confection
Deep fat frying mixtures
Dentifrices

Excipients or diluents in:
  capsules
  suppositories
  tablets
  vitamins

Flour, bleached
Foods, fried
French dressing
Fritos®
Frostings
Fruits
Frying fats

Gelatin capsules
Gelatin dessert
Gin
Glucose products
Graham crackers
Grape juice
Gravies

Grits
Gum on envelopes, stickers,
  stamps, tapes, labels
Gums, chewing
Gummed papers

Ham, cured or tenderized
Harvard beets
Holiday-type stickers
Hominy

Ice creams
Ices
Inhalants
  bath powders
  body powders
  cooking fumes from fresh corn

Jams
Jellies
Jell-O®

Kremel

Leavening agents
  baking powders
  yeasts
Liquors
  ale
  beer
  gin
  whiskey
Lozenges

Margarine
Meat
  bacon
  bologna
  cooked, with gravies
  frankfurters
  ham, cured or tenderized
  lunch ham
  sausages, cooked

weiners
Milk, in paper cartons
Monosodium glutamate
Mull-Soy

Nescafe®™

Ointments

Pablum
Paper containers
 boxes
 cups
 plates
 (Only when foods come in
 contact with these containers)
Pastries
 cakes
 cup cakes
Peanut butters
Peas, canned
Pies, creamed
Plastic food wrappers (the inner
 surfaces may be coated with
 corn starch)
Powdered sugar
Preserves
Puddings
 blanc mange
 custards
 Royal pudding

Rice, coated

Salad dressings
Salt
 salt cellars in restaurants
Sandwich spreads
Sauces
 sundaes
 meats
 fish
 vegetables

Seasoned salt
Sherberts
Similac®
String beans
 canned
 frozen
Soups
 creamed
 thickened
 vegetable
Soybean milks
Starch
Starch fumes while ironing
 clothes
Sugar, powdered
Syrups, commercially prepared
 glucose
 Karo®

Talcums
Teas, instant
Toothpaste (some)
Tortillas

Vanillin
Vegetables
 canned
 creamed
 frozen
Vinegar, distilled
Vitamins

Whiskies
 bourbon
 scotch
Wines, American*
 dessert
 fortified
 sparkling

*Some brands are corn-free

Foods Containing Eggs

Baking powder
Batters for french frying
Bavarian cream
Boiled dressings
Bouillon
Bread
Breaded foods
Cake flour
Cakes
French toast
Fritters
Frosting
Glazed rolls
Griddle cakes
Hamburger mix
Hollandaise sauce
Ice cream
Ices
Icings
Macaroni
Macaroons
Malted cocoa drinks
  Ovaltine®
Marshmallows
Meat jellies
Meat loaf

Meat molds
Meat patties
Meringues
Noodles
Pancake flour
Pancakes
Pastes
Pretzels
Pudding
Salad dressing
Sauces
Sausages
Sherberts
Souffles
Soups
  consommes
  mock turtle
  noodle
Spaghetti
Spanish creams
Tartar sauce
Timbales
Waffle mixes
Waffles
Wines

Foods and Materials Containing Formaldehyde

Formaldehyde is a formic aldehyde, a powerful disinfectant gas produced by the oxidation of methyl alcohol. The aqueous solution is a colorless, volatile fluid used as a surgical and general antiseptic as well as a preservative. It is also utilized as a reagent, a substance used in the detection or analysis of another substance by chemical, microscopic, or other means.

Common Uses of Formaldehyde Include:

Intermediates in the synthesis of
  alcohols, acids, and chemicals
Tanning agent
A rodent poison

The formulation of slow-release
  nitrogen fertilizers and in destroying micro-organisms responsible for plant disease

An added agent to make concrete, plaster, and related products impermeable to liquids

Antiperspirants and antiseptics in dentifrices, mouthwashes, and germicidal and detergent soaps

Hair-setting lotions, shampoos, and detergent soaps

Air deodorant in public places and in industrial environments

Destroying bacteria, fungi, molds, and yeasts

Disinfecting equipment in the fermentation industry and the manufacture of antibiotics

Disinfecting sickrooms and surgical instruments

Synthesis of dyes, stripping agents, and various specialty chemicals in the dye industry

The manufacture of embalming fluids when combined with alcohol, glycerol, and phenol

Preserving products such as waxes, polishes, adhesives, fats, oils, and anatomical specimens

The synthesis of explosives

Preparing fireproofing compositions to apply to fabrics in conjunction with other chemicals

Insecticidal solutions for killing flies, mosquitoes, and moths

The synthesis of Vitamin A and to improve the activity of Vitamin E preparations

Improving set strength and water resistance in paper products

Preserving and accelerating photographic developing solutions

Making natural and synthetic fibers crease-resistant, wrinkle-resistant, crushproof, water-repellent, dye-fast, flame-resistant, water-resistant, shrinkproof, moth-proof (wool), and more elastic (wool)

Making synthetic resins, wood veneer (for wall paper) and artificial aging, and reduction of shrinkage in wood preservation

One of the component parts of wallboard in construction of houses and apartments

Resin in nail polish and undercoating of nail polish

Formaldehyde accounts for about fifty percent of the estimated total aldehydes in polluted air. The major sources of aldehyde pollution are in the incomplete combustions of hydrocarbons in gasoline and diesel engines, burning of fuels, and incineration waste. Formaldehyde is believed to be the principal agent responsible for burning of the eyes in smog. Aldehydes can also react further to form additional products such as ozone.

Foods and Materials Containing Hydrocarbons

Hydrocarbons are organic compounds comprised of hydrogen and carbon. If the geological concept that conifer forests are the precursors of the original sources of the hydrocarbons—coal, oil, gas—is valid, then we should consider these materials as well. Such an interpretation is indicated by the similar clinical effects of pine and its combustion products with those of coal, oil, and gas and their combustion products and derivatives.

Common Uses of Hydrocarbons Include:

Alcohol

Artificially colored foods and drugs

Burning green wood containing considerable oil and resin

Cements and other adhesives

Cleaning fluids and lighter fluids

Creosote impregnated wood

Evaporating oil from mechanical devices

Evaporating paints, varnish, and other solvents

Foods exposed to gas for ripening, roasting, or clarifying through bone char that is reactivated in gas-fired ovens

Fuel: coal, oil, gas, diesel and nondiesel, and their combustion

Garage odors fouling the air of living quarters

Industrial and agricultural chemicals contaminating water supplies

Insecticides

Mineral oil

Miscellaneous odors: detergents, soaps containing naphtha, am-

monia, bleach, cleansing powders containing bleach, window washing compounds, certain silver and brass polishing materials, and deodorants and disinfectants (especially pine-scented)

Newsprint

Oil-soluble food sprays that permeate the cooking surface to which they are applied and cannot be removed by washing, peeling, soaking in water or vinegar, or by cooking

Paraffins used in coating and scaling, in candles, in rubber compounding, in pharmaceuticals, and in cosmetics

Pine exposure

Plastics

Plastics produced by chemical condensations

Refrigerants (freon) and spray containers

Roofing and road construction compounds

Sponge rubber

Foods Containing Milk

Baker's bread

Baking powder biscuits

Bavarian cream

Bisques

Blancmange

Boiled salad dressings

Butter
Buttermilk
Butter sauces
Cakes
Candies
Cheeses
Chocolate
Chowders
Cocoa drinks, mixtures
Cookies
Cream
Creamed foods
Cream sauces
Curds
Custards
Doughnuts
Eggs, scrambled
Flour mixtures
Foods fried in butter (fish, poultry, beef, pork)
Foods prepared au gratin
Fritters
Gravies
Hamburgers
Hard sauces
Hash
Hot cakes
Ice creams

Junket®
Malted milk
Margarine
Mashed potatoes
Meat loaf
Milk Chocolate
Omelets
Ovaltine
Pie crust (some)
Prepared mixes
  biscuits
  cakes
  cookies
  doughnuts
  muffins
  pancakes
  pie crust
  waffles
Rarebits
Salad dressings
Sausages, cooked
Scalloped dishes
Sherberts
Soda crackers
Souffles
Soups
Whey
Zwieback

Foods and Materials Containing Soybeans

Foods Containing Soybeans or Made from Soybeans:

Automobile Parts: Some automobile manufacturers are using soybeans to make a plastic from which window frames, steering wheels, gear shift knobs, distributors, and other parts are made. They also make an upholstery fabric from soybeans.

Bakery goods: Soybean flour containing only one percent oil is now used by many bakers in their dough mixtures for breads, cakes, rolls, and pastries. This keeps baked goods moist and salable several days longer. The roasted nuts are used in place of peanuts on breakfast rolls. Biscuits and several crisp crackers have soybean flour in them.

Candies: Soy flours are used in hard candies, fudge, nut candies, custards, and caramels. Lecithin

is invariably derived from soy-beans for use in candies, particularly chocolate, to prevent drying out and to emulsify the fats.
Cereals
Industrial and Other Contacts:
Soy products are used in varnish, paints, enamels, printing ink, massage creams, candles, celluloid, linoleum, adhesives, paper finishes, blankets, cloth, nitroglycerine, urease, pet food, soaps, fertilizers, and automobile parts. It is also used for fodder, textile dressing, glycerine, coffee substitutes and to make lubricating and illuminating oil. Soybeans are used to make rubber substitutes and its lecithin is used as a stabilizer in leaded gasoline.

Meats: Pork link sausage and lunch meats can contain soybeans. The allergic individual should buy only pure meat products.

Milk Substitutes: Some bakeries use soy milk instead of cow's milk in recipes.

Miscellaneous: Soy products are used in some ice creams and in many soups. Fresh green soy sprouts are served as a vegetable, especially in Chinese dishes. Soybeans are roasted, salted, and used in place of peanuts. They are also used to make soy noodles, macaroons, and spaghetti. Some seasonings contain soy, as do a number of frying fats and shortenings. Oleomargarines and butter substitutes contain the oil and bean products. It is also present in many cookies, crackers, and snacks.

Salad Dressings: Many salad dressings and mayonnaises contain soy oil but only show on the label that they contain vegetable oil. When using a particular brand of dressing or mayonnaise, inquire as to the contents.

Sauces

NOTE: *Keep in mind that soybeans and their products are used as flour, oil, milk, and nuts. We are living in an era of expanding uses for soybeans, and the allergy sufferer should anticipate the many possible contacts. Additionally, as new food combinations become popular, many new contacts can be expected. When undergoing an NAET treatment for soybeans, eat only foods in their original form. Avoid baked, processed, and packaged foods. Wear cotton or leather gloves and a mask when handling or coming in close proximity (less than four feet) with the products on the above list.*

Foods Containing "Hidden Sugars"

Beverages:
Cola drinks
Cordials
Ginger ale
Orange ade
Root beer
Seven-Up®
Soda pop
Sweet cider
Whiskey sour
Cakes and Cookies:
Angel food
Applesauce cake
Banana cake
Brownies (plain)
Cheese cake
Chocolate cake (iced)
Chocolate cake (plain)
Chocolate cookies
Chocolate eclairs
Coffee cake
Cream puff
Cup cake (iced)
Donuts (glazed)
Donuts (plain)
Fig Newtons
Fruit cake
Gingersnaps
Jelly roll
Macaroons
Nut cookies
Oatmeal cookies
Orange cake
Pound cake
Sponge cake

Strawberry shortcake
Sugar Cookies
Candies
Chewing gum
Chocolate (cream filling)
Chocolate mints
Fudge
Hard candy
Hershey's® bar
Lifesavers®
Peanut brittle
Canned Fruits and Juices:
Apricots
Apricot syrup
Fruit cocktail
Fruit juice (sweetened)
Fruit syrup
Peaches
Stewed fruits
Dairy Products:
Ice cream
Ice cream bar
Ice cream cone
Ice cream soda
Ice cream sundae
Milk shake
Jams, Jellies, and Desserts:
Apple butter
Apple cobbler
Custard
French pastry
Jell-O®
Jelly
Orange marmalade
Strawberry

Foods Containing Wheat

Beverages:
Beer
Cocomalt
Gin (any drink with grain-
  neutral spirits)
Malted milk
Ovaltine
Postum
Whiskey
Breads:
Biscuits
Breads
  corn
  gluten
  graham
  rye (rye products are not
    entirely free of wheat)
  soy
  wheat
Crackers
Muffins
Popovers
Pretzels
Rolls
Cereals:
All wheat cereals
Bran flakes
Corn Flakes®
Cream of Wheat®
Farina®
Grapenuts®
Other malted cereals
Puffed Wheat®
Rice Krispies®
Shredded Wheat®™
Triscuits®
Wheatena®
Flours:
Buckwheat
Corn

Gluten
Graham
Lima Bean
Patent
Rye
White
Whole wheat
Pastries and Desserts:
Cakes
Candy bars
Chocolate candy
Cookies
Doughnuts
Frozen pies
Pies
Puddings
Wheat Products:
Bread
Dumplings
Macaroni
Noodles
Rusk
Spaghetti
Vermicelli
Zweiback
Miscellaneous:
Bouillon cubes
Chocolate candy
Chocolate (except bitter cocoa
  and bitter chocolate)
Cooked mixed meat dishes
Fats that have been used for
  frying
Foods rolled in flour (including
  meat)
Gravies
Griddle cakes
Hot cakes
Ice cream cones
Matzos

Mayonnaise
Most cooked and prepared meat
including sausages, wieners,
bologna, liverwurst, luncheon
ham, and hamburger
Pancake mixes
Sauces

Synthetic pepper
Some yeasts
Thickening in ice cream
Wheat cakes
Wheat germ
Waffles

Foods Containing Yeast

The following foods contain yeast as an additive ingredient during preparation (often called leavening):

Breads
Cake and cake mixes
Canned icebox biscuits
Cookies
Crackers
Hamburger buns
Hot dog buns

Meat fried in cracker crumbs
Milk fortified with vitamins from
yeast
Pastries
Pretzels
Rolls, homemade or canned

The following substances contain yeast or yeast-like substances because of their nature or the nature of their manufacture or preparation:

Buttermilk
Cheeses of all kinds including
cottage cheese
Citrus fruit juices, frozen or
canned (only home-squeezed
are yeast-free!)
Fermented beverages including
whiskey, wine, brandy, gin, rum,
vodka, and root beer
Malted products including cereals,
candy, and malted milk drinks
Mushrooms

Truffles
Vinegars (apple, pear, grape, and
distilled). These may be used
alone or in such foods as catsup,
mayonnaise, olives, pickles,
sauerkraut, condiments,
horseradish, French dressing,
salad dressing, Bar B-Q sauce,
tomato sauce, chili peppers,
mince pie, and Gerber's® Oatmeal and Barley Cereal

The following contain substances that are derived from yeast or have their source in yeast. READ ALL LABELS!

Capsules or tablets containing Vi-
tamin B made from yeast
Multiple vitamins
Some enzyme supplements con-

taining brewer's yeast
Vitamin B capsules or tablets
made from yeast

Drugs Containing NO Corn, Wheat or Milk

Acetaminophen
Accutane Capsules®
Allerest Children's Chewable
 Tablets®
Allerest Eye Drops®
Allerest Nasal Spray®
Amphojel Suspension®
Amphojel Suspension without
 Flavor®
Anaprox®
Ancef Injection®
Aspirin Uniserts

Bacitracin Sterile®
Bacitracin Topical Ointment®
Bactrim Suspension™
Bactrim Tablets™
Basaljel Suspension®
Basaljel Suspension Extra
 Strength®
Benadryl Steri-Vial®™
Berocca Plus Tablets®
Berocca Tablets®
Bisacodyl (Dulcolax)®
Brexin L. A. Capsules®

Cafergot Suppositories®
Calciferol Drops™
Castor Oil
Casufru Liquid
Cedilanid-D Injection
Cerose Compound Capsules
Cerubidine Injectable®
Chardose Powder
Chloromycetin® Cream, 1%
Chloromycetin® Opthalmic
 Ointment
Chloromycetin® Palmitate Oral
 Suspension
Chloromycetin® Sodium
 Succinate Steri-Vial

Chromagen® Capsules
Claforan® Injection
Codeine Sulfate
Cod Liver Oil
Coly-Mycin M Parenteral®
Coly-Mycin S Oral Suspension®
Comhist LA Capsules®
Compazine Syrup®
Cortenema (Hydrocortisone
 Retention Enema)®
Cortril Hydrocortisone Topical
 Ointment

Dallergy Syrup®
Dantrium Intravenous®
Debrox Drops®
DHE 45 Injection®
DiaBeta Tablets®
Diapid Nasal Spray
Dilantin–30/Pediatric
 Dilantin–125®
Dilor G Liquid and Tablets®
Dimetane Ten®
Ditropan Syrup®
Docusate Sodium Capsules®
Docusate Sodium with
 Casanthranol Capsules®
Dopram Injectable®

Elase®
Emcyt Capsules®
Endep Tablets®
Entex LA Tablets®
Entex Liquid®
Equagesic Tablets®

Festal II Digestive Aid Tablets®
Festalan Tablets®
Flagyl I.V.®
Flagyl I.V. RTU®
Flagyl Tablets®

Fluogen®
Fumerin Tablets®
Furacin Products-Topical Cream®
Furadantin Oral Suspension®
Furosemide Injection®

Gantrisin Pediatric Suspension®
Gantrisin Syrup®
Gaviscon®™

Histatapp Elixir®
Hydergine LC Liquid Capsules®
Hydergine Oral Tablets,
  Sublingual Tablets, and Liquid

Ipsatol DM®
Isordil Chewable Tablets®
Isordil Tembids Capsules®
Isordil Tembids Tablets®
Isordil Titrados Tablets®

Kie Syrup®
Klor-Con Powder®
Klor-Con 8/Klor-Con 10®
Klor-Con/25 Powder®
Klor-10%®
Klorvess Effervescent Granules®
Klorvess Effervescent Tablets®

Lactocal-F Tablets
Laraodopa Tablets®
Lasix Oral Solution®
Levsin Drops®
Levsin Elixir®
Levsin PB Drops®
Levsin PB Elixir®
Lidex (Cream, Gel, Ointment,
  Topical Solution)®
Lidex-E Cream®
Lidex Ointment®
Lidex Topical Solution®
Lithonate Capsules®
Lithotabs Tablets™

Lomotil Tablets and Liquid®

Medihaler-Epi™
Medihaler Ergotamine Aerosol™
Mestinon Syrup®
Metamucil (Powder Contains
  Dextrose)®
Methergine Injection®
Milk of Magnesia
Mineral Oil
Mycelex Troches®
Mycostatin Oral Suspension®
Mytrex Cream & Ointment®

Nitro-Bid® (IV, Ointment, 2.5
  Plateau Caps, 6.5 and 9 Plateau
  Caps)
Nitrostat Injection®
Nitrostat Ointment 2%®
Nitrostat Tablets®
Nydrazid Syrup®

Omnipen for Oral Suspension®
Omnipen Pediatric Drops®

Pamelor Solution®
Penicillin G Potassium
  for Injections®
Penicillin G Potassium Tablets®
Pen Vee K Tablets®
Pen Vee K Oral Solution®
Pfizerpen Capsules and Oral
  Suspension®
Pfizerpen-AS®
Pfizerpen VK Tablets and Oral
  Suspension®
Polymyxin B Sulfate®
Procan SR®
Prolixin Decanoate®
Prolixin Elixir®
Prolixin Enanthate®
Prompt®

Reglan Injectable®
Rid (topical)®
RMS (Suppositories) Uniserts®
Robaxin Injection®
Robinul Injectable®
Robicillin for VK Oral Solution®
Rocaltrol Tablets®
Roniscol Timespan Tablets®

Saccharin Tablets
Secobarbital Sodium Capsules®
Silvadene Cream (topical)®
Sinarest 12 Hour Nasal Spray®
SK Chloral Hydrate Capsules®
SK Potassium Chloride Oral
 Solution®
Sorbitol
Star-Otic
Stelazine Concentrate®
Stoxil Ophthalmic Ointment®
Stoxil Ophthalmic Solution®
Streptase®
Streptomycin Sulfate
Sumycin Syrup
Surmontil Capsules®
Sweeta Liquid®
Synacort Cream®
Synalgos Capsules®
Synalgos DC Capsules®
Synalar HP Cream®
Synalar Ointment®
Syntocinon Injection®
Syntocinon Nasal Spray®

Tagamet Liquid®
Terra Cortril Opthalmic
 Suspension®
Terra Cortril Topical Ointment®

Terramycin IM®
Terramycin IV®
Terramycin Ophthalmic
 Ointment®
Terramycin Topical Ointment®
Theo-Dur Sprinkle®
Theo-24 Capsules®
Theolair-Plus Liquid™
Theolair-Plus Tablets™
Theragran Liquid®
Thorazine Concentrate®
Thorazine Syrup®
Topicort Cream®
Topicort Gel®
Topicycline®
Trecator-SC Tablets®
Tuss-Ornade Liquid
Tylenol Children's Chewable
 Tablets®

Urolene Blue®
Urtex®

Vi Penta F Chewables®
Vi Penta F Drops®
Virilon®
Vistaril®

Wygesic Tablets®
Wymox Capsules®
Wymox Oral Suspension®

Yeast Tablets
Yeast X®

Zantac®
Zarontin Syrup®
Zaroxolyn Tablets®

SPECIFIC DIETS RELATED TO DIETARY STRESS

The following diets are based on individual dietary stresses. The four different dietary stresses are sugar, complex carbohydrate, fat, and protein. People generally fall into one of these specific food intolerances. This concept was discussed throughout this book and more specifically in Chapter 13.

The determination of one's specific intolerance is based on a thorough case history, a complete abdominal diagnostic palpation examination, and a twenty-four hour urine evaluation as taught by Dr. Howard Loomis. To locate a practitioner in your area, contact 21st Century Nutrition at 1-800-614-4400.

After a complete evaluation, one of these diets will be recommended to promote optimum health, weight management, and overall good energy levels. I have also included the Candida/yeast avoidance diet and the gastric diet in this section.

For additional dietary recommendations, consult the following books:

> *Eat More, Weigh Less* by Dean Ornish, M.D.
> *The New Pritikin Program* by Robert Pritikin
> *Enter the Zone* by Barry Sears, Ph.D.

DIET FOR COMPLEX CARBOHYDRATE INTOLERANCE—LOWER LEFT QUADRANT

Individuals who are carbohydrate intolerant usually crave fatty foods and have an irritable bowel. For these individuals, I recommend a diet that includes:

- liberal quantities of protein, certain cooked vegetables (see list below), water, any type of mineral water, and selected herbal teas

- moderate quantities of lipids as well as polyunsaturated vegetable oils, plant protein, fruits, and refined carbohydrates

- minimal consumption of whole grains, nuts, seeds, raw vegetables, and vegetables with seeds

- limited intake of salt including soy sauce and spicy foods that contain large amounts of salt

- limited intake of alcohol which acts as pure sugar is high in calories, void of nutrients, and can cause cravings

- avoidance of all artificial sweeteners and caffeinated beverages

Proteins: *(3–5 servings per day)*
2 egg whites	4 oz. beef (3 servings or less
2 oz. skim mozzarella cheese	2 oz. skim ricotta cheese
1 egg	per week)
4 oz. protein soy powder	1 oz. spirulina
4 oz. fish, shellfish, poultry	4 oz. veal
1 cup low or nonfat yogurt	3 oz. tofu
2 oz. low fat cottage cheese	4 oz. lamb

Carbohydrates: *Unlimited amounts of the following vegetables*
cooked cauliflower	cooked onions
cooked yellow squash	cooked yellow or green beans
cooked eggplant	cooked okra
cooked zucchini	cooked mushrooms
cooked artichoke	celery
all types of lettuce	onions
radishes	endive
spinach	escarole
kale	cabbage
jicama	bok choy

Limited amounts of the following vegetables (3–4 servings per week)
4 oz. sweet peas	4 oz. yam
4 oz. cooked carrots	4 oz. sweet potato
4 oz. cooked corn	4 oz. cooked pumpkin
4 oz. potatoes	

Vegetables to avoid
tomatoes	cucumber
sprouts	

Fruits: *(2 servings per day)*
1 apple	fruit juices
1 peach	1 nectarine
2 apricots	1 pear
½ honeydew	1 cup grapes
10 cherries	2 plums

1 cup berries | 1 cup watermelon
½ cup fresh pineapple | ½ cup cantaloupe
1 cup papaya | ½ banana

Limited fruits (3–4 servings per week)
1½ dried figs | ½ cup raisins
1½ dates | ½ cup cranberries

Complex carbohydrates:

Legumes, grains, and grain products (1–2 servings per day)
1 slice whole grain bread | ½ cup brown rice
½ cup bulgur | ½ cup oatmeal
½ cup quinoa | ¼ bagel
½ cup pasta | ½ English muffin
⅓ cup dried beans | ½ waffle
1 rice cake | ½ pita bread
1 corn tortilla | ½ cup spelt or kamut
½ cup white rice

Avoid
popcorn | granola
tortilla chips

Fats: *(1–2 servings per day)*
⅓ tsp. canola oil | ½ tbsp. avocado
⅓ tsp. olive oil | ½ tbsp. tahini
⅓ tsp. peanut oil | 1 tsp. olive oil and vinegar dressing

Limited fats (3–4 servings per week)
1 tsp. mayonnaise | ½ tsp. sesame oil
⅓ tsp. soybean oil | 2 tsp. bacon bits
⅓ tsp. butter | ½ tbsp. cream
1 tsp. cream cheese | ½ tbsp. sour cream
⅓ tsp. lard | ⅓ tsp. margarine

Avoid
nuts | seeds

DIET FOR FAT INTOLERANCE—UPPER RIGHT QUADRANT

Individuals who are fat intolerant usually have a deficiency in fatty acids and possibly an exhausted thyroid. Those individuals tend to crave sugars and often suffer from eczema, liver, and gallbladder disease. For these individuals, I recommend a diet that includes:

- liberal quantities of vegetables (raw or cooked without fat or salt—see list below), fruits, legumes, protein, water, any type of mineral water, hot grain beverages, vegetable juices, fruit juices, and selected herbal teas

- moderate quantities of higher fat protein sources such as seafood, low fat dairy, whole grains (see list below under complex carbohydrates) and starchy vegetables such as potatoes, yams, and winter squashes

- avoidance or minimal consumption of animal fats, tropical oils, hydrogenated oils, butter, cocoa butter (found in chocolate), margarine, mayonnaise, shortening, meats, whole dairy products, nuts, egg yolks, fried foods, nondairy creamers, refined grains, and grain products

- using olive oil, canola oil, avocado oil, sesame oil, peanut oil, corn oil, cottonseed oil, sunflower oil, soybean oil, safflower oil, and walnut oil sparingly (1 tsp. 1–2 times per day)

- limited intake of olives and avocados because they contain high amounts of fat

- limited intake of salt including soy sauce and spicy foods that contain large amounts of salt because fat-intolerant individuals tend to be water retentive

- limited intake of alcohol because it is irritating to the liver and the upper right quadrant, can cause cravings, acts as pure sugar, is high in calories, and is void of nutrients

- avoidance of nuts, all nut butters, cream cheese, sour cream, bacon, artificial sweeteners, and caffeinated beverages

Proteins: *(1–3 servings per day)*

2 egg white	$^2/_3$ cup soybeans
3 oz. fish, shellfish	3 oz. tofu
3 oz. lean poultry	3 oz. lean beef (no more than 3
2 oz. nonfat powdered milk	times per week)
2 oz. low fat or nonfat cottage cheese	3 oz. lean lamb (no more than 3 times per week)
6 oz. nonfat yogurt	

Carbohydrates:

Unlimited amounts of the following vegetables

beets	bok choy
broccoli	cabbage
cauliflower	celery
cucumbers	eggplant
endive	escarole
jicama	kale
leeks	lettuce
mushrooms	okra
onions	parsley
radishes	rutabagas
sprouts	squash
water chestnuts	watercress
green or yellow beans	

Limited amounts of the following vegetables (3–4 servings per week)

artichokes	carrots
sweet peas	corn
potatoes	sweet potatoes
yams	pumpkins

Complex carbohydrates:

Legumes, grains, and grain products (4 servings per day)

$1/3$ cup dried beans	$1/3$ cup cooked lentils
$1/3$ cup brown rice	$1/2$ bagel
1 slice whole wheat bread	$1/2$ (6 inch) pita bread
$1/3$ cup cooked wild rice	$1/2$ cup barley
$3/4$ oz. rice cakes	$1/2$ cup whole wheat macaroni
$1/2$ cup cooked grits	$1/2$ cup cooked oatmeal
$1/2$ cup cooked noodles	$1/2$ cup steel cut oats
1 (6-inch) corn tortilla	

Fruits: *(3 servings per day)*

1 small apple	4 medium fresh apricots
$1/2$ banana	$3/4$ cup berries
$1/3$ cantaloupe	12 cherries
$1^1/2$ dried figs	$2^1/2$ medium dates
$1/2$ grapefruit	$1/4$ honeydew melon
10 grapes	1 orange
1/2 mango	1 peach
1 cup papaya	$3/4$ cup pineapple
1 small pear	2 medium fresh prunes
2 plums	2 small tangerines
$1^1/4$ cups strawberries	

PROTEIN INTOLERANCE—LOWER RIGHT QUADRANT

Individuals who are protein intolerant usually crave sugar and tend to experience anxiety, osteoporosis because of poor calcium absorption, and possibly hypoglycemia. For those individuals, I recommend a diet that includes:

- liberal quantities of vegetables (raw or cooked without fat or salt—see list below), fruits, water, any type of mineral water, hot grain beverages, vegetable juices, fruit juices, and selected herbal teas

- moderate quantities of whole grains (see list below) and starchy vegetables such as potatoes, yams, and winter squashes

- minimal consumption of all proteins, legumes, animal fats, tropical oils, hydrogenated vegetable oils, fried foods, whole dairy products, and nuts such as coconut and macadamia

- limited intake of salt including soy sauce and spicy foods that contain large amounts of salt

- limited intake of alcohol that acts as pure sugar, is high in calories, is void of nutrients, and can cause cravings

- avoid all artificial sweeteners and caffeinated beverages

Proteins: *(1–2 serving per day)*

2 eggs (3 servings or less per week)	3 oz. tofu
3 oz. low-fat cottage cheese	3 oz. lean poultry
2 oz. skim mozzarella cheese	4 oz. fish, shellfish
4 oz. protein powder	2 oz. skim ricotta cheese
1 cup nonfat yogurt	1 oz. spirulina
no red meat	2/3 cup soybeans

Carbohydrates:

Unlimited amounts of the following vegetables

beets	bok choy
broccoli	cabbage
cauliflower	celery
cucumber	eggplant
endive	escarole

jicama	kale
leeks	lettuce
mushrooms	okra
onions	parsley
radishes	rutabagas
sprouts	squash
water chestnuts	watercress
beans, green or yellow	

Limited amounts of the following vegetables (3–4 servings per week)

artichokes	carrots
sweet peas	corn
potatoes	sweet potatoes
yams	pumpkin

Complex carbohydrates:

Legumes, grains, and grain products (3–4 servings per day)

$\frac{1}{3}$ cup dried beans	$\frac{1}{3}$ cup cooked lentils
$\frac{1}{3}$ cup brown rice	$\frac{1}{2}$ bagel
1 slice whole wheat bread	$\frac{1}{2}$ cup cooked wild rice
$\frac{1}{2}$ (6 inch) pita bread	1 rice cake
$\frac{1}{2}$ cup barley	$\frac{1}{2}$ cup cooked grits
$\frac{1}{2}$ cup whole wheat macaroni	$\frac{1}{2}$ cup cooked noodles
$\frac{1}{2}$ cup cooked oatmeal	1 (6-inch) corn tortilla
$\frac{1}{2}$ cup steel cut oats	$\frac{1}{2}$ cup millet

Fruits: *(3 servings per day)*

1 small apple	4 medium fresh apricots
$\frac{1}{2}$ banana	$\frac{3}{4}$ cup berries
$\frac{1}{3}$ cantaloupe	12 cherries
$1\frac{1}{2}$ dried figs	$2\frac{1}{2}$ medium dates
$\frac{1}{2}$ grapefruit	$\frac{1}{4}$ honeydew melon
10 grapes	1 orange
$\frac{1}{2}$ mango	1 peach
1 cup papaya	$\frac{3}{4}$ cup pineapple
1 small pear	2 medium fresh prunes
2 plums	2 small tangerines
$1\frac{1}{4}$ cups strawberries	

Fats: *(2 servings per day)*

7 almonds or $\frac{1}{2}$ tsp. almond butter	$\frac{1}{2}$ tbsp. avocado
$\frac{1}{3}$ tsp. canola oil	$\frac{1}{2}$ tbsp. tahini
$\frac{1}{3}$ tsp. olive oil	1 tsp. olive oil and vinegar dressing
3 olives	$\frac{1}{2}$ tsp. peanut butter
$\frac{1}{3}$ tsp. peanut oil	6 peanuts

Limited fats (3–4 servings per week)

1 tsp. mayonnaise	$\frac{1}{2}$ tsp. sesame oil
$\frac{1}{3}$ tsp. soybean oil	$\frac{1}{2}$ tsp. walnuts
$\frac{1}{2}$ tsp. brazil nuts	2 tsp. bacon bits
$\frac{1}{3}$ tsp. butter	$\frac{1}{2}$ tbsp. cream
1 tsp. cream cheese	$\frac{1}{2}$ tbsp. sour cream
$\frac{1}{3}$ tsp. lard	$\frac{1}{3}$ tsp. margarine

DIET FOR SUGAR INTOLERANCE— UPPER LEFT QUADRANT

Individuals who are sugar intolerant tend to crave protein and to suffer from depression, malabsorption, bloating, hyperactivity, asthma, chronic constipation, and severe food allergies. They usually have low blood sugar and exhausted adrenal glands. For those individuals, I recommend a diet that includes:

- liberal quantities of vegetables (see list on the next page), raw or cooked

- moderate quantities of lipids (fats), polyunsaturated vegetable oils, plant protein, eggs, animal protein, and fresh vegetables

- minimal consumption of sugars, fruits, grains, and dairy products

- avoidance of refined grains, refined grain products, and sweet vegetables such as potatoes, carrots, and corn

- taking protein within an hour of having the carbohydrate to balance the intake of foods

- limited intake of salt including soy sauce and spicy foods that contain large amounts of salt

- limited intake of alcohol because it weakens and stresses the adrenal glands, acts as pure sugar, is high in calories, is void of nutrients, and can cause cravings

- avoidance of all artificial sweeteners, sugars, and caffeinated beverages

Proteins: *(3–5 servings per day)*

2 egg whites	1 egg
4 oz. fish or lean poultry	3 oz. tofu

2 oz. low-fat cottage cheese
2 oz. skim ricotta cheese
1 oz. spirulina
4 oz. veal
4 oz. lamb

2 oz. skim mozzarella cheese
4 oz. soy protein powder
1 cup low or nonfat yogurt
4 oz. beef (3 or less servings per week)

Carbohydrates:

Unlimited amounts of the following vegetables

all types of of lettuce
celery
radishes
onions
cauliflower
yellow squash
spinach
endive
beans, yellow or green
eggplant
kale

bell peppers
mushrooms
sprouts
tomatoes
zucchini
cabbage
cucumbers
jicama
bok choy
escarole
okra

Limited amounts of the following vegetables (3–4 servings per week)

1 small artichoke
4 oz. potatoes
4 oz. carrots
4 oz. sweet potatoes

4 oz. sweet peas
4 oz. yam
4 oz. corn
4 oz. pumpkin

Fruits: *(2 servings per day)*

1 apple
1 peach
2 apricots
½ honeydew
10 cherries
1 cup berries
½ cup fresh pineapple

1 nectarine
1 pear
2 plums
10 grapes
2 plums
1 cup watermelon
½ cantaloupe

Limited amounts of the following fruits (3–4 servings per week)

½ banana
½ mango
1½ dried figs
1½ dates

1 cup papaya
½ cup raisins
8 oz. fruit juices
½ cup cranberries

Complex carbohydrates:

Legumes, grains, and grain products (2 servings per day)

1 slice whole grain bread
½ cup bulgur

½ cup brown rice
½ cup oatmeal

½ cup quinoa
½ cup cereal
½ cup pasta
½ oz. tortilla chips
1 rice cake
½ pita bread
½ cup spelt or kamut

¼ bagel
½ English muffin
½ cup granola
½ waffle
2 cup popped popcorn
1 corn tortilla
⅓ cup dried beans

Fats: *(2 servings per day)*
7 almonds or ½ tsp. almond
 butter
⅓ tsp. canola oil
⅓ tsp. olive oil
3 olives
⅓ tsp. peanut oil

½ tbsp. avocado
½ tbsp. tahini
1 tsp. olive oil and vinegar dressing
½ tbsp. peanut butter
6 peanuts

Limited amounts of the following fats (3–4 servings per week)
1 tsp. mayonnaise
⅓ tsp. soybean oil
½ tsp. brazil nuts
⅓ tsp. butter
1 tsp. cream cheese
⅓ tsp. lard

½ tsp. sesame oil
½ tsp. walnuts
2 tsp. bacon bits
½ tbsp. cream
½ tbsp. sour cream
⅓ tsp. margarine

CANDIDA YEAST AVOIDANCE DIET

After being treated with NAET for Candida and yeast, I recommend my patients follow this diet for ten days. I also prescribe a natural antifungal enzyme to take for eight to ten weeks.

Avoid eating the following foods:

- dairy products excluding unsweetened yogurt

- yeast products such as bread, baked goods, pastries, crackers, beer, and wine

- substitute lard, Crisco, margarine, hydrogenated vegetable oils, safflower, soybean, cottonseed, and corn oils with extra virgin olive oil, grapeseed, flax, canola, or sesame oils

- pasta, corn, and corn oils

- fruits or juices

- apple cider vinegar, hops, malts, and other fermented products

- peanuts, peanut butter, and other seeds (nuts and nut butters are permitted as long as they are roasted)

- mushrooms

- marbled meats, all processed meats, bacon, sausage, corned beef, and ham

- potato chips, other fried snack foods, and fried foods in general

- all forms of simple sugars, sucrose, fructose, malt sugar, honey, date sugar, molasses, turbinado sugar (this includes candy, soda pop, and desserts)

- condiments such as soy sauce, catsup, mayonnaise, barbecue sauce, and MSG

- leftover food in general

- rice or rice cakes

- regular coffee, instant coffee, and teas of all sorts including herbal teas

Foods you can eat:

- lean cuts of meat including beef, veal, pork, lamb, wild game, eggs, chicken, turkey, shellfish, and fish (not breaded)

- unlimited amounts of low carbohydrate vegetables, seeds, and grains (see list below)

- moderate amounts of high carbohydrate vegetables (1 serving per day)

- very limited amounts of whole grains (3–4 servings per week—see list below)

Low carbohydrate vegetables:

Asparagus	Greens such as spinach, mustard,
Beets	beets, collards, kale
Broccoli	All types of lettuce
Brussel sprouts	Okra
Cabbage	Onions
Carrots	Parsley

Cauliflower
Celery
Cucumbers
Eggplant
Green peppers

Radishes
Soybeans
String beans
Fresh tomatoes
Turnips

Nuts, seeds, and oils (unprocessed and roasted):
Almonds
Brazil nuts
Cashews

Filberts
Pecans
Pumpkin seeds

High carbohydrate vegetables:
Beans and peas (dried and
  cooked)
Lima beans
Peas

Sweet corn
Sweet potatoes
Winter squash (acorn, butternut)
White potatoes

Whole gains:
Barley
Millet

Oats

Gastritis Diet

I recommend to individuals who are suffering from epigastric irritation to avoid the following gastric irritants:

Alcohol
Aspirin
Amino acids
Bile salts
Caffeine, caffeinated tea
Calcium
Chocolate
Cloves
Coffee, decaffeinated coffee
Mustard

Niacin
Nicotine
Nutmeg
Peppermint oil
Peppers (black, red, and chili)
Progesterone
Spearmint oil
Tomatoes
Vinegar

FOODS CONTAINING OXALIC AND URIC ACID

Foods Containing High Oxalic Acid

Beans in tomato sauce
Beets
Blackberries
Black raspberries
Blueberries
Celery
Chocolate
Cocoa
Collards
Concord grapes
Dandelion greens
Eggplant
Escarole
Green gooseberries
Green peppers
Grits
Lager beer

Leeks
Lemon peel
Lime peel
Okra
Parsley
Peanuts
Pecans
Red currants
Rhubarb
Rutabagas
Soybean crackers
Spinach
Summer squash
Sweet potatoes
Swiss chard
Tea
Wheat germ

Foods Containing Low Oxalic Acid

Apple juice
Avocados
Bananas
Barley water
Bottled beer
Broccoli
Brussels sprouts
Butter
Cabbage
Cauliflower
Cheese
Cherries
Chicken noodle soup
Chives
Cider
Cocoa-Cola®
Cornflakes
Cucumbers
Dry sherry

Eggs
Fish (except sardines)
Grapefruit juice
Jelly with permitted fruit
Lemon juice
Lettuce
Lime juice
Macaroni
Mangoes
Margarine
Meats
Melons
Milk
Mushrooms
Nectarines
Oatmeal
Onions
Orange juice
Peaches

Peas

Pepsi®

Pineapples

Plums

Poultry

Radishes

Red plum jam

Rice

Seedless grapes

Turnips

White potatoes

Wine

Foods Containing High Uric Acid

Asparagus

Beef

Breads and cereals

Cauliflower

Chicken, duck, and turkey

Crab, lobster, and oysters

Eel

Fish, fresh and saltwater

Game meats

Green peas

Herring

Kidney

Lamb, pork, veal, and beef

Legumes, beans, lentils, and peas

Liverbreads and cereals

Mackerel

Meat

Meat extracts

Meat soups and broths

Mushrooms

Oatmeal

Sardines

Scallops

Spinach

Sweetbreads

Wheat germ and bran

Whole grains

Foods Containing Low Uric Acid

Cheese

Coffee, tea, and sodas

Eggs

Fats

Fruits and fruit juices

Gelatin

Milk

Nuts

Other vegetables beside the
   ones listed above

Sugars, syrups, sweets

ACID- AND ALKALINE-FORMING FOODS

Alkaline-Forming Foods

Fruits:

Apples

Apricots

Bananas

Berries

Cranberries

Currants

Grapefruit

Grapes

Lemons

Melons

Oranges

Pears

Persimmons

Pineapple

Plums

Prunes
Ripe olives
Vegetables:
Artichokes
Asparagus
Beets
Brussel sprouts
Cabbage
Carrots
Cauliflower
Celery
Cucumbers
Beans:
Dried peas
Nuts:
Almonds
Dairy:
Milk

Tangerines

Endive
Fresh peppers
Lettuce
Mushrooms
Onions
Parsley
Parsnips
Peas
Sweet potatoes

Lima beans

Fresh coconut
Roasted chestnuts
Yogurt

Acid-Forming Foods

Starches:
Barley
Bran
Cornstarch
Crackers
Dried corn
Proteins:
Bacon
Baking powder
Beef
Cheese
Chicken
Clams
Crab
Duck
Eggs
Dairy Products:
All cheese
Butter

Pastries
Rye bread
Spaghetti
White bread
White flour
Whole wheat bread
Fish
Lamb
Liver
Lobster
Oysters
Pork
Scallops
Shrimp
Veal

Ice cream
Malted milk

Neutral

Corn oil
Cottonseed oil
Olive oil

Peanut oil
Sesame oil
Soybean oil

MOST COMMON INFECTANTS FOR IMMUNE DISORDERS

Bacteria

Aerobacter aerogenes
Aerobacter cum Coli
Bac. Acidophilus
Bac. Coli (E. Coli)
Bac. Dysenteriae
Bac. Faecalis alkaligenes
Bac. Gaertner
Bac. Morgan
Bac. Proteus
Bac. Pyocyaneus
Bac. Subtilis
Bach Polyvalent
Bacillinum
Bacteroides
Banti
Bladder Tbc
Borrelia burgdorferi-LYME
Brucella abortus (Bang)
Camplyobacter pylori
Camplyobacter jejuni
Catarrhal mixed flora
Chlamydia trachomatis
Clostridium cadaveres
Clostridium dificile
Clostridium innocuum
Edwardsiella tardia
Enterococcinum
Gaertner
Gonococcinum
Hemophilus influenzae

Hemophilus infl. Serotyp.B
Hemophilus vaginal
Klebsiella
Klebsiella pneumoniae
Leptospirosis
Morgan(Pure & Gartner)
Morganella morganii
Neisseria meningitides
Paratyphus A,B/Salm.
Peptococc./Micrococc
Pertussin(Bordetella)
Pneumococcinum
Pneumococcinum M
Proteus
Proteus(Bach)
Salmonella
Salmonella typimurium
Salmonella typhus
Staphlococcus abdom.
Staphlococcus aureus
Staphlococc. Saproph.
Staphylococcinum
Strep. Haemolyticus
Strep. Pneumoniae
Strep. Pyogenes
Strep. Viridans
Sycotic coli
Thermibact. Intestinalis
Thermibact. Bifidus
Yersinia
Yersinia enterocolitica

Fungi

Actinomyces israelii
Aflatoxin
Alternaria
Alternaria tenuis
Aspergillus fumigatus
Aspergillus flavus

Aspergillus glaucus
Aspergillus nidulans
Aspergillus terreus
Blastomycosis
Blastomyces dermatoides
Candida albicans

Candida parapsilosis
Candida stellatoidea
Candida tropicalis
Candida guilliermondii
Candida lusitaniae
Candida pseudotropicalis Candida
 rugosa
Cladosporium cladospor.
Cladosporium herbarum
Epidermophyton
Epicoccum purpurascens
Epidermophyton floccosum
Malassezia furfur
Mold Mix A
Mold Mix B
Mold Mix C
Mucor mucedo
Mucor plumbeus
Mucor racemosus
Mycetoma

Nos Vaginitis
Penicillium camemberti
Penicillium chrysogenum
Penicillium digitatums
Penicillium italicum
Penicillium notatum
Penicillium roqueforti
Penicillium rubrum
Peniccillium spp.
Rhizopus nigricans
Saccharomyces cerevisiae
Schimmelpilz I
Schimmelpilz II
Sporotrichosis
Stemphylium botryosum
Stemphylium solani
Stemphylium sarcinforms
Tetracoccosporium
Trichophyton rubrum
Trichothecium roseum

Parasites

Entamoeba histolytica
Giardia lamblia
Blastocystis hominis
Cryptosporidium
Dientamoeba fragilis
Endolimax nana
Entamoeba gingivalis
Pneumocystis carinii
INTESTINAL NEMATODES:
Anisacis marina
Ascaris lumbricoides
Ascaris suum
Necator americanus
Toxocara canis
Toxocara mystax
TISSUE NEMATODES:
Dracunculus medinensis
Filariosis

Onchocerca volvulus
Mansonella ozzardi
Mansonella perstans
Mansonella streptocera
CESTODES (TAPEWORMS)
Taenia solijm
Echinococcus granulosus
Echinococcus multilocaris
Multipceps multiceps
TREMATODES:
LIVER FLUKES:
Opistorchiasis felineus
Opistorchiasis viverrini
INTESTINAL FLUKES:
Heterophyes heterophyes
Metagonimus yokogawai
BLOOD FLUKES:
Bilharziasis (Schistosoma)
Schistosoma haematobium
Schistosoma intercalatum

Viruses

Adenovirus
Coronovirus
Coxsackie virus A7
Coxsackie virus B1
Coxsackie virus B2
Coxsackie virus B3
Coxsackie virus B4
Coxsackie virus B5
Coxsackie virus B6
Cytomegaloviurs (CMV)
Distemperinum
Enteric R.R. Virus
Enterovirus
Epstein-Barr virus (EBV)
Hepatitis A
Hepatitis B
Hepatitis C nos
Herpes Simplex I
Herpes Simplex II
Herpes zoster
Herpes type VI
HPV
Infectious mononucleosis
Morbillinum (Measles)
Para influenza virus
Parotidinum (Mumps)
Poliomyelitis
Rhinovirus
Rubeola (Rubella)
Vaccininum
Varicella

Variola
FLU VIRUS
Grippe A (Asian)
Grippe V
Grippe V2
Grippe V3
Grippe V4
Grippe V5
Grippe VA2
Grippe VA2L
Grippe VAPCH
Grippe V'75
Grippe V'76
Grippe V'78
Grippe V'79
Grippe V'80
Grippe V'83
Grippe V'84
Grippe V'86
Grippe V'87
Grippe V'88
Grippe V'89
Grippe V'90
Grippe V'91
Influenzinum
Inf. Vesiculosis
Inf. Vesiculosis NW
Inf. Vesiculosis SW
Influenzinum AB
Influenzinum toxicum
Influenzinum Berlin
Swine Flu
Hong Kong Flu

ALLERZYME™ By Ellen W. Cutler, D.C., formulated by Enzyme Formulations.

This section includes the selected enzyme formulas that I use for certain allergy treatments and conditions. The enzymes have been a profound adjunct to allergy elimination, detoxification, immune enhancement, and regeneration. I generally supplement with an enzyme or enzymes after some major treatments; therefore, immediately following the allergy elimination and the

25 hours, a person will begin the enzyme formulas. These are the suggested dosages, but your doctor may choose others. The enzymes below are the professional names and products to be ordered by the doctor. There is a companion list of enzymes for the public that can be ordered from Enzyme Formulations. The AllerZyme list carries the same names for doctors and the public.

1. After treating the allergy to calcium, one should supplement with para—2 capsules after meals, or trauma 4 two to three times a day between meals.

2. After treating the allergy to Vitamin C, one should supplement with opt—3 capsules on rising and at bedtime. If the person has accompanying nasal congestion, use nasal in addition to opt.

3. After treating for minerals, one should supplement with thy—2 capsules inbetween meals.

4. After completing the top ten allergies, one should supplement with elixir 2 capsules after meals.

5. After Vitamin E allergy clearing, one should supplement with ribs—2 capsules in between meals.

6. After treating the allergy to Vitamin B, one should supplement with adrenal—3 capsules two times a day on rising and mid-afternoon.

7. If the patient becomes overly sensitive to other allergens after starting NAET treatments (for example, they notice they are more sensitive to perfumes, pollen, or some foods), they need to use liver enzyme—2 capsules after or between meals, kdy enzyme 2 capsules between meals.

8. If a patient experiences emotional symptoms during the treatments and also concurrently experiences insomnia, use calm—4 capsules one hour before bedtime and 4 capsules at bedtime.

9. After treating for amino acids, one should supplement with IVD 2 capsules after meals, and SRB powder.

10. Patients who crave sugars, and are very allergic and intolerant to sugars, should supplement with digest or pan—2 capsules before meals, and SVG—2 capsules two to three times in between meals.

11. Kidney enzyme is an excellent enzyme to use in the beginning of NAET treatments because it helps those allergic individuals feel some relief from environmental allergies, including pollen and mold.

ENZYME THERAPY

The use of enzyme therapy and NAET (allergy elimination treatment) work concurrently in the successful treatment of immune disorders. I will always supplement with the following enzyme formulas immediately upon beginning treatment. They are my formulations that I have developed in conjunction with Enzyme Formulations, Inc.

AllerZyme V (Virus): This formula is used whenever one is treating for viruses (with NAET) as well as treatment for saliva as explained in Chapter 5.

AllerZyme CFS (Chronic Fatigue Syndrome or Fibromyalgia): This formula is used for individuals with chronic fatigue syndrome and fibromyalgia.

AllerZyme H (Herpes): This formula is used for herpes outbreaks as well as prevention of herpes. (Includes all Herpes I, II, and shingles.)

AllerZyme C (Candida): This formula is used for all fungus and Candida infections and related symptoms.

AllerZyme B (Bacteria): This formula is used for bacterial infections and can be used ongoing as a preventive formula for infections as well as a support for the immune system.

AllerZyme P (Parasites): This formulas is used for parasites and as a detoxification program.

AllerZyme A (Asthma): This formula is used for all asthmatics as well as for anyone with respiratory problems.

AllerZyme Thy (Thyroiditis): This formula is used with individuals with thyroid problems, including hypothyroid, Hashimoto's thyroiditis, and Graves Disease.

AllerZyme IB (Colitis and Irritable Bowel): This formula is used for colitis, Irritable Bowel Syndrome, and Crohn's Disease.

ENZYME PRODUCTS

The following enzyme products are available from Enzyme Formulations, Inc., 1-800-614-4400.

Professional Products and Consumer Products
AllerZyme V Virus:

AllerZyme CFS
(or Fibromyalgia)

AllerZyme H Herpes

AllerZyme C Candida

AllerZyme B Bacteria

AllerZyme P Parasites

AllerZyme A Asthma

AllerZyme Thy Thyroiditis

AllerZyme IB (colitis,
Crohn's Disease, Irritable
Bowel Syndrome)

Other enzymes available from Enzyme Formulations, Inc., and mentioned throughout the text, include:

Professional Products (for doctors only)	Consumer Products
TheraZyme SYM— Parasympathetic	Enzyme & Herbal Formula #01
TheraZyme VSCLR—Vascular	Enzyme & Herbal Formula #02
TheraZyme OPT—Optical	Enzyme & Herbal Formula #03
TheraZyme NSL—Nasal	Enzyme & Herbal Formula #04
TheraZyme IVD—Disc	Enzyme & Herbal Formula #05
TheraZyme SVG—Salivary Gland	Enzyme & Herbal Formula #06
TheraZyme THY—Thyroid	Enzyme & Herbal Formula #07
TheraZyme RBS—Ribs	Enzyme & Herbal Formula #08
TheraZyme CIRC—Circulation	Enzyme & Herbal Formula #09

TheraZyme RSP—Respiratory	Enzyme & Herbal Formula #10
TheraZyme BIL—Biliary	Enzyme & Herbal Formula #11
TheraZyme STM—Stomach	Enzyme & Herbal Formula #12
TheraZyme ADR—Adrenal	Enzyme & Herbal Formula #13
TheraZyme PAN—Pancreas	Enzyme & Herbal Formula #14
TheraZyme SPL—Spleen	Enzyme & Herbal Formula #15
TheraZyme LVR—Liver	Enzyme & Herbal Formula #16
TheraZyme SMI—Small Intestine	Enzyme & Herbal Formula #17
TheraZyme KDY—Kidney	Enzyme & Herbal Formula #18
TheraZyme SKN—Skin	Enzyme & Herbal Formula #19
TheraZyme LGI—Large Intestine	Enzyme & Herbal Formula #20
TheraZyme IRB—Bowel	Enzyme & Herbal Formula #21
TheraZyme MAL—Male	Enzyme & Herbal Formula #22
TheraZyme FEM—Female	Enzyme & Herbal Formula #23
TheraZyme URT—Urinary Tract	Enzyme & Herbal Formula #24
TheraZyme PARA—Sympathetic	Enzyme & Herbal Formula #25
TheraZyme CLM	Enzyme & Herbal Formula #26
TheraZyme MSCLR	Enzyme & Herbal Formula #27
TheraZyme TRMA	Enzyme & Herbal Formula #28
TheraZyme Challenge	Enzyme & Herbal Formula #29
TheraZyme DGST	Enzyme & Herbal Formula #30
TheraZyme ELXR	Enzyme & Herbal Formula #31
TheraZyme HCL	Enzyme & Herbal Formula #32
TheraZyme SRB	Enzyme & Herbal Formula #33
TheraZyme LAC	Enzyme & Herbal Formula #34
TheraZyme OSTEO	Enzyme & Herbal Formula #35

EMDR: A NEW BREAKTHROUGH IN THERAPY

By Stephen Bodian, M.A.

What is EMDR?

EMDR (eye movement desensitization and reprocessing) is an important new psychotherapeutic technique developed by Francine Shapiro, Ph.D., a psychologist in Palo Alto. EMDR has been used with unprecedented success in the "desensitization and reprocessing" of traumatic memories.

Initially Dr. Shapiro and others had dramatic results with people suffering from the painful after-effects of rape, childhood sexual abuse, and traumatic Vietnam War experiences, a condition known as post-traumatic stress disorder (PTSD). In some cases, veterans who had suffered from nightmares and flashbacks for many years were cured of these symptoms in a few sessions. More recently, EMDR has been used successfully in treating a range of problems from phobias and free-floating anxieties to mild depression, relationship difficulties, eating disorders, low self-esteem, and grief.

How Does EMDR Work?

Dr. Shapiro discovered the technique serendipitously while noticing how she naturally processed her own unpleasant recurring memories. Although she does not claim to fully understand how it works, she offers the following tentative explanation:

> In REM (dream) sleep, we process the unpleasant experiences of the preceding day with "rapid eye movements," somehow "metabolizing" them so they do not continue to disturb us. When experiences are traumatic, however, REM sleep is insufficient to process them through. As a result, we store them in the nervous system as highly charged memories, usually associated with strong feelings and beliefs about ourselves and the world. Using eye movements similar to those of REM sleep, EMDR facilitates the reemergence and reprocessing of these memories; they no longer haunt us in the present as unwanted negative emotions and beliefs, but take their appropriate place in the perspective of the past, where they belong.

What is EMDR therapy like?

Most psychotherapists use EMDR, along with a variety of other methods, in the context of a caring, supportive, therapeutic relationship. Although it can be very effective, EMDR is not a magic elixir, and it does not seem to be equally effective with everyone.

In EMDR therapy itself, clients focus on a traumatic memory and/or a strong feeling or negative belief. If no memory is available, a feeling or belief will often be sufficient. While holding this focus, clients follow with their eyes the side-to-side motion of the therapist's fingers. After 30 or 40 such "passes," clients are asked to stop, take a deep breath, and report on what they have experienced.

Feelings may intensify (and sometimes discharge) before waning or even disappearing entirely. New memories may surface and/or old memories may become more vivid and detailed. And most significant of all, one's beliefs about oneself and the world—usually based on how one holds, or interprets, one's past experiences—may change dramatically. By the end of a session or series of sessions, painful memories and negative beliefs lose some or all of their charge, and present events no longer seem so difficult or threatening.

For each client and each problem, the approach used and the results obtained differ substantially. In many cases, EMDR ultimately roots out and reprocesses the feelings, memories, and unresolved issues that are keeping clients from moving forward in their lives.

Who can benefit from EMDR?

Clinical experience suggests that people with a range of problems can benefit from the use of EMDR. In particular, those whose difficulties are the direct result of traumatic or otherwise painful past experiences respond especially well to EMDR. If a person was physically, sexually, or emotionally mistreated as a child, experienced unresolved grief for the loss of a loved one, suffered the trauma of physical injuries or accidents, or been the victim of a natural disaster or a violent crime, EMDR is the treatment of choice. Guilt, fear, anxiety, low self-esteem, relationship difficulties, and depression have also responded well to EMDR, and continued investigation is constantly yielding new applications for the technique.

If you have any further questions about EMDR please call (415) 454-6149.

Stephan Bodian, M.A., is a psychotherapist in San Rafael, California, and an experienced practitioner of EMDR. In the context of a caring, supportive, therapeutic relationship, he has used the technique effectively for more than four years, with both men and women, in treating a range of client problems. He is the former editor of the Yoga Journal *and author of* Timeless Visions, Healing Voices.

MISCELLANEOUS RESOURCES

For information on NAET/enzyme therapy workshop (Winning the War workshop series), contact: Ellen Cutler, P.O. Box 5356, Larkspur, CA 94977

Allergy Control Products
96 Danbury Road.
Ridgefield, CT 06877
203-438-9580

Allergy Home Care Products
P.O. Box 2471
Silver Spring, MD 20915
800-327-4382
email ahcp@aol.com
http://www.ahcp.com

Laboratory for Loomis' 24-Hour
  Urinalysis
Metabolic Research Labs, Inc.
6620 West 110th Street, Suite 102
Overland Park, KA 66211
913-345-0088

Priorities
(A Common Sense Guide to Allergy
  and Asthma Managements)
70 Walnut Street
Wellesley, MA 02181-2175
1-800-553-5398
Fax: 617-239-7559
Web Site: www.priorities.com

Rocky Mountain FMS/CFIDS Support
  Foundation
980 W. 7th Avenue Drive
Broomfield, CO 80020
303-388-0727

For Enzyme Therapist Referral
  Contact:
Enzyme Formulations
6421 Enterprise Lane
Madison, WI 53719
800-614-4400

For Catalog of Natural Household
  Products Contact:
7th Generation Products for a
  Healthy Planet
1 Mill Street, Suite 826
Burlington VT 05401-1545
800-456-1177

For Information on NAET Seminars
  Contact:
Nambudripad's Allergy Research and
  Relief Foundation
614 Beach Boulevard
Buena Park, CA 90621
714-523-8900

Great Smokies Diagnostic Laboratory
63 Zillicoa Street
Asheville, NC 28801-9801
704-253-0621

Eco-Home: Home evaluation, water,
and air filtration, non-toxic products.
Call: 1-800-818-4592. Proceeds go
toward N.A.R.F. research studies
(research in NAET).

BIBLIOGRAPHY

Barnes, Broda O., M.D., and Galton, Lawrence. 1976. *Hypothyroidism: The Unsuspected Illness.* Toronto, Canada: Harper & Row, Publishers.

Berne, Katrina, Ph.D. 1995. *Running on Empty.* Alameda, CA: Hunter House Inc., Publishers.

Bland, Jeffrey S., Ph.D. 1995. *Applying New Essentials in Nutritional Medicine.* Gig Harbor, WA: HealthComm International, Inc.

Cichoke, Anthony J., M.A., D.C., D.A.C.B.N. 1993. *New Look At Enzyme Therapy.* Portland, OR: Seven Seas Publishing.

Crook, William G., M.D. 1995. *Chronic Fatigue Syndrome and the Yeast Connection Illustrated.* Jackson, TN: Professional Books, Inc.

Crook, William G., M.D. 1986. *The Yeast Connection.* New York, NY: Vintage Books.

Cutler, Ellen W., D.C. 1998. *Winning the War Against Asthma and Allergies.* Albany, NY: Delmar Publishers.

Dunne, Lavon J. 1990. *Nutrition Almanac, 3rd ed.* New York, NY: McGraw Hill.

Feiden, Karyn. 1990. *Hope and Help for Chronic Fatigue Syndrome.* New York, NY: Fireside of Simon & Schuster Inc.

Guyton, Arthur C., M.D. 1991. *Textbook of Medical Physiology.* Philadelphia, PA: W. B. Saunders Company, 8th ed.

Kirschmann, Gayla J., and Kirschmann, John D. 1996. *Nutrition Almanac, 4th ed.* New York, NY: McGraw-Hill.

Loomis, Howard F., Jr., D.C. 1996. *Introduction to Enzyme Nutrition.*

Loomis, Howard F.Jr., D.C. 1996. *The Physiology of Enzyme Nutrition.*

Murray, Michael T., N.D. 1994. *Chronic Fatigue Syndrome.* Rocklin, CA: Prima Publishing.

Nambudripad, Devi S., D.C., L.Ac., Ph.D., O.M.D. 1993. *Say Goodbye To Ilness.* Buena Park, CA: Delta Publishing Co.

Ornish, Dean, M.D. 1993. *Eat More, Weigh Less.* New York, NY: Harper Collins Publishers, Inc.

Pennington, Jean, A.T. 1989. *Food Values.* New York, NY: Harper Collins Publishers, Inc.

Pritikin, Robert. 1990. *The New Pritikin Program.* New York, NY: Simon & Schuster Inc.

Rosenthal, Sara M. 1993. *The Thyroid Sourcebook.* Los Angeles, CA: Lowell House.

Sears, Barry, Ph.D. 1995. *Enter The Zone.* New York, NY: Harper Collins Publishers, Inc.

Stoff, Jesse A., M.D., and Pellegrino, Charles R., Ph.D. 1988. *Chronic Fatigue Syndrome: The Hidden Epidemic.* New York, NY: HarperCollins Publishers, Inc.

Strang, Virgil V. 1984. *Essential Principles of Chiropractic.* Davenport, IA: Palmer College of Chiropractic.

REFERENCES

Antibodies in Thyroid Autoimmune Disease: Peter Bodlaender, Ph.D.

Aspartame and Phenylalanine: Smart Drug News Vol. 6, No. 2 Sep. 2, 1997: Pg. 7-8

Common treatments for CFS: (cdc.gov/ncidod/diseases) Oct. 21, 1996 The CFS FAQ (alternatives)

Chronic Fatigue Syndrome: (Well-Connected)

Chronic Fatigue Syndrome: Questions and Answers (medaccess)

Chronic Fatigue Syndrome: (medaccess)

Chronic Fatigue Syndrome: Paul F. Howard, M.D. (National sjogren's syndrome association)

The Chronic Fatigue Syndrome: A Comprehensive Approach to its Definition and Study: (lifelines)

Chronic Fatigue Syndrome Pathophysiology: NIH Guide, Vol 25, Number 28, August 16, 1996

Cichoke, Anthony T., D.C., D.A.C.B.N. 1993 *New Look at Enzyme Therapy*. Portland, OR: Seven C's Publishing

Crohn's Disease and Ulcerative Colitis: Ronald Hoffman, M.D., Conscious Choice Sep/Oct 1995

Chronic Fatigue Syndrome: Judith A. DeCava, Ph.D., L.N.C.: Nutrition News and Views Jan/Feb 1997 Vol.1, No. 1

Fibromyalgia: Notes From our Users : Colorado Health Net

Enzyme Therapy Effective On Inherited Immune Deficiency; Robert

Luciano, Ralph J. 1978. Direct Observation and Photography of Electroconductive Points on Human Skin. *American Journal of Acupuncture* No. 4, Vol. 6, October-December.

Steinbrook, Times Medical Writer: Los Angeles Times March 5, 1987.

Fats The Inside Story: Edward Kane

Fatty Acid Metabolism and the Impact of Trans Fatty Acids on Health: Mary G. Enig, Ph.D., F.A.C.N., C.N.S.

Feeling the Pulse: Rocky Mountain FMS/CFIDS Support Foundation Vol II n. 3 Oct. 1996

Fibromyalgia: Stephen J. Gislason., M.D. Environmed Research Inc.

Guyton, Arthur C., M.D., *Textbook of Medical Physiology*, 7th Ed. Philadelphia, PA: R. Saunders.

Immune Response: (familyinternet)

Idiopathic Autoimmune Syndromes: (members tripod. Com) March 1997

Inflammatory Bowel Disease: Exploration of the Problem, Identification of the Causes and Approaches to Recovery: Paul Goldber, M.P.H., D.C. Today's Chiropractic July/August 1997 pg. 24-28

Licorice Root-Potential Early Intervention for Chronic Fatigue Syndrome D. Brown Herb Review Summer 1996 pg. 95

Osteoporosis, hrmful calcification, and nerve/muscle malfunctions: Ray Peat's newsletter June, 1997

Screening tests for detecting common exclusionary conditions: (cdc.gov/ncidod/diseases)

Serotonin Precursors and Reuptake Inhibitors in Depressive Illness: Ward Dean, M.D, and Steven Wm. Fowkes: Smart Drug News Vol.6, No.1 August 1, 1997. P1-9

Steroid Fails to Adequately Relieve Symtpoms of Chronic Fatigue Syndrome: (abridged from an NIH news release) (cdc.gov/ncidod)

Summary of Research Conference Presentations at the 1996 San Francisco Meeting of the AACFS Scientific Session 1: Epidemiology; Session II Microbiology and Immunology; Session III: Interdisciplinary Studies; Session IV: Physiology; Session V: Clinical Studies; Workshop Summary: Neuropsychologica Functioning in CFS.

The Omega Factor: Our Nutritional Missing Link: Donald O. Rudin, M.D.

Tryptophan and Tourette's Syndrome: Steven Wm. Fowkes: Smart Drug News Vol5, No.v Oct. 23, 1996. Pg. 1-3

Unsaturated Vegetable Oils: Toxic: Ray Peat's Newsletter

Vimy, Murray J. *Toxic Teeth: The Chronic Mercury Poisoning of Modern Man.* International DMAS Newsletter, Vol. V, Issue 2. Albuquerque, NM: Murlene Brake.

GLOSSARY

Abdominal Palpation   A physical diagnostic test used to determine digestive competence, inflammation, and nutrient deficiencies.

Allergen   Any substance—physical, nutritional or emotional—which causes an allergic response in an individual. An allergen is a special type of antigen which causes an IgE antibody response.

Allergy   Inappropriate or exaggerated reactions of the immune system to substances that in the majority of people cause no symptoms.

ANA   A specific blood test for Lupus.

Anaphylaxis   Also known as anaphylactic shock, a severe and life-threatening allergic reaction. The reaction, which is rare, can be triggered as a reaction to a drug, insect bite or less commonly after ingesting certain allergic foods.

Antibody   A protein, also called an immunoglobulin, manufactured by lymphocytes (a type of white blood cell) to neutralize an antigen or allergen.

Antigen   A substance that can trigger an immune response, resulting in production of an antibody as part of the body's defense mechanism, against allergies, infections, and disease.

Antihistamine   A group of drugs that block the effects of histamine, a chemical released in body fluids during an allergic reaction.

Antioxidants   Free radical scavengers that remove dangerous free radical particles from the tissue, strengthening the immune system, building up tissue, and regenerating the body.

Autoimmune reaction   An allergic reaction within or to one's own body and systems. There are numerous auto-immune disorders that exist.

Basal Body Temperature Test   The resting temperature of the body, taken upon awakening in the morning. Done by taking the temperature under the armpit and recording it for a few days in a row. It is a very useful test for determining a hypothyroid condition.

B Cells   Blood cells that are produced by the immune system which are the main warriors that defend the body against invaders of any kind, including bacteria, viruses, cancer, and others. The B Cells produce antibodies or immunoglobulins.

Candida Albicans A common saprophyte of the digestive tract and the female urogenital tract. It can cause disease in patients with depressed immune systems.

Candidiasis Also known as Candida, or yeast infections. A common infection in Asthmatics. There are numerous symptoms, including bloating, fatigue, and possible vaginal infections.

Celiac Disease A deficiency disease of young children caused by faulty absorption of food in the intestines and characterized by diarrhea and malnutrition.

Chronic Fatigue Syndrome (CFIDS) Also known as Chronic Fatigue Immune Dysfunction Syndrome. A syndrome of multiple symptoms, most commonly associated with fatigue and low energy.

Circulating Immune Complexes (CICs) Tiny immune complexes that float freely in the blood or the lymph, comprised of antigens and antibodies, which can be eaten by the large macrophages of the immune system

Contact Allergens Any substance which when contacted physically will cause an allergic reaction. These can include chemicals, fabrics, plants, dyes and others.

Corticosteroids A group of anti-inflammatory drugs used extensively in medicine for the treatment and control of asthma, allergies, and immune disorders.

Crohn's Disease An intestinal disorder associatied with colitis and irritable bowel syndrome. One of the auto-immune diseases.

Cytomegalovirus (CMV) One of the eight known human herpesviruses, also known as human herpesvirus 5 (HHV-5). It can cause severe problems in patients with immune deficiency.

Dental Amalgams Various material used in dental corrective procedures, primarily comprised of mercury.

Desensitization To change one's reaction to an allergen, or to make one less sensitive to something that is causing a reaction in the body.

Enzymes Complex proteins in the body that cause chemical changes in other substances in order to provide the labor force and energy necessary to keep us alive. They help convert food into chemical substances that can be used by cells to perform our everyday functions. They keep the immune system strong in order to fight disease. Enzymes help nourish and clean the body. Life could not be sustained without enzymes.

Eosinophil   A white blood cell whose chief role is to combat parasites in the body.

Epinephrine   A naturally occurring hormone also called adrenaline. It is released by the adrenal glands. Epinephrine dilates the airways to improve breathing and narrows blood vessels in the skin and intestine so that an increased flow of blood reaches the muscles and allows them to cope with the demands of exercise. It is the drug used in the treatment of anaphylaxis.

Epstein Barr Virus (EBV)   One of the eight know types of human herpesviruses, also known as herpesvirus 4 (HHV-4). It commonly causes acute mononucleosis, and less commonly chronic mononucleosis.

Fibromyalgia   An immune disorder often confused with Chronic Fatigue Syndrome. It is characterized by pain all the different quadrants and the 18 trigger points of the body.

Free Radicals   Solo molecules that steal other molecules anywhere they can find them in the body. They are oxygen molecules that have split from their original form and in their quest for mates they cause damage to health tissue and cells. The results can be inflammation, cataracts, accelerated aging, depressed immune function, heart disease, or even cancer.

Gastric Reflux   A hyperacidic condition of the stomach also known as gastritis which can irritate the mucous membranes of the stomach or small intestines. Commonly known as heartburn.

Genetic   Passing from one generation to the next. Allergies and immune disorders can be genetic based.

Gulf War Syndrome   A condition experienced by some Gulf War veterans resembling Chronic Fatigue and Multiple Chemical Sensitivities syndromes.

Hashimoto's disease   An auto-immune disorder of the Thyroid gland causing hypothyroid.

HDL   A good form of cholesterol.

HEPA Filter   The most effective high efficiency particulate filter to filter the air in the home to remove airborne allergens which can be harmful to asthmatics.

Herpesvirus   A family of large DNA viruses. Eight distinct types have been associated with a variety of human diseases.

Histamine   A chemical present in cells throughout the body that is released during an allergic reaction. It is one of the substances responsible for the symptoms of inflammation, including sneezing and itching in allergic rhinitis. It also stimulates production of acid by the stomach and narrows the bronchi or airways in the lungs.

Homeopathic   A natural system of medicine that uses small doses of medicines to cure illness.

Homeostasis   A state of balance or equilibrium in the human body.

Hypersensitivity   Extreme sensitivity to some substance, either physically, nutritionally or emotionally, which can cause symptoms in the body.

Hypoadrenal   A condition in the body where the Adrenal glands are weak and are not functioning normally.

Hypothyroidism   A condition where there is diminished production of thyroid hormone leading to thyroid gland insufficiency.

IgE (Immunoglobulin E)   When exposed to allergens, allergic individuals develop an excess of the antibody called IgE. These antibodies react with allergens to release histamines and other chemical from cell tissues, producing allergic symptoms.

Immune System   A collection of cells and proteins that works to protect the body from potentially harmful, infectious microorganisms, such as bacteria, viruses, fungi, and other disease processes.

Immunosuppressor   Anything that suppresses the ability of the immune system to function normally.

Inflammation   Inflammation is the redness, swelling, heat, and pain in tissue due to chemical or physical injury or to infection. It is a characteristic of allergic reactions in the nose, lungs, and skin.

Inflammatory Bowel Diseases (IBDs)   Diseases of the bowel, most commonly ulcerative colitis and Crohn's Disease.

Kinesiology   A system of healing, developed by George Goodheart, D.C., as a means of evaluating the human body by means of muscle testing and analysis. It draws on the relationship between the muscles and organs of the body.

LDL   The harmful form of cholesterol in the body.

Lymphocytes   Any group of white blood cells of crucial importance to the adaptive part of the immune system. The adaptive portion of the immune system mounts a defense when dangerous invading organisms penetrate the body's defenses.

Malaise   A feeling of general discomfort or uneasiness, an out of sorts feeling, often the first sign of an infection.

Multiple Chemical Sensitivity Disorder   An allergic sensitivity to a broad range and number of substances. There is some doubt as to its existence.

Multiple Sclerosis (MS)   A slowly progressive Central Nervous System disease characterized by disseminated patches of demyelination in the brain and spinal cord.

Muscle Response Testing   A technique based on kinesiology to test a muscle or group of muscles in the body, in relation to allergens. The NAET system of Allergy Elimination, uses this form of testing in its analysis.

Myalgic encephalomyelitis   A synonym for chronic fatigue syndrome in common usage in the United Kingdom and Canada.

NAET (Nambudripad Allergy Elimination Technique)   A technique to permanently eliminate allergies from the body, developed by Dr. Devi Nambudripad, and practiced by over 1000 health practitioners worldwide. This technique is completely natural and drug-free, and has been effectively used in the treatment of immune disorders and allergies.

Neuro Mediated Hypotension (NMH)   An abnormal condition in the Central Nervous System where the heart gets a signal to slow down, causing a decrease in the blood pressure.

Neurotransmitters   Biochemical substances, such as norepinephrine or acetylcholine, which transmit nerve impulses from one nerve cell to another.

Nystatin   A drug used to control the proliferation of yeast infection in the body.

Pathogen   Any microorganism that can cause disease or allergies.

pH   The acid-alkaline balance of the body important in the maintenance of overall health.

PMS (Pre Menstrual Syndrome)   A common female disorder that occurs prior to the menstrual cycle characterized by multiple symptoms of discomfort and agitation.

Polymyalgia Rheumatica (PMR)   A syndrome characterized by aches in muscles of the neck, shoulders, and hips, especially in the morning on rising.

Premarin   An estrogen replacement drug which has estrogen-like effects on women, but is not natural to the human body.

Rotation Diet   A system of treating allergies whereby a person rotates the foods he or she eats every few days, never eating any of the same foods more than one day in a row. It is usually a 4-5 day rotation in order to detect and eliminate food allergies.

Sick Building Syndrome   Also referred to as building related illness. These terms are used when one or more occupants of a building develop similar symptoms that are apparently related to some indoor pollutant(s). Many of these symptoms involve hypersensitivity of the lungs and respiratory system.

SOD   Superoxide dismutase, a copper/zinc containing enzyme found in all body cells which is a primary defender against free radicals. SOD eliminates destructive superoxide molecules, a common free radical produced in the body, and soaks up free radical oxygen molecules in the bloodstream which would otherwise destroy healthy tissue. Some people are deficient in this enzyme and may need to take it in supplement form. SOD is found in green vegetables, yeast, sprouted seeds, and grains.

Synthroid   Synthetic thyroid replacement hormone.

T Cells   Lymphocytes produced by the thymus gland which play a cardinal role in the regulating of the immune system.

Thymus   The major gland of the immune system. It release several hormones which regulate the immune system functions. These hormone levels are often low in the elderly.

Twenty-Four Hour Urinalysis   A diagnostic urine test, gathered over a 24-hour period and analyzed in the laboratory for any abnormalities. Used in this context to determine the need for enzyme therapy in the patient.

Thyroid Stimulating Hormone (TSH)   A hormone of the anterior pituatary gland that stimulates and regulates the development and secretory activity of the thyroid gland.

ABOUT THE AUTHOR

Ellen W. Cutler, D.C., is a well-established NAET Practitioner, Enzyme Therapist, Chiropractor, and Nutritionist who brings a wealth of expertise to the areas of allergies, asthma, women and children's health, nutrition, weight loss, immune disorders and chronic diseases. She has been practicing chiropractic and nutrition for 18 years, and has more than ten years of clinical experience with enzyme therapy and NAET. More than ninety-eight percent of her practice is dedicated to the treatment of allergies related to a wide array of illnesses. She has developed a national reputation for her work with NAET and enzyme therapy.

Since she focused her work on the treatment of allergies, Dr. Cutler has been a regular lecturer on topics ranging from allergies, asthma, children's health, and migraines to women's health, including hormonal imbalances, thyroid dysfunction, menopause, endometriosis, and PMS. She has appeared on numerous radio and TV programs, including "Alternative Medicine for Total Health." Her work has been published in the *Alternative Medicine Digest* and *Natural Health Magazine*, and northern California newspapers and others throughout the country.

Dr. Cutler earned her Chiropractic degree from Western States Chiropractic College in Portland, Oregon, after completing a BA in Psychology at the University of Buffalo, New York. She went on to do post graduate work in Kinesiology, Directional Nonforce Chiropractic, Chiropractic Orthopedics, Visceral and Cranial Manipulation, Women's Health, Nutrition, Enzyme Therapy and NAET (Nambudripad Allergy Elimination Technique).

She is a member of the American Chiropractic Association, California Chiropractic Association, North Bay Chiropractic Association, Mothers of Asthmatics, the advisory board of NAET, and is an associate member of the American Holistic Medical Association. She founded the Tamalpais Pain Clinic in northern California, where she lives with her husband, Steven, and two children, Aaron and Gabrielle.

WORKSHOPS

Dr. Cutler is offering an ongoing series of "Winning the War Workshops" throughout the year, given on both the east and west coasts. For a schedule of workshops, or for further information, call (415) 927-0741.

Dr. Cutler's "Winning the War Against Allergies Series" newsletter is published bi-monthly. The subscription rate is $79.00/yr. The newsletter serves to update and inform NAET practitioners and other health professionals of Dr. Cutler's progress and latest research. To order the newsletter, please write to P.O. Box 5356, Larkspur, CA 94977.

In order to be placed on Dr. Cutler's NAET Referral List, a subscription to her newsletter is recommended, as well as attendance at her workshops.

To order the latest NAET Referral List, please send $4.95 to: Dr. Ellen Cutler, P.O. Box 5356, Larkspur, CA 94977; or refer to: http://www.allergy2000.com (on the internet).

TAKE ACTION AND RECLAIM YOUR HEALTH

The Problem: Allergy and illness today is on the rise. The American Cancer Society reports that one out of three Americans will get cancer and one out of five will die from it. The degradation of our environment through toxic waste, generated by our chemically based society has overloaded our bodies' ability to maintain optimal health. The Center for the Study of Responsive Law found that U.S. drinking water contains 2,000 substances for which the EPA has issued a health advisory. Chemicals in our water, pollutants in our air, and pesticides, herbicides and fungicides on our food impact our health and our world with devastating effect.

The Solution: Prevention is the solution. NAET is the cure. We can take responsibility for our personal environment by arming ourselves with state-of-the-art air and water filtration. By using non-chemically based products, we lessen our exposure and enhance our bodies' ability to cope. Treating with NAET and taking action to reclaim our personal environment is the solution to preventing illness and to ensure health in our future.

To find out how you can reclaim your personal environment and take charge of your health beginning today, please call Eco-Home at 1-800-818-4592.

INDEX